STUDY GUIDE

The Nursing Assistant
Essentials of Holistic Care

by

Renae Boydston
Whitewater, WI

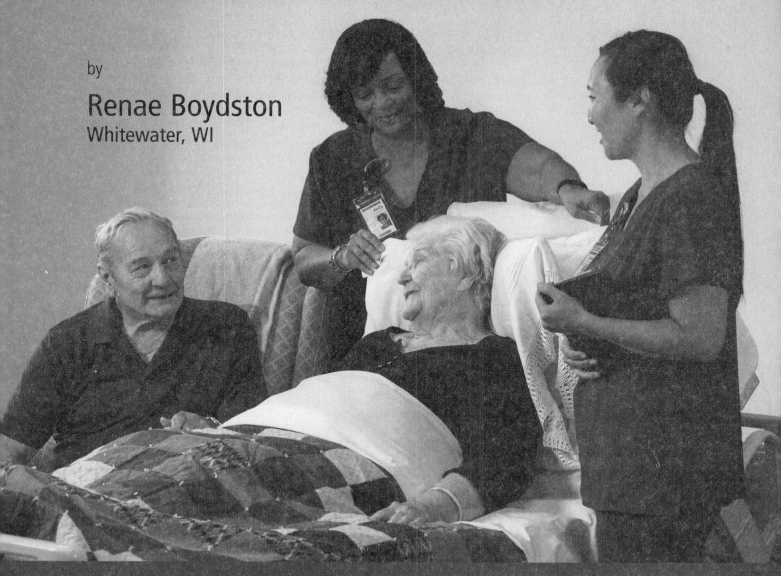

Publisher
The Goodheart-Willcox Company, Inc.
Tinley Park, IL
www.g-w.com

Contents

Name: _____   Date: _____

Matching Section 1.1 Key Terms

Match each definition with the key term.

A. activities of daily living (ADLs)
B. ambulating
C. certification
D. certified nursing assistant (CNA)
E. compassion
F. contaminated
G. empower
H. holistic care
I. hospice
J. infection control
K. job description
L. licensed nursing staff
M. licensed practical/vocational nurse (LPN/LVN)
N. patients
O. registered nurse (RN)
P. residents
Q. scope of practice
R. vital signs

_____ 1. nursing staff members who have passed state licensing examinations that allow them to perform healthcare tasks within their scope of practice

_____ 2. a healthcare facility that provides supportive care for those who are terminally ill and their families

_____ 3. care that is sensitive to a person's values and desires and that integrates a person's physical (body), emotional (mind), and spiritual (spirit) needs to help achieve the highest level of well-being possible

_____ 4. a licensed staff member who delivers nursing care that includes assessment; providing nursing diagnoses; and planning, implementing, and evaluating care

_____ 5. the rates or values of a person's temperature, pulse, respiration, and blood pressure

_____ 6. people staying in a long-term care facility, often for a long period of time, due to age, illness, or inability to care for themselves at home

_____ 7. walking

_____ 8. a credential earned when a person has completed the designated education, training, and testing that prepares him or her for a specific field, discipline, or professional advancement

_____ 9. policies and procedures used to minimize the risk of spreading infection

_____ 10. a licensed nurse who provides care under the supervision of a registered nurse (RN)

_____ 11. the specific responsibilities, procedures, and actions of a healthcare provider, as permitted by state regulation

_____ 12. a person who has successfully completed the nursing assistant education and training needed to take and pass a state certification competency examination

_____ 13. actions such as bathing, walking, eating, dressing, and toileting

_____ 14. soiled or dirty as a result of contact or mixture with something that is not clean

_____ 15. a written document used by facilities to describe the duties, responsibilities, and qualifications required for a particular position

_____ 16. people who are in a healthcare facility, such as a hospital, due to illness or disease

_____ 17. the desire to help another person who is suffering or in pain

_____ 18. to give a person the power to control his or her own destiny and decision making

Name: _____ Date: _____

Becoming a Nursing Assistant

Identify whether each statement is true or false.

_____ 1. The *Omnibus Budget Reconciliation Act (OBRA)* standardized minimum requirements for certified nursing assistant education and training.

_____ 2. Nursing assistant education and training programs are the same in each state.

_____ 3. The certification competency examination only tests the individual's knowledge in a written exam.

_____ 4. All nursing assistant training programs include hospital or clinical experience.

_____ 5. Each state must maintain a *registry*, or list, of certified nursing assistants.

_____ 6. A graduate must pass only one part of the examination with a state-determined score to be on the registry.

_____ 7. To maintain active status on the registry, a nursing assistant cannot have any findings of abuse, neglect, or theft.

_____ 8. Nursing assistants must renew their registration every four years.

Understanding Holistic Care

Select the *best* answer.

_____ 1. Holistic care is care that
   A. focuses on the disease process
   B. integrates the body, mind, and finances
   C. integrates the body, mind, and spirit
   D. focuses on rehabilitation of the resident

_____ 2. The essential knowledge and skills of a holistic nursing assistant include
   A. being independent instead of valuing team relationships
   B. being professional, using critical thinking, caring, and effectively communicating
   C. not exercising cultural humility
   D. focusing on shortening procedures to save time

_____ 3. The framework of holistic care
   A. illustrates factors that affect nursing assistant well-being
   B. does not consider the workplace environment
   C. is not concerned with policies and procedures of the facility
   D. illustrates the interactions and support between nursing assistants, residents, residents' families and friends, and the healthcare environment

_____ 4. Holistic nursing assistants establish an environment that
   A. addresses a resident's emotional needs, if there is time
   B. responds primarily to the resident's physical needs
   C. focuses on the resident's disease
   D. supports the whole person

_____ 5. Holistic nursing assistants must not only respond to physical needs, but should also
   A. focus on the resident's attitude
   B. try to give the resident anything he or she wants
   C. educate the resident on religion
   D. consider the resident's spirit, or *higher self*

Elements of Holistic Care

The Providing Holistic Care Framework illustrates the different facets of holistic care. Identify the missing elements in each section of the framework.

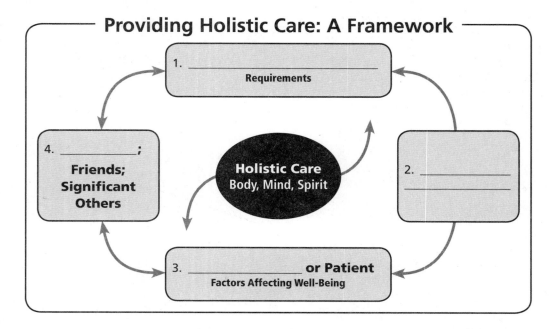

Providing Holistic Care: A Framework

1. _____ Requirements

4. _____; Friends; Significant Others

Holistic Care Body, Mind, Spirit

2. _____

3. _____ or Patient
Factors Affecting Well-Being

FIRST CHECK Procedural Checklists

Each procedure in your textbook is broken down into different components—the rationale, preparation, procedural steps, follow-up, and reporting and documentation. Steps are repeated throughout most of the procedures to ensure the nursing assistant continually delivers safe, competent care. Understanding and remembering these steps is vital when preparing for the certification competency examination. You will be expected to perform these as part of the hands-on portion of the exam.

Using the acronym *FIRST CHECK*, you can easily remember each of these steps to ensure you are completing each step properly and in the correct order. If you are consistent, using this tool will help you memorize the important preparation, follow-up, and reporting and documentation steps included in nearly every procedure a nursing assistant is expected to perform.

There are five letters in *FIRST* and five letters in *CHECK*. During practice, simply count the preparation FIRST steps on the fingers of your left hand. Then, count the follow-up and reporting and documentation CHECK steps on the fingers of your right hand.

For this activity, write the letters of the *FIRST CHECK* acronym in the spaces below. Then, use this reference as you practice the procedures you will perform as a nursing assistant.

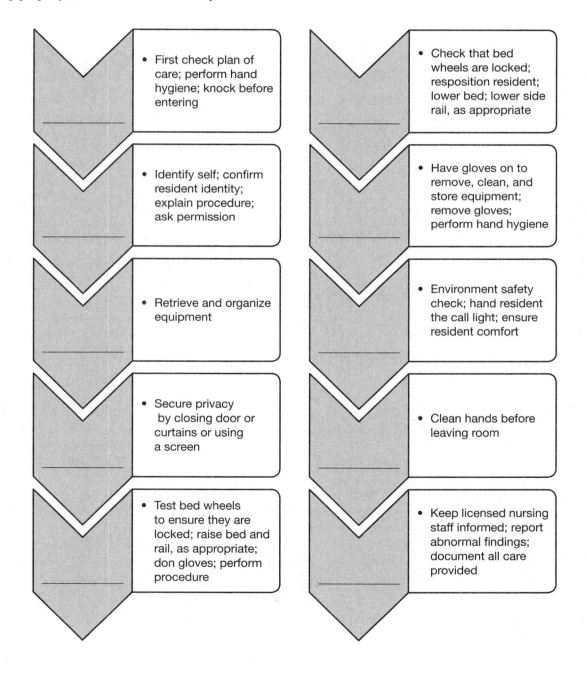

- First check plan of care; perform hand hygiene; knock before entering

- Identify self; confirm resident identity; explain procedure; ask permission

- Retrieve and organize equipment

- Secure privacy by closing door or curtains or using a screen

- Test bed wheels to ensure they are locked; raise bed and rail, as appropriate; don gloves; perform procedure

- Check that bed wheels are locked; resposition resident; lower bed; lower side rail, as appropriate

- Have gloves on to remove, clean, and store equipment; remove gloves; perform hand hygiene

- Environment safety check; hand resident the call light; ensure resident comfort

- Clean hands before leaving room

- Keep licensed nursing staff informed; report abnormal findings; document all care provided

Nursing Assistant Responsibilities

Fill in the blanks of the following matrix showing the important responsibilities of a nursing assistant.

Important Responsibilities of the Nursing Assistant
Measurement and _____ (vital signs, fluid intake and output, changes in condition)
_____ (with residents and their significant others, the healthcare team, and the licensed nursing staff)
Activities of _____ (assistance with bathing, grooming, dressing, eating, and toileting)
_____ (standardized steps for performing care)
_____ Control (hand hygiene, appropriate handling of contaminated objects, personal protective equipment)
_____ Care and Safety (clean, safe room conditions and response to emergencies)
_____, Movement, and Exercise (lifting, moving, transferring, and walking)
_____ Collection (collection of sputum, urine, or feces)

Using the Key Terms

Complete the following sentences using key terms from the chapter.

1. _____ are ways of thinking or feeling about a person, situation, or object.
2. Accepted and expected limits on behavior or actions are called _____.
3. The _____ is a US federal agency that seeks to prevent and control the spread of infectious diseases and responds to health threats.
4. A nursing assistant who has achieved _____ possesses the knowledge and skills needed to do something well.

5. _____ encompasses the traditions, beliefs, rituals, customs, and values that are specific to a group of people.
6. A person who possesses strong moral principles and professional standards has _____.
7. _____ is an attitude that is supportive and accepting of others.
8. A nursing assistant who is _____ demonstrates an expected level of excellence and competence.
9. _____ are beliefs or ideals that set a standard of what is good or bad.
10. _____ actions are not in line with accepted rules of conduct.
11. _____ is a belief in the importance of work and can strengthen a person's character.

Analyzing Nursing Assistant Behaviors

Identify whether the following nursing assistant behaviors are appropriate (A) or inappropriate (I).

_____ 1. A nursing assistant states, "You are my favorite resident."

_____ 2. A resident asks why the nursing assistant appears tired, and the nursing assistant responds, "I had a wild date last night."

_____ 3. A nursing assistant accepts a piece of candy from a resident, knowing that facility policy approves of this practice.

_____ 4. A nursing assistant calls to speak with a specific resident after leaving work.

_____ 5. A nursing assistant asks to change assignments with another nursing assistant so she can care for a particular resident.

_____ 6. A nursing assistant spends extra time with a resident who is not part of his or her assignment.

_____ 7. A nursing assistant uses offensive language when talking with a resident.

_____ 8. A nursing assistant accepts a gift from a resident.

_____ 9. A resident asks a nursing assistant for financial advice, but the nursing assistant suggests the resident ask a family member instead.

_____ 10. Two nursing assistants make jokes of a sexual nature at the nurse's station.

Name: _____ Date: _____

Matching Section 2.1 Key Terms

Match each definition with the key term.

A. acute care
B. chronic care
C. co-payment
D. deductible
E. dementia
F. diabetes mellitus
G. epidemic
H. healthcare
I. healthcare facility
J. healthcare services
K. immunization
L. managed care
M. Medicaid
N. Medicare
O. premium
P. primary care provider (PCP)
Q. private insurance
R. Social Security
S. stem cell
T. subacute care
U. trauma
V. vaccine
W. wellness

_____ 1. screening, diagnostic, and evaluative activities that assist and support the restoration, maintenance, or improvement of health

_____ 2. a US law passed in 1965 that supplies federal funds to deliver healthcare to people 65 years of age or older

_____ 3. serious, critical, or surgical care; typically delivered in hospitals

_____ 4. an outbreak of an infectious disease that spreads quickly and makes many people sick

_____ 5. a mixture given by injection or taken orally that is used to protect a person against a specific disease; contains a very mild form of that disease so the body builds antibodies against the disease to increase or create immunity

_____ 6. a doctor, nurse practitioner, or physician assistant whose legal scope of practice allows him or her to be the first contact for a person's healthcare needs

_____ 7. a form of insurance in which there are contracts with specific healthcare providers who will deliver care at a reduced cost

_____ 8. a severe loss of mental capacity that interferes with a person's ability to lead a normal life

_____ 9. a fixed fee for specific medical services not covered by health insurance

_____ 10. a state of health and well-being, including all aspects of health

_____ 11. care provided to a person who has a moderate-to-severe illness, injury, or recurrence of disease, but who does not require acute care in a hospital

_____ 12. the amount of money paid, usually on a schedule, to an insurance company for a specific insurance policy

_____ 13. a method of providing protection against certain diseases; usually involves a vaccine

_____ 14. a building in which healthcare is delivered

_____ 15. care given to those who have long-term diseases or illnesses

_____ 16. a disorder in which there are excessive amounts of glucose in a person's blood due to an insufficient production of insulin or insulin resistance

_____ 17. the amount of money that a health insurer program or employer requires people to pay out of pocket as their share of the cost for health insurance coverage

_____ 18. a plan for payment of healthcare services; may be purchased by an employer on the employee's behalf or by an individual

_____ 19. a US law passed in 1965 that provides a combination of federal and state financing to offer healthcare at the state level for those with low incomes

_____ 20. a serious or life-threatening injury or shock to a person's body

_____ 21. a human cell capable of renewing, dividing, and changing to become a specific tissue or organ cell

_____ 22. the prevention, diagnosis, and treatment of diseases; the management of acute and chronic illnesses; and the promotion of wellness

_____ 23. a US law established in 1935 that provides retirement benefits, disability coverage, dependent coverage, and survivor benefits

The Advancement of Healthcare and Medicine
Select the *best* answer.

_____ 1. In the mid-1800s, Hungarian doctor Ignaz Semmelweis introduced the practice of
A. using penicillin
B. vaccinating people to prevent disease
C. pasteurization
D. hand washing between patients to prevent the spread of infection

_____ 2. The discovery of _____ as the cause of disease was made in the 1800s.
A. vaccines
B. germs
C. immunization
D. blood

_____ 3. English doctor Edward Jenner successfully administered the first vaccine against _____ in 1796.
A. polio
B. cholera
C. smallpox
D. cowpox

_____ 4. _____ advocated for sanitary medical facilities, better hygiene, and proper nutrition in the 1800s.
A. Edward Jenner
B. Elizabeth Blackwell
C. Louis Pasteur
D. Florence Nightingale

_____ 5. Vaccines against diseases such as _____ were developed during the 1900s.
A. polio, smallpox, and cholera
B. whooping cough, diphtheria, and smallpox
C. whooping cough, measles, and mumps
D. mumps, rubella, and cowpox

_____ 6. During the 1900s, _____ was discovered as a treatment for bacterial infections.
A. penicillin
B. insulin
C. glucose
D. aspirin

_____ 7. Cardiopulmonary resuscitation was developed in the
A. 1700s
B. 1800s
C. 1900s
D. 2000s

_____ 8. The development of _____ ensured the standardization of policies and procedures and more accurate documentation.
A. paper charts
B. robotics
C. the human genome
D. electronic health records (EHRs)

_____ 9. Research involving _____ offers new possibilities in disease treatments that replace diseased cells with healthy ones.
A. robotics
B. the human genome
C. immunization
D. stem cells

_____ 10. Today, medical decisions are consistently made using
A. intuition
B. evidence-based research
C. untested hypotheses
D. actions based on theories

Categories of Care
Correctly identify the category of care in each description.

Primary	Acute
Secondary	Subacute
Tertiary	Chronic

1. _____ care is highly specialized care, such as treating trauma, burns, or cancer. This type of care is found in hospitals or medical centers.

2. _____ care is provided to a person who has a moderate-to-severe illness, injury, or recurrence of a disease, but who does not require the level of care given at a hospital.

3. _____ care is the initial medical care a person receives at a doctor's office or a medical clinic to treat an illness or disease.

4. _____ care applies to people who have a long-term disease or illness that may never go away.

5. _____ care is serious, critical, or surgical care that is usually received in a hospital.

6. _____ care focuses on the prevention of disease or the promotion of health and wellness. This might include immunization, health education, or health screening in a public health clinic or a pharmacy.

Understanding Healthcare Facilities
Identify whether each statement is true or false.

_____ 1. People who need around-the-clock care and rehabilitation for conditions such as a stroke, fractured hip, or knee-replacement surgery can be cared for at a skilled nursing facility.

_____ 2. Stays at skilled nursing facilities are often lifelong.

_____ 3. The goal of skilled nursing facilities is to help patients become well enough to return home and function effectively.

_____ 4. Residential care facilities provide services 24 hours per day, seven days a week.

_____ 5. Residential care facilities never need to be licensed by the state or have licensed nursing staff.

_____ 6. Residents living in independent living facilities do not need to be independent in all ADLs, but must be mentally alert.

_____ 7. Continuing care communities offer care that changes over time, depending on the resident's needs.

_____ 8. In assisted living facilities, residents may live in their own apartments, which are equipped with emergency devices to alert licensed nursing staff if help is needed.

_____ 9. Residential care is for people who require only moderate assistance and supervision.

_____ 10. Long-term care facilities are designed to care for residents who can take complete care of themselves.

Describing Healthcare Facilities

Select the *best* answer.

_____ 1. Hospice is care that
   A. focuses primarily on grief counseling
   B. provides for people who have a life expectancy of 12 months or less
   C. may be provided at a residential hospice center, in the home, or in a long-term care facility
   D. does not provide family caregiver support

_____ 2. Home healthcare services
   A. do not include cooking or running errands
   B. may include companion care, which involves performing light housekeeping, escorting patients to appointments, or reading and playing games
   C. employ only RNs
   D. cannot provide respite care for family caregivers

_____ 3. Pharmacies are facilities that
   A. are responsible for paying for prescriptions
   B. employ unlicensed pharmacy staff members
   C. cannot provide information about medications, side effects, and drug interactions
   D. are responsible for filling, dispensing, and refilling prescriptions

_____ 4. Laboratories and medical imaging facilities
   A. provide assistance with the diagnosis of a disease or condition
   B. check a resident's blood using X-rays
   C. never offer services within a hospital, clinic, or doctor's office
   D. typically send licensed staff to the resident's home to conduct diagnostic procedures

_____ 5. Surgical centers are facilities that
   A. offer a wide range of surgical procedures
   B. do not perform biopsies
   C. are always located within a hospital
   D. offer both surgical and diagnostic procedures

_____ 6. Outpatient clinics are facilities that
   A. never offer free services or use a sliding scale when setting fees
   B. have a specific purpose, or focus of care
   C. provide preventive and wellness care
   D. do not offer dental care

_____ 7. Hospitals are facilities that
   A. may be not-for-profit, for-profit, or public
   B. are never funded by the government
   C. have a specific number of licensed beds, which is determined by the federal government
   D. only provide nursing, medical, surgical, and critical care services

_____ 8. Doctors' offices are facilities that
   A. do not employ RNs
   B. are staffed with primary care providers (PCPs)
   C. do not have laboratory or diagnostic and supportive care staff
   D. do not rely on nurse practitioners or physician assistants to give care

_____ 9. Urgent-care centers are facilities that
   A. are only open in the nights and on the weekends
   B. treat people with long-term care needs
   C. provide emergency care, including minor surgeries
   D. address acute-care needs

_____ 10. Which of the following healthcare facilities provides inpatient, tertiary care for people with a severe illness or trauma?
   A. skilled nursing facility
   B. urgent-care centers
   C. hospitals
   D. surgical centers

Healthcare Funding

Consider the following scenarios related to healthcare funding. Identify which type of funding would best apply in each case.

Medicare	Patient Protection
Social Security	and Affordable Care
Medicaid	Act (ACA)
	private insurance
	managed care

1. A father works at a factory full time and has health benefits for himself and his children through his job. He chose a plan with a high co-payment to keep the monthly costs lower. This _____, paid ahead of time, ensures that he and his family are covered in case they need to use healthcare services.

2. A 24-year-old man works six days a week in the food industry. Minimum wage barely covers the cost of his apartment, utilities, and food expenses. He is overall healthy, but concerned that he cannot afford healthcare coverage in the event of a change in his health. Under the _____, he may be eligible for coverage under a parent's healthcare plan.

3. A doctor contracted with an insurance company to perform consults at a reduced cost as part of their _____ network. One of his former patients, a 50-year-old woman, decided to see a different doctor outside the network. She may have to pay for all, or most, of her care.

4. A US citizen worked over 10 years at a glass factory and now qualifies for _____, a program that provides retirement benefits, disability coverage, dependent coverage, and survivor benefits.

5. A 21-year-old woman with schizophrenia missed a week of work without notifying her supervisor and lost her job. She may be eligible for health coverage in her state through _____.

6. A surgeon has informed a 66-year-old woman that it is necessary to remove her diseased gallbladder. The surgeon's payment for services will come from _____ and will be a fixed amount, even if the surgeon charges more than that amount for gallbladder removal.

Matching Section 2.2 Key Terms

Match each definition with the key term.

A. chain of command   D. nursing unit
B. charge nurse   E. orientation
C. delegate   F. shift

_____ 1. an area within a healthcare facility where care is delivered; is typically designated by a floor name, area, or type of illness

_____ 2. the RN or LPN/LVN who is the leader of a particular nursing unit

_____ 3. to transfer duties to another competent person

_____ 4. a period of time that a staff member works

_____ 5. on-the-job training given to new employees

_____ 6. the levels of staff in a facility with regard to authority

Sample Healthcare Facility Organizational Structure

Place each of the following positions in the appropriate place within this sample healthcare facility organizational chart. Note that some positions may be used more than once.

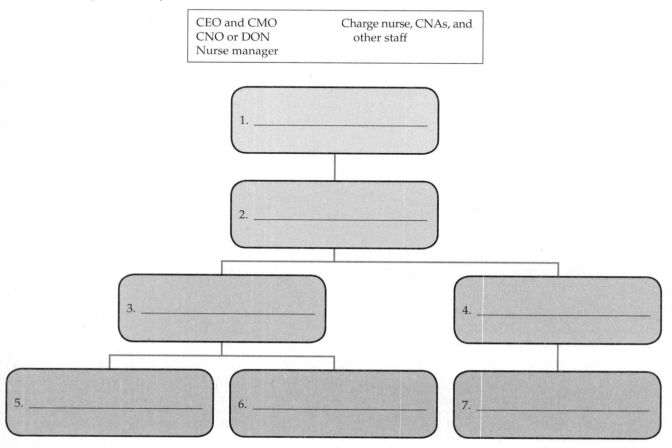

| CEO and CMO CNO or DON Nurse manager | Charge nurse, CNAs, and other staff |

1. _____

2. _____

3. _____

4. _____

5. _____

6. _____

7. _____

Working on a Nursing Unit

Read each of the following scenarios about working on a nursing unit. Then determine whether or not each scenario represents professional, holistic care and explain your answer.

1. Healthcare facilities divide the 24 hours in a day into 8-, 10-, or 12-hour shifts. These are often described as *day*, *evening*, or *night shifts*. A nursing assistant refuses to help the night shift assist a resident to the bathroom because his shift has not started yet. Is he demonstrating professional, holistic care?

   _____

   _____

   _____

   _____

2. An eight-hour day shift begins at 7:00 a.m. and ends at 3:00 p.m. The day-shift nursing assistant wakes up at 5:00 a.m. and arrives ready to work at 6:30 a.m. Is she demonstrating professional, holistic care?

   _____

   _____

   _____

   _____

3. A 12-hour night shift starts at 7:00 p.m. and ends at 7:00 a.m. The nursing assistant arrives at 7:00 p.m. and changes into her uniform. Is she demonstrating professional, holistic care?

   _____

   _____

   _____

   _____

4. The structure of work shifts is determined by facility policy, services provided, and the needs of residents. Another nursing assistant called in sick 30 minutes prior to the end of your shift, and your supervisor asks you to stay until a replacement arrives. You refuse. Does this demonstrate professional, holistic care?

   _____

   _____

   _____

   _____

5. There are usually requirements for how many weekends and holidays nursing assistants must work. You are required to work Thanksgiving Day, but many of your coworkers are sick with the flu, leaving you short-staffed. Instead of being angry, you make the best of the situation and smile at the residents enjoying their feast. Does this demonstrate professional, holistic care?

   _____

   _____

   _____

   _____

Name: _____ Date: _____

Matching Section 3.1 Key Terms

Match each definition with the key term.

A. abuse
B. accreditation
C. assault
D. battery
E. civil law
F. confidentiality
G. criminal law
H. defamation of character
I. elder abuse
J. false imprisonment
K. informed consent
L. liability
M. libel
N. licensure
O. malpractice
P. neglect
Q. negligence
R. regulation
S. rehabilitation
T. self-determination
U. slander
V. The Joint Commission (TJC)

_____ 1. the legal process of securing written permission prior to giving care or conducting procedures

_____ 2. unintentional failure to act or provide necessary care that a reasonably prudent, or sensible, person would

_____ 3. a rule or requirement that healthcare facilities and staff must follow

_____ 4. false statements made about a person that damage his or her reputation; written or spoken

_____ 5. the act of keeping personal information that has been shared with healthcare staff private

_____ 6. failure to provide necessary care that meets a resident's daily needs

_____ 7. a private regulatory agency that accredits various healthcare facilities

_____ 8. a period of recovery in which healthcare staff members help patients regain their strength and mobility with the goal of patients learning to function independently

_____ 9. false spoken statements made about a person that damage his or her reputation

_____ 10. legal responsibility

_____ 11. a form of negligence in which a caregiver in a healthcare discipline does not comply with the standards set by his or her discipline's regulatory body, resulting in injury

_____ 12. the process of making choices and decisions based on one's own preferences and interests

_____ 13. recognition that a person or facility has permission to deliver care

_____ 14. a deliberate action (physical, verbal, financial, or sexual) that causes harm to a senior

_____ 15. a type of law that imposes a fine or prison sentence to keep offenders and others from acting unlawfully again

_____ 16. any words or actions that a person finds threatening or that cause a person to fear harm

_____ 17. the act of touching a person without his or her permission

_____ 18. a deliberate action that causes harm

_____ 19. a type of law that deals with disagreements between individuals and organizations

_____ 20. illegal confinement in which a person is held against his or her will by another, resulting in restraint of movement

_____ 21. an official recognition indicating that a healthcare facility meets predetermined professional and community standards that promote safety and quality

_____ 22. false written statements made about a person that damage his or her reputation

Laws and Regulations

Complete the following sentences.

1. _____ are formal rules enforced by a legal authority such as the US government, a state, a county, or a city.

2. _____ law is a system of laws that governs a nation, such as those laws found in the US Constitution.

3. _____ law, or *case law*, is a system of laws established as a result of decisions usually made in a court of law.

4. _____ laws, such as laws regarding income tax, affect everyone in the United States.

5. _____ laws affect those who live in that state and address areas such as healthcare, patient rights, safety, and licensure.

6. _____ are rules or requirements that are based on laws and that healthcare facilities and staff must follow.

Understanding Healthcare Laws, Regulations, and Scope of Practice

Identify whether each statement is true or false.

_____ 1. Healthcare facilities can choose whether to follow accreditation and licensure rules and regulations.

_____ 2. Healthcare facilities receive accreditation from the federal government.

_____ 3. Licensure of healthcare facilities is usually handled by agencies within a state's health department.

_____ 4. Legal scope of practice determines what nursing assistants can and cannot do.

_____ 5. Nursing assistants are supervised by LPNs/LVNs, but not by RNs.

_____ 6. Nursing assistants may use the title CNA without achieving certification.

_____ 7. Nursing assistant regulations are defined by the Omnibus Budget Reconciliation Act (OBRA).

_____ 8. All nursing assistants are allowed to deliver medications.

_____ 9. Each state determines the legal scope for a nursing assistant's practice in that state.

_____ 10. If a nursing assistant works outside her legal scope of practice, she may be disciplined by the facility and state.

Determining Your Scope of Practice

List the three questions a nursing assistant should ask to determine if a responsibility is within his or her scope of practice. Then answer the question that follows.

1. _____

_____

2. _____

_____

3. _____

_____

4. Whom should you ask if you do not know the answers to these questions?

_____

Working Outside the Scope of Practice

Select the *best* answer.

_____ 1. When you work within the legal scope of practice,
A. you are less likely to get caught by the charge nurse
B. disciplinary action will be severe
C. you know the limitations of your position and are aware of your liability
D. ethical problems will not happen

_____ 2. Violations of criminal law
A. are legal if they protect the resident
B. are always felonies
C. are not reported to the state board of nursing or health department
D. result in criminal actions

_____ 3. Which of the following is true of misdemeanors?
A. They include petty theft, trespassing, and public intoxication.
B. They are more serious crimes than felonies.
C. They never have penalties because they are less serious.
D. They include homicide, trespassing, and theft.

_____ 4. Felonies are
A. unlikely to result in prison time
B. more serious crimes, such as homicide
C. less serious crimes, such as trespassing
D. actions that cause reasonable doubt

_____ 5. Civil actions
A. are called *torts* because they never cause physical or emotional injury
B. do not address negligence or malpractice
C. will not occur if the nursing assistant works outside the scope of practice
D. deal with disagreements between individuals and organizations for failing to deliver proper care

_____ 6. Which of the following is true of negligence?
A. It is the unintentional failure to act or provide care.
B. It occurs when professional standards are not followed, resulting in injury.
C. It is a violation of criminal law.
D. It does not occur if you work within your scope of practice.

_____ 7. Which of the following is true of malpractice?
A. It is a violation of criminal law.
B. It occurs when professional standards are not followed, resulting in injury.
C. It results in a prison sentence, rather than monetary compensation for the injury.
D. It is the unintentional failure to act or provide care.

_____ 8. To prevent negligence and avoid malpractice, you should
   A. avoid alerting the licensed nursing staff if you make a mistake
   B. not document negligent care
   C. continue performing a procedure, even if you are unsure of the next step
   D. give care only within your legal scope of practice

HIPAA and Bills of Rights

Match the definition with the appropriate healthcare law or regulation.

A. Health Insurance Portability and Accountability Act (HIPAA)
B. Nursing Home Resident Rights
C. Patient Bill of Rights

_____ 1. ensures that personal medical information is stored and shared securely, maintaining confidentiality

_____ 2. guarantees privacy of information, a safe environment, fair treatment, and the ability to make medical decisions

_____ 3. ensures that resident rights are protected and promoted and emphasizes individual dignity and self-determination

Protecting Residents' Rights

Determine whether each of the following scenarios is an example of protecting a resident's rights by indicating *yes* or *no*.

_____ 1. Mr. S begins to cry after a nursing assistant states, "I can't believe you need to use the bathroom again."

_____ 2. A nursing assistant locks the wheelchair to keep Mr. L from leaving his room.

_____ 3. A nursing assistant applies a bath blanket prior to giving a back rub.

_____ 4. A nursing assistant asks permission to touch Ms. P's personal care items prior to assisting her.

_____ 5. A nursing assistant knocks before entering the Mr. and Mrs. R's shared room.

_____ 6. A nursing assistant tosses Mr. K's junk mail into the garbage before he receives it.

_____ 7. Mrs. G receives a walker from physical therapy, but has not been given any information about it.

_____ 8. A nursing assistant schedules her tasks so Mr. A can visit with friends from his former workplace.

_____ 9. A nursing assistant is running late, so she decides to skip repositioning Mr. F, even though it has been two hours since he was last repositioned in bed.

_____ 10. A nursing assistant reports Ms. O's input about her plan of care.

Understanding Informed Consent, Neglect, and Abuse

Identify whether each statement is true or false.

_____ 1. Residents must sign an informed consent form before certain procedures can be performed.

_____ 2. Important procedures may be performed even if the resident refuses care.

_____ 3. Failure to meet a resident's daily hygiene needs is not considered neglect.

_____ 4. If abuse or neglect is suspected, the licensed nursing staff must be alerted.

_____ 5. Nursing assistants are not responsible for determining if a resident is being abused.

_____ 6. Nursing assistants are not responsible for observing and reporting any signs or symptoms of abuse.

_____ 7. If signs of abuse are not reported, the nursing assistant will not be legally liable.

_____ 8. Reporting information related to abuse is required by federal and state laws.

_____ 9. Performing a procedure without a resident's consent may be considered battery.

_____ 10. Elder abuse may be physical, verbal, or sexual, but *not* financial.

Acting Ethically

Complete the following paragraph.

(1.) _____ are principles that guide our conduct; they help us determine what is the right or wrong thing to do. (2.) _____ influence a person's attitudes and behavior and are the basis of ethics and a person's ethical practice. It is important to know and understand your values so you can determine how they might affect your ability to practice (3.) _____ caregiving.

Principles of Ethical Caregiving

Explain how the following principles should be observed and followed to ensure healthcare staff members practice ethically.

1. Autonomy: _____

   _____

   _____

2. Freedom: _____

   _____

   _____

3. Confidentiality:_____

   _____

   _____

4. Beneficence:_____

   _____

   _____

5. Nonmaleficence:_____

   _____

   _____

6. Veracity: _____

   _____

   _____

7. Fidelity: _____

   _____

   _____

8. Justice: _____

   _____

   _____

The Problem-Solving and Decision-Making Process

Insert the steps of the problem-solving and decision-making process into the appropriate locations in the diagram. Also identify which side of the diagram includes problem-solving steps and which side includes decision-making steps.

| Decision making | Evaluate | Identify the problem | Problem solving |
| Determine alternatives | Examine the problem | Implement | Select an alternative |

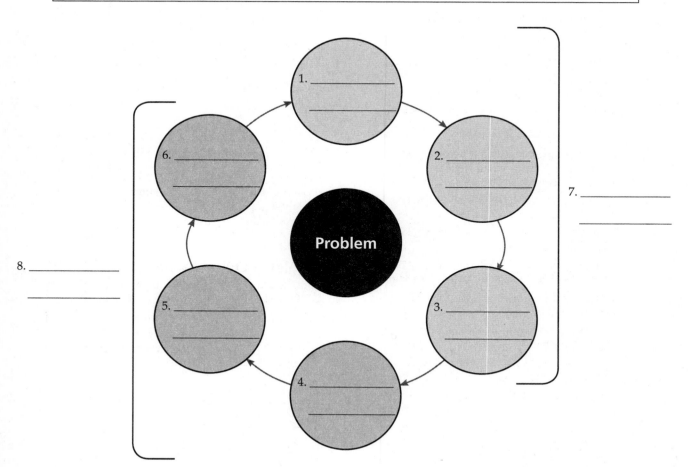

Name: _____   Date: _____

Matching Section 4.1 Key Terms

Match each definition with the key term.

A. census
B. level of care
C. ratio
D. staffing
E. staffing plan
F. turnover

_____ 1. the number of residents on a nursing unit

_____ 2. the number of staff members who leave a healthcare facility and are replaced by new employees during a specific period of time

_____ 3. a formal document that shows the mix and types of healthcare staff members who will work on each shift in the nursing unit

_____ 4. the process of determining the numbers and types of healthcare staff needed to take care of a group of patients or residents on a nursing unit

_____ 5. the number of patients or residents in a facility or unit assigned to each member of the healthcare staff

_____ 6. a type of care needed for a particular resident; typically higher for a resident with a serious illness and lower for a resident who needs assistance only with ADLs

The Healthcare Team

For each sentence, fill in the correct member of the healthcare team working closely with nursing assistants to provide care.

1. Similar to a case manager, a(n) _____ has a specialized graduate degree that emphasizes the psychological, social, and economic aspects of healthcare.

2. A(n) _____ is also called a physician, primary care provider (PCP), medical doctor (MD), or doctor of osteopathic medicine (DO).

3. _____ therapists work with residents during recovery to improve flexibility and mobility and help residents achieve the highest levels of function possible.

4. _____ are responsible for creating special diets residents require due to illness or disease.

5. _____ work within their legal scope of practice and take directions from the licensed nursing staff.

6. A(n) _____ leads the nursing team and is accountable for the coordination of healthcare services and nursing care.

7. The _____ staff includes housekeeping staff and transport aides.

8. A(n) _____ therapist might help a resident learn how to swallow and speak again after a stroke.

9. A(n) _____, or unit secretary or unit clerk, is trained to coordinate the administrative and support responsibilities of a nursing unit or healthcare facility.

10. _____ therapists work with residents who have trouble performing daily tasks due to injury or illness.

Developing Successful Teams

Describe the six qualities a team must possess to function at its best.

1. _____

   _____

2. _____

   _____

3. _____

   _____

4. _____

   _____

5. _____

   _____

6. _____

   _____

Common Team Roles

When working with a team, you may discover that team members fulfill common roles. Match the following statements with the role that best fits the speaker's personality and attitude.

A. the clarifier
B. the dominator
C. the energizer
D. the gatekeeper
E. the harmonizer
F. the information seeker or giver
G. the initiator
H. the optimist
I. the skeptic
J. the summarizer
K. the timekeeper

_____ 1. "It's better that we avoid this angry conversation about workload and just keep the peace."

_____ 2. "We all need a chance to share our opinions and give input about why we are having trouble completing these tasks on time."

_____ 3. "So far, we have information about the thermometer, have raised ideas about timeliness, and have discussed the flu."

_____ 4. "It is 9:00. If we don't speed things up, we'll never get to lunch."

_____ 5. "We're getting a lot of exercise today. Look at the residents smile!"

_____ 6. "I have further information that will help us understand the problem with the electronic thermometer."

_____ 7. "I know nobody asked for my opinion, but I have even more information to give about why the resident is angry."

_____ 8. "My way of getting the residents to supper on time is better. I've been here longer."

_____ 9. "You may think that's a good idea, but what about residents who take longer to bathe? I don't think that plan will work."

_____ 10. "The flu outbreak seems grim, but at least the healthcare staff is staying healthy."

_____ 11. "I thought of a new idea for how to get four baths done before breakfast."

Matching Section 4.2 Key Terms

Match each definition with the key term.

A. anxiety
B. bias
C. deduction
D. engagement
E. humility
F. intuitive
G. journal
H. meditation
I. mindfulness
J. nonverbal communication
K. rational
L. self-reflection
M. stress
N. systematic
O. verbal communication

_____ 1. the use of spoken words to convey a message

_____ 2. having insight

_____ 3. an unfair belief that some people, objects, or situations are better than others

_____ 4. using a specific method

_____ 5. the use of specific assumptions to reach a conclusion

_____ 6. a feeling of worry, uneasiness, or nervousness

_____ 7. the practice of looking at one's self in an honest and truthful way and being open to any changes that may be needed

_____ 8. the practice of being aware and mentally present in every situation by focusing on what is being said, what you are doing, or what is happening in the environment around you

_____ 9. the quality of not putting one's self first

_____ 10. a physical or psychological response to a situation that causes worry or tension

_____ 11. the practice of being fully involved and committed

_____ 12. having the ability to think clearly and make decisions based on facts

_____ 13. a written record of observations and experiences

_____ 14. the use of gestures, facial expressions, or body movements to convey a message

_____ 15. the practice of emptying the mind of thoughts, feelings, and emotions to reach a state of relaxation through concentration

Understanding Engagement and Critical Thinking

Identify whether each statement is true or false.

_____ 1. Being mindful is the only way to achieve engagement.

_____ 2. Being engaged as a holistic nursing assistant means focusing your attention completely on those in your care.

_____ 3. Critical thinking is a cognitive process that helps you examine your thinking and the thinking of others.

_____ 4. Mindfulness can only be integrated into daily living through meditation.

_____ 5. Critical thinking requires the ability to be purposeful, rational, and systematic, when examining a situation.

_____ 6. Critical thinking does not require the use of deduction or intuition.

_____ 7. Nursing assistants who practice self-reflection examine the work they have done and how it can be improved.

_____ 8. Critical thinking requires focus, presence, and the ability to form conclusions and make decisions.

_____ 9. Critical thinking does not require an attitude of inquiry and the capacity to reflect on one's thinking.

_____ 10. Journaling is a helpful tool for self-reflection.

Verbal and Nonverbal Communication

Identify whether verbal (V) or nonverbal (N) communication is used in the following scenarios.

_____ 1. A nursing assistant tells the licensed nursing staff that a resident has foul-smelling urine.

_____ 2. A nursing assistant rolls her eyes when the charge nurse walks past her.

_____ 3. The charge nurse says to the nursing assistant, "Let's talk in private when you have time."

_____ 4. A nursing assistant walks away without replying to the charge nurse.

_____ 5. The charge nurse scowls and crosses her arms.

_____ 6. An anxious resident glances at the door.

_____ 7. The dietitian's eyes narrow when a nursing assistant offers dessert to a resident before the rest of the resident's meal.

_____ 8. The respiratory therapist informs the resident that years of smoking have damaged his lungs.

_____ 9. A family member hears laughter and loud talking coming from the activity room and slams the resident's door shut.

_____ 10. The director of nursing reiterates the importance of accurate, timely documentation during a staff meeting.

Name: _____ Date: _____

Matching Chapter 5 Key Terms
Match each definition with the key term.

A. accountable
B. assessing
C. cognitive status
D. continuity
E. discharge plan
F. evidence-based practice
G. nursing diagnosis
H. nursing process
I. philosophy
J. plan of care
K. priorities
L. pulse oximeter
M. sphygmomanometer
N. standards of care
O. tracheostomy

_____ 1. the identification of a health problem or the cause of a health problem; does not identify a specific disease

_____ 2. an uninterrupted connection or sequence of events

_____ 3. a set of instructions given to the patient at the time of discharge

_____ 4. a method of problem solving that includes assessing, identifying, and organizing nursing knowledge, judgments, and actions to provide safe, quality care

_____ 5. the ability to understand, think clearly, and remember

_____ 6. a surgical opening in the trachea

_____ 7. examining a situation so it can be evaluated

_____ 8. the process of locating and using research findings to guide decisions made about care delivery

_____ 9. a medical device used to measure blood pressure

_____ 10. fundamental beliefs and values

_____ 11. responsible; able to explain any actions taken

_____ 12. reasonable and sensible processes or actions healthcare providers follow when addressing certain medical conditions

_____ 13. a written plan that provides directions and serves as a guide to delivering individualized, holistic care

_____ 14. a medical device, usually applied to a fingertip, that indirectly measures the amount of oxygen in the blood

_____ 15. items or actions that are ranked as having high importance

Levels of Care
Complete the following sentences.

1. _____ describe the types and amounts of care that patients and residents require to achieve the best result or outcome.

2. Providing the right level of care helps ensure that a resident in a long-term care facility remains as _____ as possible.

3. Knowing the level of care a resident requires helps healthcare staff members evaluate the resident's _____ to determine if the care is covered financially.

4. Personal care needs, such as the amount of assistance required to complete _____, are a factor in evaluating level of care.

5. A patient's or resident's _____ status and self-care abilities also influence the level of care.

Assigning Levels of Care
Identify whether each statement is true or false.

_____ 1. Level-of-care assignments may change over time.

_____ 2. Levels of care change more frequently in long-term care facilities than in hospitals.

_____ 3. When people seek long-term care, they should consider current and future needs and choose a facility that meets both.

_____ 4. Long-term care facilities offer only skilled and supportive care.

_____ 5. Skilled care is intermittent care provided over a long period of time.

Understanding Levels of Care
Select the *best* answer.

_____ 1. Which of the following is true of skilled care?
   A. It is fully paid for by Medicare for the duration of need.
   B. It does not offer therapy.
   C. It requires 24-hour, hands-on care in a healthcare facility.
   D. It focuses on curing the resident so the resident can return home.

_____ 2. Intermediate care is
  A. provided for those who require assistance with ADLs, such as bathing
  B. mostly provided by doctors and registered nurses
  C. a type of care in which needs are assessed by the nursing assistant
  D. not provided in a person's home or in assisted living

_____ 3. Which of the following is true of supportive care?
  A. It does not involve special rehabilitation.
  B. It could include end-of-life care.
  C. It never addresses multiple medical problems.
  D. It is not provided in a person's home.

_____ 4. End-of-life care
  A. typically excludes the healthcare team
  B. does not require a doctor's orders
  C. provides for a person's physical, emotional, and spiritual needs
  D. excludes ADLs

_____ 5. Nursing care delivery has
  A. no relationship to the medical condition of the resident
  B. no relationship to the numbers and type of nursing staff available
  C. the goal of matching resident needs with the cheapest care possible
  D. a relationship with the healthcare facility's philosophy

Nursing Care Delivery
Identify and describe the six types of nursing care delivery.

1. _____
_____
2. _____
_____
3. _____
_____
4. _____
_____
5. _____
_____
6. _____
_____

Delegation
Identify whether each statement is true or false.

_____ 1. Delegation occurs when licensed nursing staff members ask a nursing assistant to take the responsibility of performing specific tasks.
_____ 2. Delegated tasks must be routine and not require special knowledge or skill.
_____ 3. A delegated task must always be part of the nursing assistant's scope of practice.
_____ 4. When in doubt, a nursing assistant may delegate a task to another nursing assistant.
_____ 5. When an RN delegates a task to a nursing assistant, he or she also transfers the responsibility for performing that task.
_____ 6. Upon accepting a delegated task, a nursing assistant becomes responsible for performing the task correctly.
_____ 7. A fundamental part of delegation is distrust.
_____ 8. Delegation is a legal act within a licensed nursing staff member's scope of practice.
_____ 9. Nursing assistants can delegate a task.
_____ 10. Licensed nursing staff members are accountable for the completion of delegated tasks.

Five Rights of Delegation
Complete the five rights of delegation by filling in the blanks with the correct words.

1. The right _____ is delegated.
2. The delegation occurs under the right _____.
3. The task is delegated to the right _____.
4. The right _____ and _____ are given.
5. The right _____ and _____ are provided.

Standards of Care
Complete the following paragraph.

One fundamental of delivering care is using a set of criteria and guidelines to direct the care you give. These guidelines are established by the nursing profession and are called (1.) _____ of care. Standards of care are methods, processes, and actions. In nursing, one standard of care is the five-step nursing (2.) _____. In the 1970s, the (3.) _____ Nurses Association recognized the nursing process as an important standard of care for guiding nursing practice. By the 1980s, state boards of nursing adopted the nursing process as part of nursing education and the licensing examination for (4.) _____ nursing staff.

Steps in the Nursing Process

Identify each step in the nursing process.

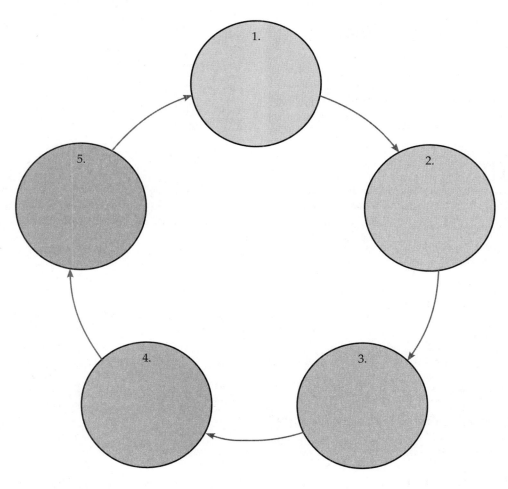

Understanding the Nursing Process

Complete the following sentences.

1. During the _____ step in the nursing process, information is gathered about the physiological, psychological, emotional, sociological, economic, lifestyle-related, and spiritual aspects of a resident.

2. Healthcare facilities have written policies and _____ that set mandatory guidelines for the care the holistic nursing assistant delivers.

3. During the _____ step, the plan of care is put into action.

4. When making a(n) _____ diagnosis, licensed nursing staff members use clinical judgment based on information collected to identify a potential or existing health problem.

5. The plan of care is developed during the _____ step.

6. The _____ step of the nursing process is ongoing throughout care to identify new goals.

7. Nursing assistants participate in the nursing process by providing timely and accurate _____ of a resident's status.

8. Policies and procedures set _____, directions, and guidelines that ensure actions taken by the healthcare staff are based on good evidence and best practice.

Understanding Admission, Transfer, and Discharge

Select the *best* answer.

_____ 1. A 78-year-old man fell at home and sustained a hip fracture. The fracture was repaired in the hospital, but the man is not able to safely go up or down steps. Which of the following is the best option for this patient?
A. discharge home with a visiting nurse twice weekly
B. transfer to a rehabilitation center for physical or occupational therapy to regain limited or lost function
C. admission to a long-term care facility since the man will not be able regain function
D. None of the above.

_____ 2. A 60-year-old woman had a cerebral vascular accident, and her doctor recommends transfer to a rehabilitation facility. She refuses the transfer. What will happen next?
   A. The doctor will refuse to write a discharge order.
   B. The doctor will write an order for admission to the rehabilitation facility, and the woman will be transferred by ambulance.
   C. The doctor will write a discharge order with documentation stating that the woman refused transfer against medical advice (AMA).
   D. None of the above.

_____ 3. A 99-year-old woman fully recovered from a septic urinary tract infection (UTI). She is excited to leave the hospital and go home to tend her vegetable garden. What will her doctor do next?
   A. write a discharge plan with information about medications, activity levels, treatments to continue at home, and follow-up appointments
   B. write an order for admission to a long-term care facility because of the woman's advanced age
   C. discharge the woman to a subacute care facility because her health has improved and she has the ability, support, and resources to take care of herself
   D. None of the above.

Performing Admission to a Healthcare Facility

It is important to follow the proper procedure for admission to ensure it is performed accurately. The following steps are part of the procedure for admitting a resident to a healthcare facility. For each set of steps, identify the proper order in which they should be completed by numbering them 1 through 5.

1. _____ Prepare the bed by pulling back the covers, placing it in a low position, and locking the bed wheels.
   _____ When the resident arrives at the room, the licensed nursing staff checks the resident's name with any admission forms.
   _____ Ensure the call light is accessible and within the resident's reach.
   _____ Bring the necessary equipment into the room and place it in an accessible location.
   _____ Wash your hands or use hand sanitizer before entering the room.

2. _____ If instructed by the licensed nursing staff, place an identification bracelet on the resident's wrist if he or she is not already wearing one.
   _____ Explain the part of the procedure you will be doing in simple terms.
   _____ Introduce yourself using your full name and title. Explain that you work with the licensed nursing staff and will be assisting with the admission.

_____ Use Mr., Mrs., or Ms. and the last name when conversing.
_____ Provide privacy by closing the curtains, using a screen, or closing the door to the room.

3. _____ A member of the licensed nursing staff or a social worker may explain the resident's rights, and a photo may be taken for identification purposes.
   _____ If the resident has a roommate, make introductions.
   _____ Let the resident stay dressed, if approved, or help the resident change into a gown or pajamas.
   _____ Access the approved admission forms for the resident.
   _____ As directed by the licensed nursing staff, ask the resident the questions on the admission forms. If the resident is disoriented or unable to answer questions, you may ask an accompanying family member.

4. _____ Help the resident into bed or into a chair, as directed by the licensed nursing staff.
   _____ Unless a family member of friend wishes to assist, put away the resident's clothes and personal items.
   _____ Complete the resident's clothing and personal belongings lists and label the resident's belongings if you are in a long-term care facility.
   _____ Provide the resident with an orientation to the room.
   _____ After an RN conducts a resident assessment, assist by measuring vital signs, height, and weight.

5. _____ If needed, provide a denture cup and label it with the resident's name, room number, and bed number.
   _____ Explain when meals are served and how to request snacks.
   _____ Explain any ordered activity limits.
   _____ Explain the facility's visiting hours and policies, provide an orientation to the facility, and explain how to identify different staff.
   _____ If fluids are allowed per the doctor's orders, fill the water pitcher and cup in the resident's room.

6. _____ Report the completion of admission. Communicate specific observations, complications, or unusual responses to the licensed nursing staff and record this information, along with the care provided, in the chart or EMR.
   _____ Wash your hands to ensure infection control.
   _____ Conduct a safety check before leaving the room. The room should be clean and free from clutter or spills.
   _____ Wash your hands or use hand sanitizer before leaving the room.
   _____ Make sure the resident is comfortable and place the call light and personal items within reach.

Name: _____   Date: _____

Matching Section 6.1 Key Terms

Match each definition with the key term.

A. empathy
B. genuine
C. homeostasis
D. motivation
E. respect
F. self-actualization
G. self-esteem
H. self-respect

_____ 1. a person's confidence and regard for himself or herself

_____ 2. honest, open, and sincere in communication and relationships

_____ 3. a person's appreciation and acceptance of himself or herself

_____ 4. a person's prompting to act in a particular way

_____ 5. a state in which someone has become everything he or she hopes to be

_____ 6. a feeling of appreciation and admiration for another person

_____ 7. understanding for another person's feelings and emotions

_____ 8. the constant or stable state of the human body and its complex body systems

Understanding Motivation

Complete the following sentences.

1. A fast-food worker decides to go back to school and become a nursing assistant. This is an example of _____ because the worker is prompted to pursue a goal.

2. A nursing assistant receives a raise of 50 cents per hour. For the next two weeks, she arrives to work 10 minutes early, but then returns to arriving right as her shift starts. This is an example of _____ motivation.

3. At the end of his shift, a nursing assistant feels exhausted, but filled with satisfaction, knowing he did a good job today. This is an example of _____ motivation.

4. Another name for intrinsic motivation is _____.

5. The first component of motivation is called _____.

6. Despite encountering numerous problems during her training, a new nursing assistant works closely with her manager to develop a plan for completing the program. This demonstrates the nursing assistant's _____.

7. A nursing assistant student is the last to leave the room on exam day. She double-checks her answers and ignores the pressure of other students who quickly complete the written exam. She is displaying the component of motivation called _____, which is the concentration and effort needed to successfully complete a goal.

8. The charge nurse gives a nursing assistant a gift card to a local restaurant as a reward for her timeliness. The nursing assistant has a history of tardiness, but hasn't been late since the reward. This is an example of _____ motivation.

9. When working toward a goal, the greater the perceived _____ are, the more strongly a person will be motivated to achieve the goal.

10. According to the _____ theory of motivation, people have strong reasons that prompt various actions for pursuing a goal.

Labeling Maslow's Hierarchy of Needs

Apply the appropriate labels to the image.

5. _____
   _____

4. _____
   _____

3. _____
   _____

2. _____
   _____

1. _____

Understanding Maslow's Hierarchy of Needs

Identify whether each statement is true or false.

_____ 1. In the 1940s, psychologist Abraham Lincoln developed a hierarchy of needs as an important way of explaining human needs and the impact of these needs on motivating action or behavior.

_____ 2. According to Maslow, human needs are ordered from the low-level basic needs of food, water, sleep, and elimination to higher-level needs, the highest of which he called self-actualization.

_____ 3. Maslow's hierarchy of needs is illustrated as a circle, with basic needs starting at the bottom and moving clockwise toward higher-level needs.

_____ 4. Maslow believed that people must satisfy needs at the bottom of the hierarchy before satisfying needs at the next level.

_____ 5. Meeting basic needs helps a person achieve a state of internal balance known as homeostasis.

_____ 6. The highest level of Maslow's hierarchy of needs is security and safety.

_____ 7. Holding a resident's hand while talking to express care and concern demonstrates empathy.

_____ 8. Needs related to love and belonging can only be achieved after a person achieves self-esteem.

_____ 9. The fourth level of Maslow's hierarchy of needs is self-esteem, which describes a person's confidence and regard for himself or herself.

_____ 10. When a person achieves self-actualization, she has fulfilled her potential.

Growth and Development

Select the *best* answer.

_____ 1. Which of the following is true of growth and development?
A. People grow taller as they age, but are born with emotional maturity.
B. People develop mentally, emotionally, and socially based on their unique characteristics.
C. People grow at the same rate through different life stages from conception until death.
D. People grow physically until they reach adolescence.

_____ 2. Which of the following is true of genetics?
A. Genetics does not affect growth and development.
B. Genetics is not affected by heredity.
C. Genetics includes heredity and affects growth and development.
D. Genetics can influence physical growth and development, but not mental development.

_____ 3. Growth charts show
A. a comparison of physical growth with specific measurements that are expected at certain ages
B. average growth patterns of a child's critical thinking ability
C. the exact weight an infant should achieve at two years of age
D. average measurements of body length or height, but not the weight of a child over time

_____ 4. Each stage of development
A. stops when a person's life span reaches the next stage
B. has a specific purpose, or task, that must be accomplished before the next stage can take place
C. is the same for every person
D. happens evenly

_____ 5. Growth and development models
A. show that critical thinking and problem-solving skills are acquired only in adulthood
B. explore the influence of growth on weight
C. prove that the simple skills of developmental stages are developed last
D. are theories that demonstrate how physical, mental, and emotional growth occur

Physical Growth Milestones

The following people are at various stages of growth and development. After reading the description of each individual, label the box with the individuals that correctly describe each growth period.

A. Mason is an outside linebacker for his school's football team. This position is a perfect fit for his stature and weight. He practices his driving skills on his way to school, with his dad in the passenger seat. People tell him that he looks identical to his dad since his last growth spurt. Mason teases that his beard is fuller than his dad's beard.

B. Aiyana neatly makes her bed, grabs her backpack, and dashes out to catch the school bus. She sits by her best friend and classmate Mari. The girls whisper about Aiyana's mom buying her a new training bra. They giggle because a cute boy sitting across the aisle is making funny faces at them.

C. Tomoko's mom worries that Tomoko is not eating enough at mealtime. Tomoko leaves the breakfast table, despite her mom's encouragement to stay and finish her toast. Tomoko would rather chase their bulldog Dozer around the living room. She points to Dozer and commands him to "Sit!" Tomoko then hides behind the curtain and waits for Dozer to find her. While hiding, she has an accident in her underpants since she is not yet fully potty trained.

D. Alejandro has doubled his weight since his last doctor's visit. His arm muscles are stronger as he lifts his head high and rolls onto his back on the living room floor. His dad is delighted at the new accomplishment. Alejandro smiles, reaches out to touch his dad's nose and says, "Dada." His dad's eyes fill with tears of joy.

E. Antoine jumps out of bed after 11 hours of sleep. He is excited about plans to play soccer at the park this afternoon. Antoine's big brother pulls him behind the door and puts a pencil mark on the wall above Antoine's head. He says, "You've grown 3 inches! I think you are going to be taller than me." This causes Antoine to smile broad, showing all 20 of his primary teeth. His big brother helps him dress for the park, but he's properly selected each piece of clothing, including his soccer shoes.

Physical Development of Children and Adolescents

Growth Period	Individual
Infancy (birth–one year)	1. _____
Toddlerhood (one–three years)	2. _____
Preschool years (three–five years)	3. _____
School-age years (six–12 years)	4. _____
Adolescence (12–18 years)	5. _____

Erik Erikson's Theory of Psychosocial Development

Apply the appropriate labels to the table.

Erikson's Stages of Psychosocial Development

Stage	Conflict
1. _____	Basic trust versus mistrust
2. _____	Autonomy versus shame
3. _____	Initiative versus guilt
4. _____	Industry versus inferiority
5. _____	Identity versus confusion
6. _____	Intimacy versus isolation
7. _____	Generativity versus stagnation
8. _____	Integrity versus despair

Matching Section 6.2 Key Terms

Match each definition with the key term.

A. behavior
B. covert
C. generation
D. generation gap
E. overt
F. stereotypes
G. taboos

_____ 1. practices determined by society or religion to be improper, unacceptable, or forbidden

_____ 2. a manner of acting; the way a person responds to stimulation

_____ 3. simplifications or biases about a group that shape the treatment of all group members

_____ 4. a lack of communication between one generation and another; often due to differences in customs, attitudes, and beliefs

_____ 5. open to view; easy to observe

_____ 6. a group of people who are born and who live during the same time

_____ 7. not shown openly

Generational Differences Affecting Behaviors and Attitudes

Identify whether each statement is true or false.

_____ 1. Most behaviors are covert, or open to view.

_____ 2. When feelings and thoughts are acted upon, they become attitudes.

_____ 3. A group of people born during the same time is a generation.

_____ 4. Concealed behavior is called overt behavior.

_____ 5. Cultural differences impact how people communicate, eat, dress, and carry out their traditions.

_____ 6. A mind gap occurs when people from different generations have trouble communicating because of differences in traditions, attitudes, or beliefs.

_____ 7. Members of the silent generation may be more patriotic than members of other generations.

_____ 8. Being aware of, but not preoccupied with, generational differences can help prevent stereotyping.

_____ 9. Stereotypes can be an unhealthy barrier within any group of diverse people.

_____ 10. The better a nursing assistant understands different generations, the harder it will be to build rapport through improved communication.

Generational Characteristics

Identify the generation born during each time period. Then interview three individuals from each generation and discuss the qualities of their generation. Ask if the individuals agree or disagree with each quality and explain their opinions.

1. _____ (1928–1945)

   Members of this generation have strong feelings of patriotism, are work oriented and quiet, are respectful of authority, and have a sense of moral obligation. They experienced economic downturn during the Great Depression and lived through World War II, causing them to be financially conservative—saving money, maintaining low debt, and pursuing secure financial investments. This generation also values security, comfort, and familiar activities and environments.

   Interview Feedback: _____

   _____

   _____

   _____

   _____

   _____

   _____

2. _____ (1946–1964)

   This generation experienced the Civil Rights Movement, the sexual revolution, several assassinations, the Korean War, and political scandals. Members have a strong work ethic, are hardworking, enjoyed good work opportunities, are driven to achieve professional goals, and define themselves by professional accomplishments. Members of this generation have also been described as self-reliant, independent, optimistic, confident, patriotic, and idolizing of youth.

   Interview Feedback: _____

   _____

   _____

   _____

   _____

   _____

   _____

3. _____ (1965–1976)

   Members of this generation have been called latchkey kids because their parents often worked. Members of this generation are entrepreneurs, are self-sufficient, focus on financial planning, are independent and educated, started a family more cautiously than parents did, and hoped to avoid raising their children the way they were raised.

   Interview Feedback: _____

   _____

   _____

   _____

   _____

   _____

4. _____ (1977–1995)

   This generation is great in numbers, sophisticated, technologically savvy, and isolated as individuals because of technology. Members of this generation ignore sales pitches because of overexposure and are less brand loyal. They've also been described as flexible, comfortable with changing fashion, and civic minded and often volunteer, value exercise, and enjoy travel.

   Interview Feedback: _____

   _____

   _____

   _____

   _____

   _____

5. _____ (1995–2004)

   This generation's environment is diverse and includes sophisticated media and technology utilized daily. Members of this generation are independent and use the Internet and social media as primary forms of communication.

   Interview Feedback: _____

   _____

   _____

   _____

   _____

   _____

   _____

Matching Section 6.3 Key Terms

Match each definition with the key term.

A. autonomy
B. conscious
C. parasympathetic nervous system (PNS)
D. rapport
E. self-image
F. subconscious
G. sympathetic nervous system (SNS)

_____ 1. the personal independence and freedom to determine one's own actions and behavior

_____ 2. not fully aware of feelings, actions, and outside surroundings

_____ 3. a component of the nervous system that controls the automatic daily functions of the cardiovascular, respiratory, and digestive systems and helps the body return to a homeostatic state after experiencing pain or stress

_____ 4. a component of the nervous system that initiates the fight-or-flight response

_____ 5. the way a person thinks about his or her self, abilities, and appearance

_____ 6. aware of feelings, actions, and outside surroundings

_____ 7. mutual understanding in a relationship

Body, Mind, Spirit

Complete the following sentences.

1. The _____ is a person's higher self, or the inner qualities that help a person feel whole and achieve a sense of inner peace and harmony.

2. The human _____ is a highly complex, integrative system with basic needs.

3. Your _____ is constantly thinking, inquiring, and directing your behavior based on your perception of the world.

Understanding the Mind

Complete the following sentences.

1. A nursing assistant smells a foul odor after a resident urinates. She suspects that the resident has a urinary tract infection. This awareness is an example of _____ thought.

2. A female resident is unaware of her prejudice against a male caregiver and is uncooperative when he provides care. This is an example of _____ thought.

3. A nursing assistant student begins to tremble and sweat prior to taking the certification competency exam. He takes in a deep breath and feels a sense of calm. This is an example of the _____ taking over and returning his body to a homeostatic state.

4. Another nursing assistant student begins to tremble and sweat prior to taking the certification competency exam. She runs out of the room. This is an example of the _____ triggering the fight-or-flight response.

5. When a nursing assistant's body, mind, and spirit are connected, he or she will feel self-assured and develop a positive _____, or view of himself or herself.

6. With an understanding of the body-mind-spirit connection, a nursing assistant can encourage residents to also maintain this connection by promoting _____, or personal independence.

Name: _____ Date: _____

Matching Chapter 7 Key Terms

Match the definition with the key term.

A. complementary and alternative medicine (CAM)
B. contraindicate
C. conventional medicine
D. disease
E. distress
F. energy
G. energy rhythm
H. eustress
I. health
J. health promotion
K. hormones
L. illness
M. integrative medicine (IM)
N. intuition
O. prioritizing
P. probiotics
Q. stress management
R. well-being
S. work-life balance

_____ 1. the state of a person's health; is influenced by balancing one's diet, exercise, relationships, financial resources, work, education, and leisure

_____ 2. the state of a person's time and energy contributions to career, work, and family commitments

_____ 3. a feeling of poor health; is not always caused by a disease

_____ 4. a condition in which an organ or body system incorrectly functions and exhibits particular signs and symptoms

_____ 5. the process of taking actions to lessen or remove reactions to stress and stressful events

_____ 6. chemical substances that are produced in the body and that control and regulate specific body processes

_____ 7. the sequence of energy peaks a person experiences over a certain time period

_____ 8. good stress; helps people become motivated and productive

_____ 9. the power and drive to make decisions and complete tasks

_____ 10. organizing responsibilities or tasks so that the most important tasks are completed first

_____ 11. bad stress; causes bodily symptoms that can lead to disease and to poor coping and decision making

_____ 12. the process of making efforts to help people improve or increase control over their health and wellness

_____ 13. a feeling that is not based on facts or evidence, but that guides actions

_____ 14. the condition of a person's physical, mental, social, and spiritual self

_____ 15. treatments performed by medical doctors, nurses, and other healthcare providers who use evidence-based scientific data to diagnose and treat diseases

_____ 16. to advise against or point out the possible dangers of a particular drug or treatment

_____ 17. treatments that take a coordinated approach to the diagnosis, treatment, and prevention of diseases; providers see people as whole individuals and focus on the energy of the body

_____ 18. treatments that are performed in addition to conventional medicine or that are entirely separate and serve as replacements for conventional medicine

_____ 19. oral dietary supplements that contain live bacteria; restore beneficial bacteria to the body

Understanding Wellness and Illness

Complete the following sentences.

1. When people experience _____, or a feeling of poor health, parts of their bodies and minds can still be well.

2. A(n) _____ is caused by an incorrectly functioning organ or body system and is usually accompanied by specific symptoms that can be diagnosed by a licensed healthcare provider.

3. A(n) _____ may be a personal interpretation of how a person is feeling.

4. A person who has a disease, but still feels well, is more likely to manage the progression of the disease in a way that has a positive impact on his or her _____.

5. The relationship between wellness and illness influences a person's sense of _____, or state of health.

6. Achieving _____ requires self-awareness, commitment to wellness strategies, and ongoing change for both the resident and nursing assistant.

Stress

Complete the following sentences.

1. _____ occurs as a result of physical, mental, or emotional pressures.

2. _____, or *good* stress, can be beneficial and can motivate you to do new or challenging tasks.

3. Stress that remains at a high level, lasts for a long time, or gets out of control can turn into bad stress, or _____.

4. When a person is stressed, his or her body releases chemical substances called _____ that regulate body processes and prepare the body for the challenges of stress.

5. When the body is stressed, the _____ triggers the fight-or-flight response.

Signs and Symptoms of Stress

Identify the following signs and symptoms of stress.

1. _____ symptoms: moodiness, short temper, agitation, loneliness, or depression

2. _____ symptoms: procrastination, isolation, nervous habits, or the use of alcohol or drugs to relax

3. _____ symptoms: aches and pains, dizziness, nausea, rapid heartbeat, or frequent colds

4. _____ symptoms: inability to concentrate, constant worry, or ability to see only the negative

Stress Management

Identify whether each statement is true or false.

_____ 1. Stress-management strategies to handle and control stress are more important for the resident than the holistic nursing assistant.

_____ 2. The first way to manage stress is to identify stressors after they cause strong stress reactions.

_____ 3. Focusing on something relaxing may help reduce stress.

_____ 4. Humor is rarely used successfully to reduce stress.

_____ 5. A solid support network of family and friends is an ineffective stress-management technique.

_____ 6. If a nursing assistant has self-awareness of personal energy levels, he will get work done and likely feel good about the accomplishment.

_____ 7. Identifying your personal energy rhythm does not help to plan work.

_____ 8. Prioritizing, or organizing responsibilities and tasks so that the most important tasks are completed first, is an important time-management strategy.

_____ 9. Prioritizing tasks is an important strategy for determining which tasks are urgent when giving care.

_____ 10. Work-life balance can help the nursing assistant feel more in control, which can reduce stress levels.

Identifying and Managing Personal Stressors

When you begin working as a nursing assistant, stress may interfere with your ability to provide quality care. Work- and career-related stress can also interfere with your home life. Respond to each of the following questions to determine how you respond to stress and how you might develop a support network to help you manage stress.

1. How do you respond to stress? (For example, does stress cause you to withdraw, lose your temper, abuse or avoid food, or seek the comfort of a loved one?)

   _____

   _____

2. Which stressors most often affect you? (For example, do you find disagreements, work or school deadlines, or even being in a crowd stressful?)

   _____

   _____

3. What makes you feel better or manage your stress? (For example, do you feel better after exercising, talking to a loved one, or journaling?)

   _____

   _____

4. Who are three people in your life you trust with this information?

   _____

   _____

5. How might the people in your support network help you manage stress?

   _____

   _____

Health Promotion

Select the *best* answer.

_____ 1. Health promotion
   A. cannot prompt large groups of people to change
   B. is the process of helping people, groups, and communities improve their control over health and wellness
   C. is usually a fixed, unchanging process
   D. is the process of helping large groups of people, not individual residents

_____ 2. What is the primary goal of health promotion?
  A. smoking cessation
  B. to create community contests to reduce overall health
  C. to place more importance on group health than individual health
  D. to share healthy ideas, beliefs, and experiences with the goal of motivating people to adopt healthy behaviors

_____ 3. Which of the following is true of health and wellness?
  A. It is unrelated to the body, mind, and spirit.
  B. It is important for you to help others achieve their health and wellness.
  C. It is not an ongoing process because people stop growing and changing.
  D. It must always be reported to the licensed nursing staff.

_____ 4. Intuition is
  A. a feeling that may not have direct evidence, but is trusted to be true
  B. a feeling based on facts
  C. never reported to the licensed nursing staff
  D. not yet observable, so there is no need to explore it further

_____ 5. The National Prevention Strategy
  A. has a goal of helping Americans lead higher-quality lives in a shorter life span
  B. sets seven priorities, which provide evidenced-based recommendations for reducing healthcare
  C. guides the United States in finding ways to promote health and well-being
  D. mandates educational minimum requirements for nursing assistants

Integrative Medicine (IM)

Complete the following sentences.

1. _____ is a coordinated approach to the diagnosis, treatment, and prevention of diseases.

2. Previously, integrative medicine (IM) was called _____.

3. Treatments performed by healthcare providers who use evidence-based scientific data are considered _____ medicine.

4. Natural products include herbs or botanicals, vitamins, minerals, and _____ (supplements that contain live, beneficial bacteria).

5. _____ products are the most popular and most used IM treatment among Americans.

6. _____ is a mind and body technique in which a person focuses his or her attention inward or outward to specific objects.

7. A mind and body technique that combines physical postures or movements, focused concentration, and breathing techniques is _____.

8. In _____ medicine, practitioners believe that each person is made of five basic elements found in the universe—space, air, fire, water, and earth.

9. _____ uses physical forces such as heat, water, light, air, and massage as primary treatments.

10. Some IM approaches may be _____ for treatments residents are currently receiving. In these cases, the licensed nursing staff should be informed of any IM approaches in use.

Identifying Mind and Body Practices

Match each definition with the appropriate mind and body practice.

A. acupuncture
B. Ayurvedic medicine
C. homeopathy
D. hypnotherapy
E. massage therapy
F. meditation
G. naturopathy
H. relaxation techniques
I. spinal manipulation
J. tai chi and qigong
K. traditional Chinese medicine (TCM)
L. yoga

_____ 1. a technique in which a practitioner provides helpful, calm, and focused suggestions that a person experience changes in sensations, perceptions, thoughts, or behavior

_____ 2. a technique in which the soft tissues of the body are manually manipulated to promote relaxation or manage pain

_____ 3. a technique in which a person learns to focus his or her attention inward or outward to help become more mindful and manage stress

_____ 4. techniques that reproduce the body's natural relaxation response like breathing exercises and guided imagery

_____ 5. a technique in which a healthcare provider applies a controlled force to a joint or the spine to treat muscle spasms of the back or neck and headaches

_____ 6. the combination of specific movements or postures, coordinated breathing, and mental focus to delay aging, prolong life, increase flexibility, strengthen muscles and tendons, and aid in the treatment of health conditions

_____ 7. a technique that combines physical postures or movements, focused concentration, and breathing techniques to integrate the body, mind, and spirit

_____ 8. practitioners use herbal compounds, special diets, and lifestyle recommendations to treat arthritis and other inflammatory conditions

_____ 9. a practice based on the principle that qi, the body's core or vital energy, flows throughout the body; a disruption of qi causes an imbalance that leads to disease

_____ 10. a technique in which a licensed practitioner inserts thin needles through the skin to stimulate specific points on the body to treat pain, headache, nausea, and fibromyalgia

_____ 11. a practice based on the concept that giving a person small amounts of a substance that causes symptoms similar to a person's illness may cure the illness

_____ 12. a system of therapy based on preventive care that uses physical forces such as heat, water, light, air, and massage as primary treatments

CHAPTER 8 The Healthy Body: Anatomy and Physiology

Name: _____ Date: _____

Matching Section 8.1 Key Terms
Match each definition with the key term.

A. acronyms
B. atrophy
C. body cavities
D. cell
E. coronal plane
F. Fowler's position
G. lateral position
H. medical terminology
I. membranes
J. neurons
K. nutrients
L. organs
M. peristalsis
N. prone position
O. sagittal plane
P. secretion
Q. supine position
R. tissue
S. transverse plane
T. tumor

_____ 1. a body position in which a patient lies on his or her abdomen with arms and hands at each side, feet comfortably positioned, and head turned to the side

_____ 2. collections of tissues that have specific structures and functions

_____ 3. a body plane that divides the body into left and right sides

_____ 4. a body position in which a patient lies flat on his or her back with the arms at each side

_____ 5. a body plane that divides the body into upper and lower halves

_____ 6. the smallest and most basic structural and functional unit of the human body

_____ 7. an abnormal growth of tissue that has no function in the body

_____ 8. spaces in the human body that contain organs

_____ 9. a body position in which a patient lies with legs extended on an examining table or bed; the head of the bed is raised to a 45° angle

_____ 10. a body position in which a patient lies on his or her side with arms free and knees slightly bent

_____ 11. the language used in healthcare

_____ 12. cells of the nervous system that transmit information throughout the body in the form of electrochemical messages (neural impulses)

_____ 13. a body plane that divides the body into front and back halves

_____ 14. the involuntary, wavelike constriction and relaxation of smooth muscles

_____ 15. substances the body needs to function normally

_____ 16. to shrink or decrease in size

_____ 17. the release of chemical substances, such as mucus or saliva, that are manufactured by cells

_____ 18. a collection of specialized cells that act together to perform specific functions

_____ 19. thin, soft, and flexible structures that cover, line, or act as boundaries for cells or organs

_____ 20. words formed from the first letters or groups of letters in a phrase

Understanding Medical Terminology
Complete the following sentences.

1. Medical _____ is the language of medicine.

2. The five _____ used in medical terminology are the root word, combining vowel, combining form (root word plus combining vowel), prefix, and suffix.

3. The _____, often derived from Greek or Latin, is the central part of a medical term.

4. A(n) _____ vowel is a vowel attached to the end of a root word to link word parts for easier pronunciation.

5. A root word plus its combining vowel is known as a(n) _____ form.

6. A(n) _____ is the part of a medical term that is attached to the beginning of a root word.

7. The _____ is the part of a medical term attached to the end of a root word and usually indicates a condition, disease, diagnosis, surgical intervention, or therapy.

8. Medical terminology includes _____, which are short combinations of letters used to represent longer words and speed up communication in healthcare facilities.

9. _____ are also used in medical terminology and are formed from the first letters or groups of letters in a phrase.

10. The acronym BP stands for _____.

Name: _____ Date: _____

Identifying Abbreviations and Acronyms

Identify the abbreviation or acronym associated with each definition.

_____ 1. as desired

_____ 2. activities of daily living

_____ 3. admission

_____ 4. ambulatory

_____ 5. basic life support

_____ 6. beats per minute

_____ 7. complains of

_____ 8. cardiopulmonary resuscitation

_____ 9. cerebrovascular accident

_____ 10. date of birth

_____ 11. family history

_____ 12. gastrointestinal

_____ 13. intake and output

_____ 14. intravenous

_____ 15. no known allergies

_____ 16. pulse

_____ 17. respiration

_____ 18. range of motion

_____ 19. signs and symptoms

_____ 20. vital signs

Understanding Body Positions

Identify whether each statement is true or false.

_____ 1. Nursing assistants place residents in different body positions for a variety of reasons, including examinations, treatments, and assistance with ADLs.

_____ 2. Anatomical lateral is the standard position for referencing anatomical structures.

_____ 3. The left and right sides of the body are not considered mirror images of each other.

_____ 4. The term *bilateral symmetry* is used when the right and left sides of the body are mirror images of each other.

_____ 5. The most common body positions nursing assistants encounter are Fowler's position, lateral position, prone position, and supine position.

_____ 6. In lateral position, the person is seated in bed, and the backrest of the bed is at a 45° angle.

_____ 7. In Fowler's position, a person lies on his or her side with arms free and knees slightly bent.

_____ 8. When in supine position, a person lies on the abdomen with arms and hands at each side.

_____ 9. When in prone position, a person lies flat on his or her back with the arms at each side.

_____ 10. Prone, supine, Fowler's, and lateral positions are the only body positions used in healthcare.

Identifying Body Positions

Apply the appropriate labels to the image.

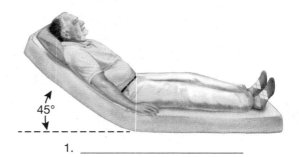

1. _____

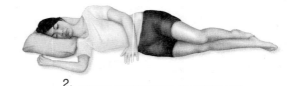

2. _____

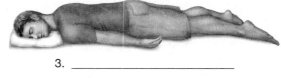

3. _____

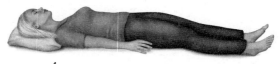

4. _____

© Body Scientific International

Identifying Body Planes

Apply the appropriate callouts to the image.

A. Coronal plane

B. Sagittal plane

C. Transverse plane

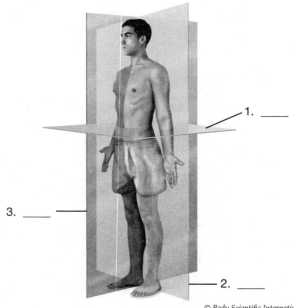

1. _____

3. _____

2. _____

© Body Scientific International

Name: _____   Date: _____

Labeling Directional Terms

Apply the appropriate callouts to the image.

A. Anterior view
B. Dorsal
C. Inferior

D. Lateral
E. Lateral view
F. Medial

G. Posterior view
H. Superior
I. Ventral

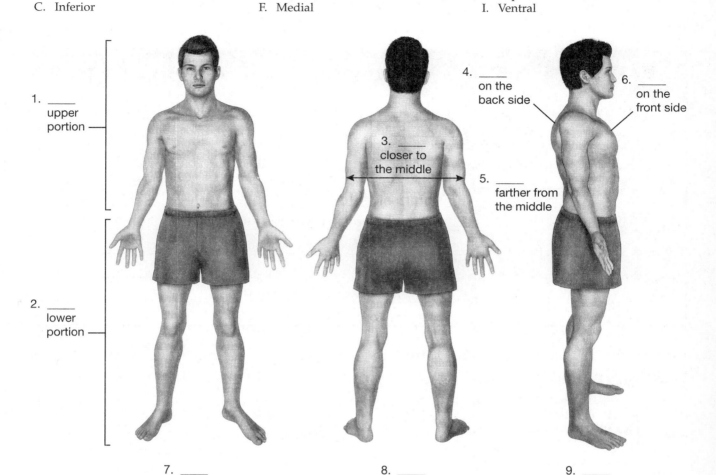

1. ____ upper portion

2. ____ lower portion

3. ____ closer to the middle

4. ____ on the back side

5. ____ farther from the middle

6. ____ on the front side

7. ____

8. ____

9. ____

© Body Scientific International

Body Cavities

Complete the following sentences.

1. The human body is divided into body _____, which are spaces in the body that contain organs.

2. _____ are collections of tissues that have specific structures and functions.

3. The two main divisions of cavities in the body are the _____ (posterior) and ventral (anterior) cavities.

4. The _____ contains the brain (cerebrum), as well as the blood vessels and nerves that support the brain.

5. The _____ contains the spinal cord, spinal column, tailbone, and vertebrae.

6. The _____ contains the lungs, heart, trachea, pharynx, larynx, and bronchial tubes.

7. The _____ contains the liver, gallbladder, stomach, pancreas, intestines, spleen, and kidneys.

8. The _____ contains the sigmoid colon, rectum, anus, urinary bladder, urethra, ureters, and male and female reproductive organs.

Name: _____ Date: _____

Describing Body Movements

Identify the appropriate body movements in the table.

Abduction	Extension	Hyperextension	Rotation
Adduction	Flexion	Pronation	Supination
Circumduction			

Body Movements	
Movement	**Description**
1. _____	The act of bending a joint
2. _____	The act of straightening a joint
3. _____	An exaggerated, or extreme, extension
4. _____	Lateral (sideways) movement away from the midline (an invisible line running vertically through the body)
5. _____	Lateral movement toward the midline of the body
6. _____	Turning of a body part around an axis, or fixed point
7. _____	Rotating a body part in a complete circle
8. _____	Rotating a body part from the body
9. _____	Rotating a body part toward the body

Cells, Tissues, and Membranes in Body Structure

Complete the following sentences.

1. Three essential internal structures are the foundation of life in the human body: _____, tissues, and membranes.

2. _____ and membranes are composed of groups of cells with similar structures and functions.

3. _____ are thin, soft, and flexible structures that support and protect body surfaces, organs, and joints.

The Cell

Identify whether each statement is true or false.

_____ 1. The organ is the structural and functional unit of the human body.

_____ 2. There are about 3,000 cells in the human body.

_____ 3. All cells begin as undifferentiated stem cells.

_____ 4. As cells mature, they produce more stem cells and undifferentiate, or evolve, into cells that perform particular functions.

_____ 5. Red blood cells defend the body against disease-causing microorganisms.

_____ 6. The structures inside cells are called organelles.

_____ 7. Mature cells exist in bone, muscle, and blood.

_____ 8. All cells use nutrients, or substances needed for normal body function.

_____ 9. When cells atrophy, they increase in size.

_____ 10. Cells can grow into unusual shapes called tumors.

Tissues

Complete the following sentences.

1. The four types of tissue include connective tissue, muscle tissue, nerve tissue, and _____ tissue.

2. _____ tissue supports body tissues, structures, and organs.

3. Connective tissue is composed of _____ (protein) fibers that provide strength and of elastin fibers that enable flexibility.

4. _____ tissue provides a covering for the external body (skin) and lines internal organs (intestines).

5. Epithelial tissue is classified by the arrangement of its _____.

6. Epithelial tissue can be simple or _____.

7. _____ tissue contracts, or shortens, to produce movement.

8. Found in the walls of the intestines and other internal organs, _____ muscle tissue moves involuntarily.

9. The involuntary movement of the intestinal muscles, called _____, moves food through the gastrointestinal system.

10. _____ muscle tissue makes up most of the heart wall, is involuntary, and causes the heart to contract.

Body Membranes
Select the *best* answer.

_____ 1. What are body membranes?
   A. thin, soft, flexible structures that support, separate, and protect body surfaces, organs, and joints
   B. bony tissues that separate cavities in the body
   C. epithelial and connective blood fibers
   D. structures that produce sensation and movement

_____ 2. Epithelial membranes
   A. protect the body, but not internal organs
   B. include cutaneous membranes, mucous membranes, and serous membranes
   C. are unique structures that do not contain cells
   D. are inflexible, rigid structures that support internal organs

_____ 3. Which of the following is true of cutaneous membranes?
   A. They exclude the skin, epidermis, and dermis.
   B. They are found deep within the respiratory tract.
   C. They cover the entire body and are commonly referred to as *skin*.
   D. They are not a major component of the integumentary system.

_____ 4. Mucous membranes
   A. only line body surfaces on the outside of the body
   B. produce a film of mucus that coats and protects underlying cells and captures disease-causing microorganisms
   C. are not found in the respiratory, gastro-intestinal, urinary, and reproductive systems
   D. are found on the soles of the feet and palms of the hands

_____ 5. Which of the following is true of serous membranes?
   A. They line the outer, open body surfaces and are composed of one layer.
   B. They contain serous fluid that helps prevent friction when organs move in the body cavities.
   C. They cover the deltoid muscle.
   D. They do not cover the abdominal organs.

_____ 6. Connective tissue membranes
   A. include the synovial membrane and the meninges
   B. drain synovial fluid from joint cavities
   C. cause friction and prevent lubrication in joints
   D. damage the brain and spinal cord

Matching Section 8.2 Key Terms, Part A
Match each key term with the definition.

A. anatomy
B. appendicular skeleton
C. autonomic nervous system (ANS)
D. axial skeleton
E. central nervous system (CNS)
F. circadian rhythm
G. endocrine glands
H. epidermis
I. exocrine glands
J. fibrous
K. gland
L. ligaments
M. peripheral nervous system (PNS)
N. physiology
O. platelets
P. receptors
Q. red blood cells
R. somatic nervous system
S. tendons
T. white blood cells

_____ 1. the part of the nervous system that consists of the brain and spinal cord
_____ 2. components of the blood that fight infection and provide protection
_____ 3. ductless glands that secrete hormones directly into the bloodstream
_____ 4. the skeletal structure that provides stability for the body; includes bones in the body's trunk
_____ 5. the physical, mental, and behavioral changes that occur in a person in a roughly 24-hour cycle
_____ 6. the outermost layer of the skin
_____ 7. the study of how the body functions
_____ 8. sensory nerve endings on or within a cell that react to various stimuli and produce an effect
_____ 9. the study of the body's structure and parts
_____ 10. a group of specialized cells that secrete substances
_____ 11. flat, circular cells in the blood that assist in the clotting process
_____ 12. fibrous cords of tissue that attach bone to bone and support organs
_____ 13. composed of tough, thin threads
_____ 14. bands of fibrous tissue that connect muscle to bone
_____ 15. the skeletal structure that enables the body to move; includes bones in the body's appendages (arms and legs)

_____ 16. glands with ducts that transport substances to other organs or to the surface of the skin

_____ 17. the components of the blood that contain hemoglobin; are responsible for oxygen and carbon dioxide exchange

_____ 18. the part of the nervous system that controls voluntary body functions and the movement of skeletal muscle

_____ 19. the part of the nervous system that controls involuntary, unconscious body functions

_____ 20. the part of the nervous system that consists of 12 pairs of cranial nerves and 31 pairs of spinal nerves

Matching Section 8.2 Key Terms, Part B

Match each definition with the key term.

A. antibodies
B. deoxyribonucleic acid (DNA)
C. dermis
D. ducts
E. enzymes
F. follicles
G. formed elements
H. hemoglobin
I. pathogens
J. plasma
K. pulse
L. sperm
M. sphincter

_____ 1. the component of a red blood cell that allows the cell to transport oxygen and that gives the cell its red color

_____ 2. disease-causing microorganisms

_____ 3. a blood protein that reduces the effects of bacteria and viruses by identifying and attacking red blood cells marked with foreign substances called antigens

_____ 4. the beat of the heart measured through the walls of a peripheral artery

_____ 5. a circular muscle that can open or close

_____ 6. the inner, thick layer of the skin

_____ 7. the liquid component of blood

_____ 8. tubes for conveying substances

_____ 9. a chemical compound containing instructions for developing and directing the growth and activities of living organisms

_____ 10. small sacs or cavities

_____ 11. the solid component of blood

_____ 12. chemical agents that can cause specific biochemical reactions

_____ 13. male reproductive cell

Body Systems

Complete the following sentences.

1. The _____ work both independently and together to ensure the body operates effectively.

2. _____ is the study of the body's structures and parts.

3. _____ is the study of how the body functions.

4. Maintaining _____ requires a balance of body system functions.

5. _____ occurs when a structure or system in the body is injured, altered, or malformed in a way that impacts its function.

The Integumentary System

Complete the following sentences.

1. The _____ system is composed of the skin, subcutaneous lipocytes, nerves, blood vessels, and accessory organs.

2. The _____ is the largest organ in the human body.

3. The skin contains the majority of the body's _____, or sensory nerve endings, for touch, pressure, temperature, pain, and itch.

4. The skin is a(n) _____ membrane and consists of two major layers.

5. The outer layer of the skin is called the epidermis, while the inner layer is called the

   _____.

6. The skin is responsible for regulating body

   _____.

7. The dermis is a(n) _____ connective tissue composed of tough, thin threads.

8. A(n) _____ is a group of specialized cells that secrete substances.

9. _____ glands secrete an oily substance called sebum.

10. The hair and fingernails are composed of the protein _____ and epithelial cells.

The Skeletal System and Body Support

Select the *best* answer.

_____ 1. At birth, the human body is composed of
   A. 270 bones
   B. 65 bones
   C. 1,840 bones
   D. primarily cartilage

_____ 2. As an infant grows, the bones
   A. become pliable and less dense
   B. atrophy
   C. store potassium and phosphoric acid needed for regulatory functions
   D. fuse together, leaving the adult skeleton with 206 bones

_____ 3. The structures of the skeletal system
   A. form plasma and platelets in the bone marrow
   B. act as levers for organ function
   C. protect internal organs by shielding them with bony structure
   D. only include sesamoid bones

_____ 4. The bones
   A. store calcium and phosphorus needed for regulatory functions
   B. excrete sebum released through ducts
   C. form the largest organ in the human body
   D. work independently of the skeletal system

_____ 5. Hematopoiesis
   A. is the process by which blood clots form
   B. provides structure and shape for the body
   C. contains the majority of the body's receptors
   D. is the production of red and white blood cells and platelets in the bone marrow

Types of Bones

Apply the appropriate labels to the image.

Flat	Long	Short
Irregular	Sesamoid	

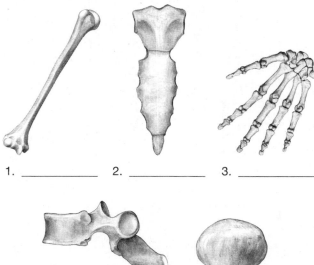

1. _____
2. _____
3. _____
4. _____
5. _____

© Body Scientific International

Bone Composition

Identify whether each statement is true or false.

_____ 1. Bones are an adipose tissue made of collagen, fiber, and minerals.

_____ 2. The two types of bone tissue are compact bone and springy bone.

_____ 3. Red blood cells, white blood cells, and platelets are manufactured in red bone marrow.

_____ 4. Red blood cells facilitate oxygen and carbon dioxide exchange throughout the body, white blood cells fight infection, and platelets aid in clotting.

_____ 5. Bones have rough, exterior processes, openings, grooves, and depressions that provide structure for the attachment of muscles and tendons.

Tendons, Ligaments, and Joints

Complete the following sentences.

1. _____ are tough, flexible bands of fibrous connective tissue that connect muscles to bones.

2. _____ are locations where two or more bones connect.

3. Bones are linked together by _____, which are also bands of connective tissue.

4. The three types of joints include _____, amphiarthroses, and diarthroses.

5. The meeting of two carpal bones is a(n) _____ joint.

6. The head of the humerus and the scapula form a(n) _____ joint.

Identifying the Bones of the Skeletal System

Apply the appropriate callouts to the image.

A. Calcaneus
B. Carpals
C. Clavicle
D. Coccyx
E. Coxal (hip) bone
F. Cranium

G. Facial bones
H. Femur
I. Fibula
J. Humerus
K. Metacarpals
L. Metatarsals

M. Patella
N. Phalanges of the foot
O. Phalanges of the hand
P. Radius
Q. Ribs
R. Sacrum

S. Scapula
T. Sternum
U. Tarsals
V. Tibia
W. Ulna
X. Vertebral column (spine)

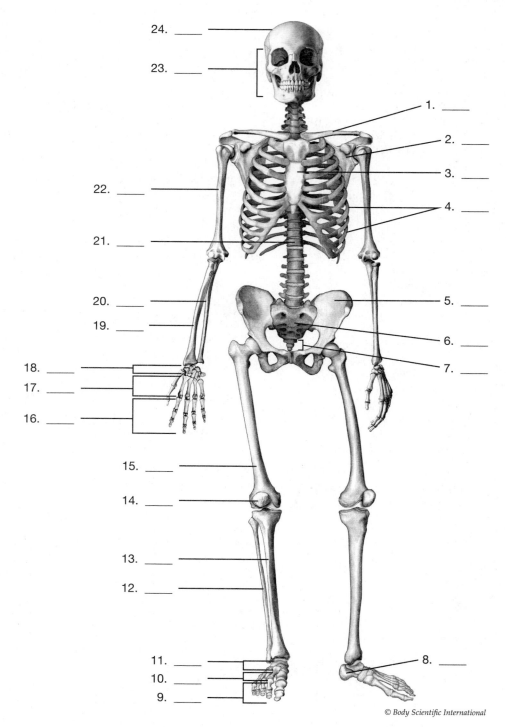

© Body Scientific International

Understanding the Muscular System

Identify whether each statement is true or false.

_____ 1. The muscular system is composed of more than 600 muscles and makes up 2 percent of the body's weight.

_____ 2. The muscular system does not respond to external stimuli.

_____ 3. The muscular system contracts and compresses to move the body's skeleton.

_____ 4. When a muscle contracts, the insertion of the muscle moves, while the origin of the muscle does not.

_____ 5. Effective muscular function requires opposition between an agonist (which contracts) and an antagonist (which relaxes).

Functions of the Muscular System

Select the *best* answer.

_____ 1. In addition to enabling movement, the muscular system also
   A. provides structure by using skeletal tone
   B. protects and covers underlying cells
   C. produces the majority of heat, through movement, to keep the body warm
   D. uses action to move food through the body's blood vessels

_____ 2. Muscle tissue
   A. has the ability to contract, must be inflexible, and must be resistant to neural messages
   B. is covered by fascia, a fibrous connective tissue that links muscles to tendons
   C. is connected to bone at six ends
   D. has thousands of muscle fibers that receive signals through the digestive system

_____ 3. Which of the following is true of skeletal, or striated, muscles?
   A. They are consciously controlled.
   B. They move the skeleton only by relaxing.
   C. They are found in the brain, face, mouth, arms, hands, abdomen, legs, and feet.
   D. They are involuntarily controlled by the brain.

_____ 4. Smooth, or visceral, muscles
   A. contract and relax with conscious control
   B. are not found in the walls of organs
   C. relax, but cannot contract, to move the contents inside an organ
   D. are part of the involuntary process of peristalsis in the gastrointestinal tract

_____ 5. Which of the following is true of cardiac muscle?
   A. It is found only in the lung and makes up most of the lung wall.
   B. It causes the heart to contract.
   C. It is smooth muscle that contracts voluntarily.
   D. It has three types: skeletal, smooth, and cardiac.

The Nervous System

Complete the following sentences.

1. The nervous system uses billions of cells called _____ to send electrochemical messages, also known as neural impulses, throughout the body.

2. Neurons send messages both consciously and unconsciously and receive information from internal and external _____ that interpret the information.

3. Voluntary responses are controlled mostly by the _____, while involuntary responses are controlled by the spinal cord.

4. The _____ nervous system consists of the brain and spinal cord.

5. The _____ nervous system consists of 12 pairs of cranial nerves and 31 pairs of spinal nerves.

6. Many neurons in a bundle are called a(n) _____.

7. Neurons are composed of a cell body, dendrites, and _____.

8. The brain and spinal cord are covered with three layers of tissue known as _____.

9. The outer layer of the meninges, called the _____, is a tough, protective membrane.

10. The middle layer of the meninges, called the _____, is a thin, transparent membrane resembling a loosely fitting sac.

11. The _____ is a thin membrane that adheres to the surface of the brain and spinal cord.

12. The _____ nervous system connects the CNS with the rest of the body.

13. Involuntary, unconscious body functions are controlled by the _____ nervous system.

14. The autonomic nervous system (ANS) is divided into the _____ and parasympathetic nervous systems.

15. The _____ nervous system controls voluntary body movements and stimulates skeletal muscle.

Regions of the Brain

Select the *best* answer.

_____ 1. The brain is divided into the
   A. central nervous system and peripheral nervous system
   B. midbrain, pons, and medulla oblongata
   C. cerebrum and brain stem
   D. cerebrum, cerebellum, diencephalon, and brain stem

_____ 2. The cerebrum
    A. is located in the anterior and lateral part
       of the brain
    B. is the smallest region of the brain
    C. controls high-level cognitive functions
    D. is divided into top and bottom hemispheres

_____ 3. The cerebellum
    A. controls the body's sense of balance and
       equilibrium
    B. is located in the anterior part of the brain
    C. coordinates involuntary muscle movements
    D. controls language

_____ 4. The diencephalon
    A. is part of the brain stem
    B. houses three glands: the thalamus, pineal
       gland, and hypothalamus
    C. houses three glands: the thymus, pineal
       gland, and hypothalamus
    D. is found beneath the cerebellum

_____ 5. Involuntary body functions such as heart rate,
    blood pressure, temperature, and digestion are
    controlled by the
    A. thymus
    B. hypothalamus
    C. cerebrum
    D. thalamus

_____ 6. The circadian rhythm is regulated by the
    A. pineal gland
    B. hypothalamus
    C. thalamus
    D. pons

_____ 7. The brain stem
    A. connects the cerebellum with the cerebrum
    B. includes the thalamus, pineal gland, and
       hypothalamus
    C. has three parts: the midbrain, pons, and
       medulla oblongata
    D. is connected to the frontal lobe of the brain

_____ 8. The midbrain
    A. is the passageway through which neural
       messages travel from the brain to the
       spinal cord
    B. is located in the cerebrum
    C. is the one area of the brain that has no
       neural receptors
    D. controls the voluntary function of digestion

_____ 9. The pons
    A. paces the heart rate
    B. connects the cerebellum to the rest of
       the brain
    C. does not play a role in breathing
    D. is located in the superior and anterior
       part of the brain

_____ 10. The medulla oblongata
    A. connects the brain to the spinal vertebrae
    B. regulates heart rate, breathing, and blood
       pressure
    C. sends messages from the sensory organs
       to the frontal lobe
    D. plays a vital role in voluntary muscle
       movement

Divisions of the Nervous System

Apply the appropriate labels to the image.

A. Autonomic nervous system
B. Central nervous system (CNS)
C. Parasympathetic nervous system
D. Peripheral nervous system (PNS)
E. Somatic nervous system
F. Sympathetic nervous system

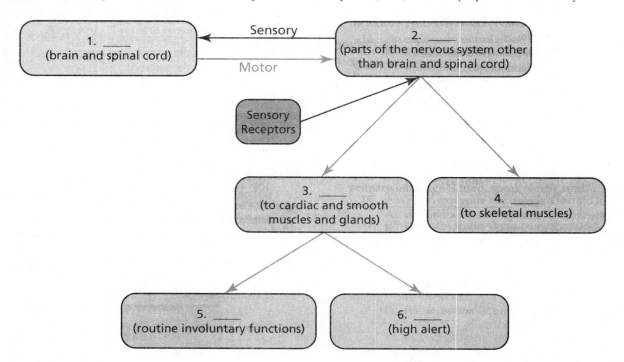

1. _____ (brain and spinal cord)

Sensory

Motor

2. _____ (parts of the nervous system other than brain and spinal cord)

Sensory Receptors

3. _____ (to cardiac and smooth muscles and glands)

4. _____ (to skeletal muscles)

5. _____ (routine involuntary functions)

6. _____ (high alert)

The Eye
Identify whether each statement is true or false.

_____ 1. The structures of the eye receive and translate light into neural messages.

_____ 2. Lacrimal glands secrete lacrimal fluid, or *tears*.

_____ 3. The eyelashes and eyebrows prevent foreign substances from leaving the eye.

_____ 4. The lacrimal canaliculi, or *tear ducts*, collect, store, and drain tears.

_____ 5. Ciliary glands secrete a protective lubricant onto the eyeball.

_____ 6. The orbital socket in the skull protects the eye.

_____ 7. The conjunctiva is a clear, colorless muscular membrane that lines the eyelid and covers the anterior portion of the eyeball.

_____ 8. The cornea protects the iris and the pupil.

_____ 9. The pupil is a colored, muscular layer of tissue.

_____ 10. Light passes through the pupil and then the lens, which is an opaque, flexible, curved structure.

_____ 11. The interior of the eye has four chambers.

_____ 12. The ciliary muscle inside the eye regulates the shape and thickness of the lens, allowing it to focus light on the retina.

_____ 13. The retina consists of light-sensitive receptor cells known as rods and cones.

_____ 14. Located at the front of the eye, the optic nerve transmits neural messages from the retina to the brain.

_____ 15. The optic nerve is also known as the *blind spot*.

The Ear
Select the *best* answer.

_____ 1. Which of the following is true of the ear?
A. It is divided into the outer ear, the middle ear, and the underside ear.
B. It plays a role in balance, but not equilibrium.
C. It consists of the auricle and the alimentary canal.
D. It is lined with hair and ceruminous glands that secrete cerumen, or earwax.

_____ 2. The middle ear
A. is separated from the nose by the tympanic membrane
B. contains three ossicles, which are the smallest bones in the body
C. contains auditory receptors connected to the optic nerve
D. is the fifth division of the ear

_____ 3. Which of the following is true of sound?
A. It comes through the auditory canal and is translated into sound waves in the eardrum.
B. It does not affect the fluid in the cochlea of the inner ear.
C. It is transmitted outside the Eustachian tube.
D. It equalizes pressure within the ear, causing pain.

Identifying Structures of the Eye
Apply the appropriate callouts to the image.

A. Ciliary gland
B. Cornea
C. Eye socket
D. Eyelashes
E. Eyelid
F. Iris
G. Lacrimal canaliculus
H. Lacrimal gland
I. Optic nerve
J. Orbital muscles
K. Pupil
L. Retina
M. Sclera

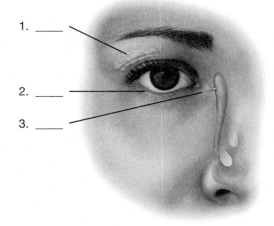

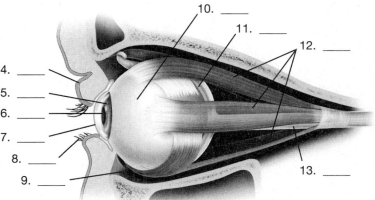

© Body Scientific International

_____ 4. The inner ear
    A. transmits neural messages using the colon nerve to determine the pitch and loudness of another person's voice
    B. contains the cochlea, a snail-shaped structure filled with earwax
    C. consists of three structures: the cochlea, the vestibule, and semicircular canals
    D. contains the organ of Corti, which is not involved in hearing

_____ 5. The cochlear nerve
    A. transmits neural messages to the auditory center of the brain
    B. contains receptors to sense dynamic equilibrium
    C. senses information regarding equilibrium and transmits the information directly to the pons
    D. has neurons that control voluntary hearing

Identifying Structures of the Ear

Apply the appropriate callouts to the image.

A. Anvil (incus)
B. Auditory canal (external acoustic meatus)
C. Auricle (pinna)
D. Cochlea
E. Eustachian tube
F. External (outer) ear
G. Hammer (malleus)
H. Internal (inner) ear
I. Middle ear (tympanic cavity)
J. Ossicles
K. Oval window
L. Round window
M. Semicircular canals
N. Stirrup (stapes)
O. Tympanic membrane (eardrum)
P. Vestibule
Q. Vestibulocochlear nerve

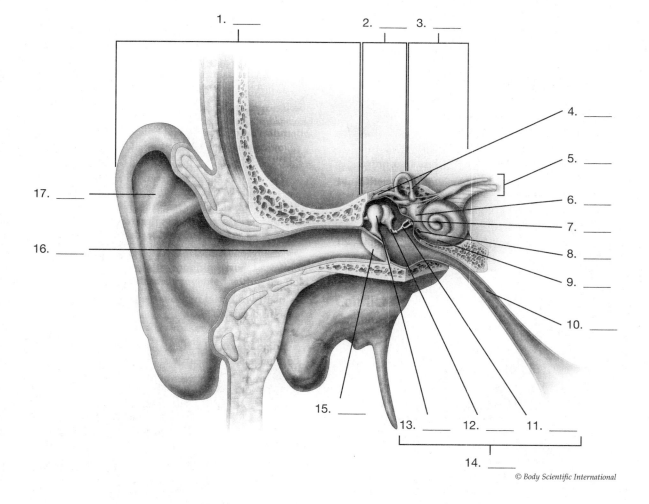

© Body Scientific International

Other Sense Organs

Complete the following sentences.

1. The nose, tongue, and skin are considered _____ organs.

2. Inside the nose are thousands of olfactory (smell) receptor cells containing _____.

3. When olfactory hairs are stimulated by smell, neural messages are transmitted via the _____ nerve to the brain, where smell is processed.

4. _____ are specialized receptors on the surface of the tongue that sense sweet, salty, bitter, sour, savory, fat, and the temperature of food.

5. The _____ contains sensory receptors responsible for touch, pressure, temperature, pain, and itch.

Hormones and the Endocrine System

Complete the following sentences.

1. The glands of the endocrine system secrete _____, or chemical messengers that initiate and regulate specific body processes.

2. _____ glands are ductless and secrete hormones directly into the bloodstream.

3. _____ glands have ducts that transport substances to other organs or to the surface of the skin.

4. The _____ is unique, as it has both an endocrine and exocrine function.

5. The _____ directly or indirectly controls all other endocrine glands and is also part of the nervous system.

6. The _____ has two lobes: the anterior pituitary and the posterior pituitary.

7. The _____ pituitary secretes adrenocorticotropic hormone, which influences the production of cortisol.

8. _____ hormone stimulates growth and development.

9. The posterior pituitary secretes _____ hormone, which controls water absorption in the kidneys.

10. Located in the thalamus, the _____ gland releases melatonin when the body is exposed to darkness.

11. The _____ is a butterfly-shaped gland that wraps around the front and sides of the trachea.

12. _____ hormone controls metabolism, regulates body temperature, and increases the rate of protein production.

13. The thyroid gland also releases _____, which regulates the amount of calcium in the blood and helps the body maintain strong, stable bones.

14. Two pairs of _____ glands are located on the back of the thyroid gland.

15. The thymus releases _____, a hormone that helps with the development and maturation of immune cells.

16. The adrenal medulla releases _____, which triggers the body's fight-or-flight response.

17. Within the pancreas, islets of _____ release the hormones insulin and glucagon.

18. The hormone _____ lowers blood sugar levels.

19. The _____ secrete estrogen and produce progesterone.

20. The testes release _____, which is essential for sperm maturation.

Identifying Endocrine Glands

Apply the appropriate callouts to the image.

Adrenal glands	Pineal gland
Hypothalamus	Pituitary gland
Ovary (female)	Testis (male)
Pancreas	Thymus gland
Parathyroid gland	Thyroid gland

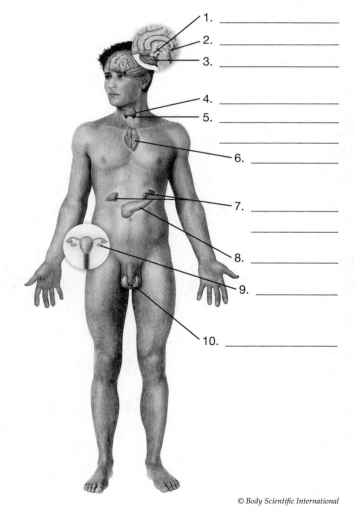

1. _____
2. _____
3. _____
4. _____
5. _____
_____
6. _____
7. _____
_____
8. _____
9. _____
10. _____

© Body Scientific International

The Cardiovascular System

Identify whether each statement is true or false.

_____ 1. The primary function of the cardiovascular system is to circulate oxygen-rich blood throughout the body and to return carbon dioxide and other waste products.

_____ 2. The heart is composed of voluntary cardiac muscle, which contracts and relaxes in a rhythmic cycle.

_____ 3. The contractions of the heart circulate blood through the heart to the rest of the body.

_____ 4. The heart sits in a sac called the perineal and has three layers of muscle: epicardium, myocardium, and endocardium.

_____ 5. The heart is divided into right and left sides by the septum.

_____ 6. Valves between the chambers of the heart cause backflow of blood.

_____ 7. The heart's muscle fibers are regulated by the somatic nervous system.

_____ 8. The heart is electrically stimulated through a process called conduction.

_____ 9. When the heart contracts, blood is forced through the arteries to the rest of the body, which is called *diastole*.

_____ 10. Between contractions, the heart relaxes and fills with blood, which is called *systole*.

_____ 11. The normal range for an adult's blood pressure is 120/80 mmHg or below.

_____ 12. The normal pulse rate for adults is 60–100 beats per minute and depends on a person's health and physical activity.

_____ 13. Pulse is most commonly felt and measured at the wrist, but is sometimes taken at the apex of the heart using a stethoscope.

_____ 14. Arteries, arterioles, and capillaries transport fully oxygenated blood from the heart to the body.

_____ 15. Veins and venules carry oxygen-poor blood from the body back to the heart.

Structures of the Heart

Apply the appropriate callouts to the image.

A. Aortic valve
B. Descending aorta
C. Endocardium
D. Inferior vena cava
E. Left atrium
F. Left pulmonary artery to left lung
G. Left pulmonary veins
H. Left ventricle
I. Mitral valve
J. Myocardium
K. Pericardium
L. Pulmonary trunk
M. Pulmonary valve
N. Right atrium
O. Right pulmonary artery to right lung
P. Right pulmonary veins
Q. Right ventricle
R. Septum
S. Superior vena cava
T. Tricuspid valve

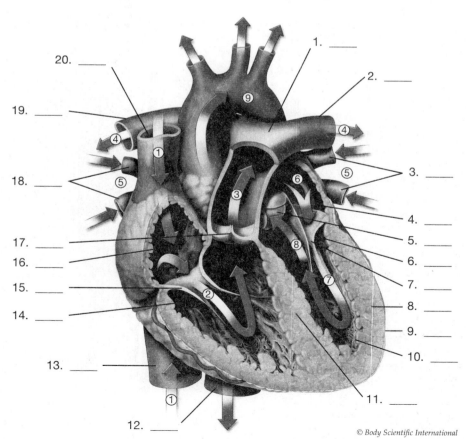

© *Body Scientific International*

Blood

Complete the following sentences.

1. The average adult has between 10 and 15 _____ of blood.

2. Blood has two basic components: blood cells and _____.

3. The _____ are the solid component of blood.

4. _____ is composed mostly of water, but also transports hormones, protein, sugar, and waste products to or from the body tissues.

5. The formed elements of the blood include _____ types of blood cells.

6. _____, or *erythrocytes*, are responsible for carrying oxygen throughout the body and removing carbon dioxide, a waste product.

7. _____ molecules on red blood cells carry oxygen from the lungs to body organs and tissues and transport carbon dioxide to the lungs.

8. _____, or *leukocytes*, defend the body against disease-causing microorganisms called pathogens.

9. Both red and white blood cells are manufactured primarily in the _____.

10. _____, or *thrombocytes*, help the blood clot.

The Respiratory System

Select the *best* answer.

_____ 1. The respiratory system
   A. contains organs for breathing in carbon dioxide and getting rid of oxygen
   B. has the primary function of breathing, or *respiration*
   C. is responsible for exhaling oxygen during respiration
   D. transports carbon dioxide to the body's cells, organs, and tissues

_____ 2. Which of the following is true of carbon dioxide?
   A. It is a waste product that is exhaled (expired) from the body.
   B. It is carried into the cells by several respiratory organs and the cardiovascular system.
   C. It is carried away from the cells through the trachea.
   D. It is oxygen-rich after leaving the heart.

_____ 3. Which of the following is true of ventilation?
   A. It includes two activities: ventilation and gas exhalation.
   B. It is measured by counting each inspiration and expiration for 30 minutes.
   C. The rate for adults is 60–100 breaths per minute.
   D. It is the movement of oxygen-rich air into the lungs and the movement of carbon dioxide out of the lungs.

_____ 4. Gas exchange occurs
   A. in the alveoli of the lungs
   B. in the heart and circulates through blood vessels to the body
   C. as carbon dioxide passes from the capillaries into the larynx
   D. when air is diffused from the alveoli into the environment

_____ 5. The respiratory system is divided into the
   A. upper and lower cardiac tracts
   B. right and left lungs
   C. upper and lower respiratory tracts
   D. right and left respiratory tracts

Structures of the Upper Respiratory Tract

Apply the appropriate callouts to the image.

A. Epiglottis
B. Esophagus
C. Frontal sinus
D. Hard palate
E. Laryngopharynx
F. Larynx
G. Lingual tonsil
H. Nasal cavity
I. Nasopharynx
J. Oropharynx
K. Palatine tonsil
L. Pharyngeal tonsil
M. Soft palate
N. Sphenoid sinus
O. Thyroid cartilage
P. Tongue
Q. Uvula
R. Vocal fold

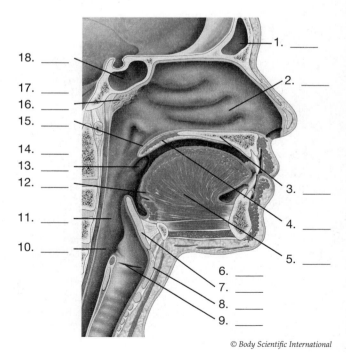

© *Body Scientific International*

The Lower Respiratory Tract

Identify whether each statement is true or false.

_____ 1. The lower respiratory tract begins with the esophagus.

_____ 2. The trachea is made of cartilage and is covered with a mucous membrane lined with cilia.

_____ 3. Midway down the chest, the trachea divides into the right and left broncos, which are the passageways into the lungs.

_____ 4. Air flows from the bronchi into smaller structures called bronchioles and finally into the alveoli.

_____ 5. Alveoli are tiny sacs in the lungs where oxygen and carbon dioxide are exchanged.

_____ 6. The lungs are the principal organs of the respiratory system.

_____ 7. There are three lobes in both the right and left lung.

_____ 8. The area between the two lungs is called the mediastinum and does not contain any organs or structures.

_____ 9. The synovial membrane covers the lungs and reduces friction during breathing.

_____ 10. At the base of the lungs is the diaphragm, a muscle that contracts to help inflate the lungs.

The Immune and Lymphatic Systems

Complete the following sentences.

1. The immune and lymphatic systems protect the body against _____.

2. The immune and lymphatic systems aid in _____, which is a person's ability to resist infection.

3. One type of immunity is _____, which is affected by a person's race, gender, genes, and cells at birth.

4. _____ is a type of immunity that humans develop through being exposed to a disease or through immunization.

5. _____ is a process in which a small or modified dose of a pathogen is injected to stimulate the production of antibodies.

6. A fetus can develop short-term _____ immunity when a mother passes antibodies through the placenta.

7. Blood proteins that reduce the effects of bacteria and viruses are called _____.

8. _____ is a colorless fluid that originates in the capillaries of the cardiovascular system and travels through the lymph vessels.

9. Organs of the lymphatic system include the _____ nodes found throughout the body, spleen, tonsils, thymus, and liver.

10. The _____ is essential for destroying worn-out red blood cells, producing lymphocytes, storing platelets, and increasing blood volume in the body.

Identifying Lymphatic Organs

Apply the appropriate callouts to the image.

A. Axillary lymph node
B. Cervical lymph node
C. Inguinal lymph node
D. Lumbar lymph node
E. Pelvic lymph node
F. Right lymphatic duct
G. Spleen
H. Thoracic duct
I. Thymus gland
J. Tonsils

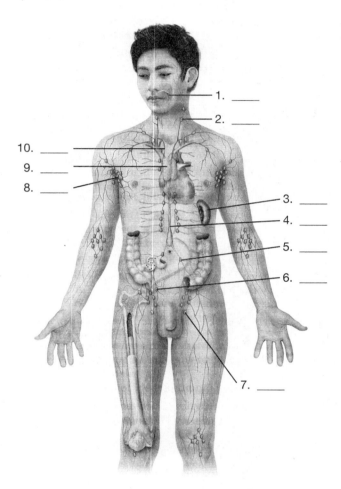

1. _____
2. _____
10. _____
9. _____
8. _____
3. _____
4. _____
5. _____
6. _____
7. _____

© Body Scientific International

The Gastrointestinal System

Select the *best* answer.

_____ 1. The gastrointestinal system
   A. has several essential functions related to the ingestion, breakdown, absorption, and elimination of food and liquid
   B. takes in food and liquid through a process called expulsion
   C. breaks down food through mastication during digestion in the stomach
   D. chemically breaks down food by chewing it into smaller components

_____ 2. Which of the following is true of peristalsis?
A. It occurs when food is liquefied into unmanageable components.
B. It stops in the stomach and aids in digestion.
C. It cannot mix food with gastric juices.
D. It involves involuntary smooth muscle contractions that break food down into manageable components.

_____ 3. The large intestine
A. is not a part of the gastrointestinal system
B. expels feces through a process called expulsion
C. eliminates undigested food from the body through the anus
D. leads into the rectum

_____ 4. The gastrointestinal tract (GI tract)
A. is also called the alimentary canal
B. leads from the mouth to the anus and includes bony structures
C. begins with the oral cavity and ends with the small intestine
D. does not include the stomach

_____ 5. Which of the following is true of the mouth?
A. It has hard and soft palates, which form the bottom of the mouth.
B. It is lined with a mucous membrane that secretes saliva produced by the salivary glands.
C. It contains the uvula, a projection that is anchored to the hard palate.
D. It cannot detect hot or cold temperatures.

_____ 6. The uvula
A. has no known purpose
B. is a fingerlike projection that aids in chewing
C. aids in the absorption of nutrients
D. hangs at the very back of the mouth to prevent liquid and food from entering nasal passages

_____ 7. Which of the following is true of the tongue?
A. It is an accessory organ attached to the epiglottis.
B. It excretes an enzyme called amylase.
C. It has tiny bumps called papillae that contain taste buds.
D. It uses muscular action to chew and move food into the trachea.

_____ 8. The teeth
A. are designed to aid in the mastication and grinding of the jaw
B. have a root surrounded by bone and a layer of soft tissue called gingivitis
C. have an outermost layer of enamel and a second layer known as gingiva
D. have a center called the pulp, which contains blood vessels and nerves

_____ 9. Salivary glands
A. reside in the oral cavity and play an essential role in digestion
B. produce 10,000 cups of saliva over a person's lifetime
C. produce an enzyme called prolase
D. provide lubrication, but do not contribute to the chemical breakdown of food

_____ 10. Which of the following is true of the pharynx?
A. It has a cardiac sphincter to prevent the esophagus from expelling air.
B. It is the passageway to the mucus-lined, muscular esophagus.
C. It is an organ of the lymphatic system.
D. It propels food by peristalsis into the small intestine.

Identifying Structures of the Stomach

Apply the appropriate callouts to the image.

A. Anterior surface
B. Antrum
C. Body
D. Cardia
E. Circular muscle layer
F. Duodenum of small intestine
G. Esophagus
H. Fundus
I. Longitudinal muscle layer
J. Oblique muscle layer
K. Pyloric region
L. Pyloric sphincter
M. Pylorus
N. Rugae (folds)

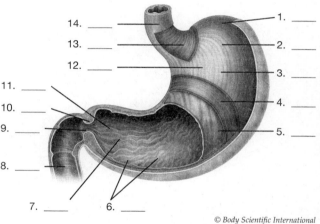

14. _____
13. _____
12. _____
11. _____
10. _____
9. _____
8. _____
7. _____   6. _____
1. _____
2. _____
3. _____
4. _____
5. _____

© Body Scientific International

The Small and Large Intestine

Complete the following sentences.

1. The small intestine continues the process of digestion and facilitates the _____ of nutrients into the blood.

2. Small extensions called _____ help move chyme along the twisted path of the small intestine and absorb nutrients.

3. The _____ is the section of the small intestine where food is digested.

4. The _____ section of the small intestine absorbs nutrients into the bloodstream.

5. In the _____ section of the small intestine, vitamin B_{12} is absorbed into the bloodstream, and unused food and waste enter the large intestine through the ileocecal sphincter.

6. The mucus-lined _____ has six sections.

7. The first section of the large intestine is the _____, which is connected to the ileum and receives unused food and waste.

8. The _____ hangs from the lower part of the cecum and has no known function.

9. The _____ colon leads into the rectum.

10. The last structure of the alimentary canal, the _____, has a muscular sphincter to control elimination of feces from the body.

Labeling the Large and Small Intestines

Apply the appropriate callouts to the image.

A. Appendix
B. Ascending colon
C. Cecum
D. Descending colon
E. Duodenum
F. Ileum
G. Jejunum
H. Rectum
I. Sigmoid colon
J. Transverse colon (cut)

10. _____
9. _____
8. _____
7. _____
6. _____
5. _____
4. _____
1. _____
2. _____
3. _____

© *Body Scientific International*

Accessory Organs of the Gastrointestinal System

Select the *best* answer.

_____ 1. The three accessory organs of the gastrointestinal system
  A. are found within the thoracic cavity
  B. include the pancreas, liver, and gallbladder
  C. all secrete glucagon and insulin
  D. are long, thin glands that produce chyme

_____ 2. Which of the following is a function of the pancreas?
  A. destroying insulin and glucagon to protect the body
  B. producing enzymes that are secreted through salivary ducts
  C. digesting enzymes to assist in homeostasis
  D. producing enzymes that assist in chemical digestion

_____ 3. The liver
  A. is divided into right and left lobes
  B. is located on the upper left side of the trunk of the body behind the rib cage
  C. produces insulin
  D. filters urine from the bloodstream

_____ 4. The key function of the liver is to
  A. make bile
  B. filter and remove waste products from the urine
  C. absorb nutrients for the body to convert into energy
  D. convert lipids into sugar

_____ 5. The gallbladder
  A. stores nutrients and removes waste products
  B. is a small organ essential to bile production
  C. stores bile produced by the liver
  D. filters waste products from the blood

The Urinary System

Identify whether each statement is true or false.

_____ 1. The urinary system is responsible for filtering the blood and eliminating liquid waste from the body in the form of urine.

_____ 2. The urinary system is composed of two kidneys, two ureters, the urinary bladder, and two urethras.

_____ 3. Gravity and peristalsis move urine through the urinary system.

_____ 4. The kidneys are two bean-shaped organs protected by adipose and connective tissue and have three regions: the renal cortex, renal medulla, and renal pelvis.

_____ 5. The outer renal pelvis is composed of microscopic nephrons that filter blood and remove waste products from the body.

_____ 6. Blood enters the kidney via the renal vein and circulates through the Bowman's capsule.

_____ 7. The glomerulus is a ball of capillaries with thin walls that allow only certain substances, such as water, waste products, and urea, to leave the bloodstream.

_____ 8. The renal medulla contains pyramid-shaped structures that carry urine from the renal cortex to the renal calyces.

_____ 9. Urine passes from the renal calyces directly into the urethra.

_____ 10. The hilum is a recessed opening in the renal medulla through which blood vessels, nerves, and the ureter pass.

Structures of the Kidney
Apply the appropriate callouts to the image.

Hilum	Renal medulla	Ureter
Renal cortex	Renal pelvis	

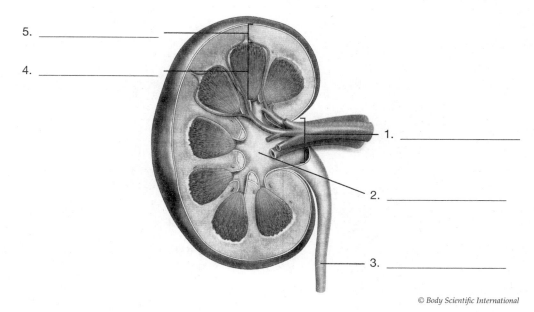

5. _____

4. _____

1. _____

2. _____

3. _____

© Body Scientific International

The Ureters, Urinary Bladder, and Urethra
Identify whether each statement is true or false.

_____ 1. The two ureters are narrow tubes that transport urine from the renal pelvis to the urinary bladder.

_____ 2. The urinary bladder stores up to 10 ounces of urine before nerves in the bladder send a message to the brain that the bladder needs emptying.

_____ 3. Two ducts control the flow of urine out of the body.

_____ 4. The internal urethral sphincter is located where the urinary bladder and the urethra meet.

_____ 5. The internal urethral sphincter moves voluntarily.

_____ 6. The external urethral sphincter is located at the end of the ureter.

_____ 7. The external urethral sphincter is controlled voluntarily.

_____ 8. Urine passes out of the body through the meatus.

The Male and Female Reproductive Systems
Complete the following sentences.

1. The male reproductive system facilitates conception by producing cells called _____.

2. The female reproductive system facilitates conception by producing cells called _____.

3. The _____ reproductive organs include the scrotum and testes, interior duct system, seminal vesicles, prostate gland, and penis.

4. The _____ reproductive organs include the ovaries, fallopian tubes, uterus, vagina, vulva, and mammary glands.

5. The _____ is a pouch covered by skin that hangs outside the male's body between the thighs and contains the testes.

6. Sperm form in small tubes called _____ tubules within the testes.

7. Luteinizing hormone (LH) and the hormone _____ are essential to the proper growth of sperm.

8. _____ is the fluid that transports sperm during sexual intercourse.

9. On the outsides of the breasts are nipples surrounded by dark areas called _____.

10. Milk is produced by lobules in the breasts and carried to the nipples via the _____ ducts.

11. The female external genitalia is called the _____.

12. Two pairs of _____ protect the vulva, vagina, and female urethra from pathogens.

13. The _____ conducts monthly menstrual flow, receives sperm during intercourse, and serves as the birth canal.

14. When a woman ovulates, an ovum is released into the _____, which will move the ovum toward the uterus.

15. The _____ is the organ that provides the home for a developing fetus.

16. The complete set of DNA is known as the _____.

Structures of the Male Reproductive System

Apply the appropriate callouts to the image.

A. Anus
B. Corpus cavernosum
C. Corpus spongiosum
D. Ductus deferens (vas deferens)
E. Ejaculatory duct
F. Epididymis

G. External urethral orifice
H. Glans penis
I. Prepuce (foreskin)
J. Prostate
K. Pubis
L. Rectum

M. Scrotum
N. Seminal gland (seminal vesicle)
O. Testis
P. Ureter
Q. Urethra
R. Urinary bladder

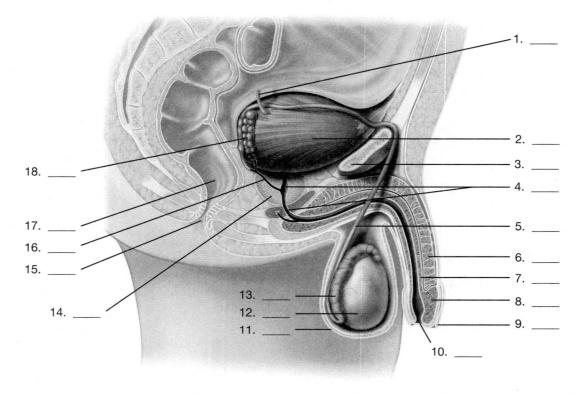

© Body Scientific International

Structures of the Female Reproductive System

Apply the appropriate callouts to the image.

A. Body of uterus
B. Cervical canal
C. Cervix
D. Fallopian (uterine) tube

E. Fundus of uterus
F. Lumen (cavity) of uterus
G. Ovarian blood vessels
H. Ovary

I. Ovum
J. Ureter
K. Uterine blood vessels
L. Vagina

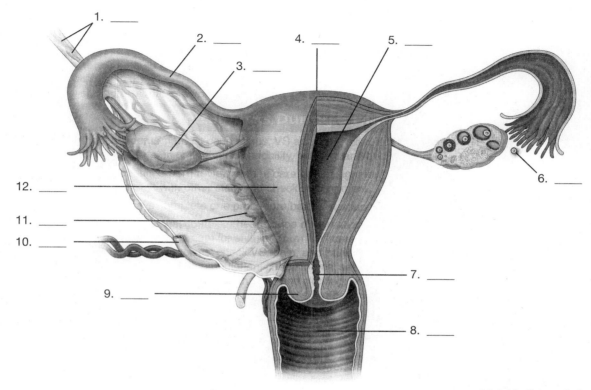

© Body Scientific International

Lifestyle Choices and Aging Body Systems

Read the scenario and complete the sentences that follow.

Mr. Carter is 84 years old. He worked for more than 30 years in an automotive factory and held multiple jobs to support his family. He has a history of smoking, but quit in his thirties. He is active and walks, works in his woodshop, gardens, and maintains the home he built. Mr. Carter's active lifestyle slows muscle atrophy and improves balance. Mr. Carter relaxes by reading and watching sports on television. He also enjoys sitting out on the porch with his wife watching the hummingbirds. His hobbies can be challenging due to arthritis in his hands and feet and an inherited cardiac disorder. Born with only one kidney, he takes extra precautions to keep his singular kidney healthy. He recently lost 15 pounds, which prompted his doctor to decrease his cardiac medication to compensate for the change in weight.

1. Older adults are responsible for their health and levels of wellness or illness and make _____ choices that ultimately affect the body's health as they age.

2. Although age is not a disease, organs change and begin to function _____ effectively as people age.

3. Over time, the most significant organ changes occur in the heart, lungs, and _____.

4. _____ aging individuals do not lose as many brain cells as unhealthy individuals.

Name: _____ Date: _____

Matching Section 9.1 Key Terms, Part A

Match each definition with the key term.

A. abrasion
B. acute disease
C. analgesic
D. chronic disease
E. condition
F. decubitus ulcer
G. flares
H. immobility
I. incontinence
J. inflammation
K. lesions
L. monotone
M. morbidity
N. mortality
O. necrosis
P. pathology
Q. plaques
R. sclerosis
S. sign
T. symptom
U. topical
V. ultrasound

_____ 1. a piece of subjective information about a disease or condition based on a person's feelings or opinions

_____ 2. a long-term or recurring disease or condition

_____ 3. abnormal spots or areas of damaged body tissue

_____ 4. the death of body tissue

_____ 5. a scraping of the outer layer of skin

_____ 6. body tissue's protective response to irritation, injury, or infection; characterized by swelling and redness

_____ 7. flat-sounding speech with no change in pitch

_____ 8. an inability to move on one's own

_____ 9. lack of bowel or bladder control

_____ 10. a collection of changes to the body's tissues or organs; occurs as a result of disease

_____ 11. sudden intensifications or escalations of a disease

_____ 12. the number of people who have a disease

_____ 13. a piece of objective, or factual, information indicating a disease or condition

_____ 14. a short-term disease or condition that usually has an abrupt onset

_____ 15. a test that uses ultrasonic waves to view the internal structures of the body

_____ 16. the number of deaths due to a disease

_____ 17. a physical or mental state of health or illness

_____ 18. on the surface of the skin

_____ 19. superficial, solid, elevated lesions

_____ 20. a type of pain medication that does not cause loss of consciousness

_____ 21. the thickening or hardening of a body part

_____ 22. a skin condition caused by continuous pressure on the skin and on bony areas, restricting blood flow and creating a sore

Understanding Diseases and Conditions

Complete the following sentences.

1. A(n) _____ occurs when an organ or body system incorrectly functions and exhibits particular signs and symptoms.

2. A(n) _____ refers to a particular physical or mental state of health or illness.

3. A genetic or _____ disorder is caused by a person's genes or by a birth event.

4. An infectious disease, also called a(n) _____ disease, is caused by microorganisms such as bacteria or viruses.

5. Pathogenic _____ can be passed from person to person, transferred by an insect bite, or ingested from contaminated food or water.

6. A(n) _____ disease is a result of cell breakdown over time, causing changes in tissues and organs.

7. A deficiency or excess in a person's diet may lead to a(n) _____ disease.

8. _____ is a disease caused by the production of abnormal or excess body cells.

9. A(n) _____ disease or condition is short-term and usually has an abrupt onset.

10. A(n) _____ disease or condition lasts more than three months or is recurring.

11. The _____ is the word part often used to form medical terms that describe diseases or conditions.

12. Each disease is associated with a particular _____, or changes that occur in the body's tissues and organs as a result of a disease.

13. A(n) _____ is a piece of objective, factual information indicating a disease or condition.

14. A piece of subjective information about a condition or disease based on a person's feelings or opinions is called a(n) _____.

Acute Versus Chronic Diseases and Conditions

Identify whether each statement is true or false.

_____ 1. A resident with arthritis may have joint damage, ongoing inflammation, and pain.

_____ 2. Eczema is an example of an acute disease.

_____ 3. Acute diseases often last a lifetime and require constant attention.

_____ 4. Many residents with chronic diseases or conditions go through periods of sadness, discouragement, hopelessness, anger, and depression.

_____ 5. Holistic nursing assistants do not need to be understanding when caring for residents with a chronic disease.

_____ 6. Holistic nursing assistants should encourage healthful habits and activities.

_____ 7. A terminal disease or condition does not result in death.

_____ 8. Acute and chronic diseases or conditions require different types of healthcare services and facilities.

_____ 9. A chronic disease or condition may become more severe over time.

_____ 10. A resident with a disease may sometimes feel defined by his or her disease.

Abbreviations and Acronyms Related to Diseases and Conditions

Complete the table by identifying the missing abbreviations and acronyms.

Abbreviation or Acronym	Meaning	Abbreviation or Acronym	Meaning
1. _____	atrial fibrillation	19. _____	hypertension
2. _____	amyotrophic lateral sclerosis	20. _____	irritable bowel syndrome
3. _____	acquired immunodeficiency syndrome	21. _____	low-density lipoprotein cholesterol
4. _____	age-related macular degeneration	22. _____	myocardial infarction
5. _____	benign prostatic hypertrophy	23. _____	magnetic resonance imaging
6. _____	cancer	24. _____	multiple sclerosis
7. _____	coronary artery bypass graft	25. _____	pulmonary embolus
8. _____	coronary artery disease	26. _____	premature ventricular contraction
9. _____	congestive heart failure	27. _____	peripheral vascular disease
10. _____	chronic obstructive pulmonary disease	28. _____	systemic lupus erythematosus
11. _____	chest pain	29. _____	sexually transmitted disease
12. _____	cerebrospinal fluid	30. _____	sexually transmitted infection
13. _____	cerebrovascular accident	31. _____	tuberculosis
14. _____	electrocardiogram	32. _____	transient ischemic attack
15. _____	gastroesophageal reflux disease	33. _____	upper respiratory infection
16. _____	hepatitis B virus	34. _____	urinary tract infection
17. _____	high-density lipoprotein cholesterol	35. _____	venereal disease
18. _____	human immunodeficiency virus	36. _____	ventricular fibrillation

Name: _____ Date: _____

Creating Flash Cards

With a partner, create a set of flash cards to help you memorize the abbreviations and acronyms related to diseases and conditions (found in Figure 9.2 in the text). One partner should write the abbreviation or acronym on one side of the card, and the other partner should write each meaning on the back side of the card. Review your flash cards until you have memorized all of the abbreviations and acronyms.

Diseases and Conditions of the Integumentary System

Complete the following sentences.

1. A(n) _____ is a doctor who specializes in treating diseases, disorders, and injuries of the skin, hair, and nails.
2. _____ is a condition in which there is too much keratin in the skin.
3. Keratosis_____ is a skin condition characterized by patches of thickened, dry skin; painless rough patches; and tiny bumps.
4. Oval-shaped growths that start as small, rough patches and develop into thick, wart-like growths are characteristics of a condition called _____ keratosis.
5. Psoriasis is a condition characterized by the excessive growth of new skin cells forming thick, red patches called _____ on the top layer of the skin.
6. _____, or intensifications of psoriasis, are usually associated with stressful situations or emotional trauma triggering the immune response.
7. Treatments for psoriasis are primarily _____, or applied to the surface of the skin.
8. Also called *herpes zoster*, _____ is a painful skin rash caused by the varicella-zoster virus.
9. Shingles is more common among people who are over 50 years of age or who have a weakened _____ system.
10. A(n) _____ is a type of pain medication that may be used to treat shingles.

Decubitus Ulcers

Select the *best* answer.

_____ 1. Which of the following is true of decubitus ulcers?
A. They are unrelated to pressure injuries.
B. They are caused by the varicella-zoster virus.
C. They are caused by continuous pressure on the skin and bony areas that restricts blood circulation.
D. They occur when a resident is too active.

_____ 2. Immobility is
A. the inability to move
B. healthy for an inactive resident's skin
C. a cause of fragile skin, which helps resist decubitus ulcers
D. important for residents who have no restrictions in their plan of care

_____ 3. Incontinence is
A. very mild with pink or red coloration
B. a condition that improves skin integrity
C. always curable
D. a lack of bowel or bladder control

_____ 4. A stage 1 decubitus ulcer
A. is open with pus
B. is not open, but appears red on people with light complexions and blue or purple on people who have darker complexions
C. looks like a crater with cellulitis and infection
D. is not serious and does not warrant reporting or documentation

_____ 5. A stage 2 decubitus ulcer
A. cannot be prevented
B. does not pose a risk for the development of cellulitis or infection
C. is difficult to detect because the skin is intact and the same color as surrounding skin
D. is still considered shallow, but is open and may form a fluid-filled blister

_____ 6. A stage 3 decubitus ulcer
A. is much shallower than stage 2 and may not break the skin
B. looks like a crater and may ooze, bleed, or contain pus
C. cannot lead to sepsis
D. cannot be treated

_____ 7. A stage 4 decubitus ulcer
A. is deep and may reach muscles, tendons, ligaments, joints, and bone
B. typically does not bleed
C. affects the epidermis, but not the subcutaneous soft tissue
D. cannot cause necrosis

_____ 8. Which of the following is true of necrosis?
A. It is not related to bone and joint infection.
B. It is a system-wide infection in the bloodstream.
C. It is tissue death.
D. It affects only unstageable decubitus ulcers.

_____ 9. Sepsis is
A. a blister caused by the chickenpox virus
B. a mass of dead tissue
C. not typically a serious infection
D. a life-threatening infection in the bloodstream that may lead to organ failure

_____ 10. Decubitus ulcers can be prevented by
A. repositioning a resident at least every three hours
B. not applying dressings to affected areas
C. discouraging a resident from ambulating
D. keeping pressure points dry and clean

Identifying Pressure Points for Decubitus Ulcers

Apply the appropriate callouts to the images.

Part A: Supine Position

A. Abdomen
B. Back of head
C. Elbows

D. Heels
E. Sacrum

F. Shoulders
G. Toes

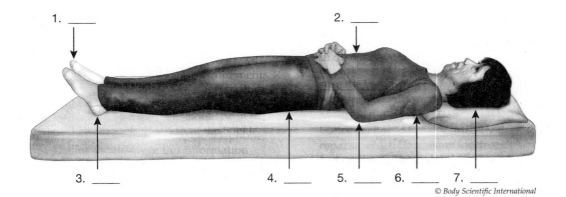

1. ____   2. ____

3. ____   4. ____   5. ____   6. ____   7. ____

© Body Scientific International

Part B: Lateral Position

A. Ankle
B. Ear
C. Heel

D. Hip
E. Knees
F. Leg

G. Shoulder
H. Side of head
I. Thigh

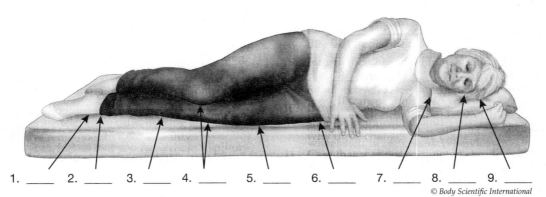

1. ____   2. ____   3. ____   4. ____   5. ____   6. ____   7. ____   8. ____   9. ____

© Body Scientific International

Part C: Prone Position

A. Anterior superior iliac spines
B. Breasts (women)
C. Cheek and ear
D. Collar bone

E. Elbows
F. Genitalia (men)
G. Knees

H. Ribs
I. Thigh
J. Toes

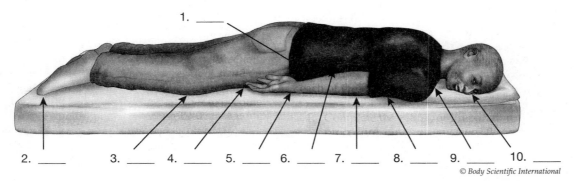

1. ____

2. ____   3. ____   4. ____   5. ____   6. ____   7. ____   8. ____   9. ____   10. ____

© Body Scientific International

Name: _____   Date: _____

Part D: High Fowler's Position

A. Back of head
B. Buttocks

C. Heels
D. Sacrum

E. Shoulders
F. Toes

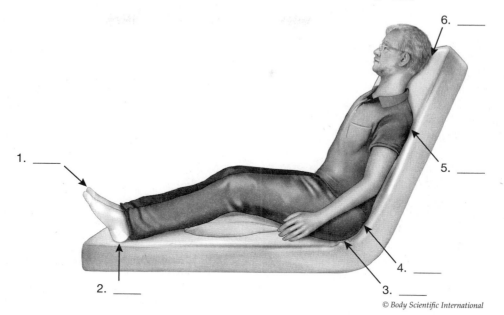

© Body Scientific International

Diseases and Conditions of the Skeletal System

Identify whether each statement is true or false.

_____ 1. Common skeletal diseases and conditions include multiple sclerosis, arthritis, and fractures.

_____ 2. Osteoporosis is a condition in which the bones are *porous*, or full of cracks.

_____ 3. Osteoporosis occurs when the body makes too little bone or starts losing bone density.

_____ 4. Arthritis describes a variety of chronic diseases and conditions characterized by joint inflammation.

_____ 5. Symptoms of arthritis include pain, aching, stiffness, swelling in or around joints, and decreased mental capacity.

_____ 6. Arthritic symptoms may appear suddenly or develop gradually.

_____ 7. For residents with arthritis, dry or wet heat may relax muscles and increase blood flow.

_____ 8. Cold compresses or ice packs increase swelling and numb the nerves to relieve pain in residents with arthritis.

_____ 9. It is the nursing assistant's responsibility to assess whether warm or cold applications are effective for a resident.

_____ 10. Nursing assistants report a resident's pain response to the licensed nursing staff and document in the resident's EMR.

_____ 11. The risk of a fracture decreases as a resident ages.

_____ 12. Fractures occur when an outside force is stronger than the bone on which the force is exerting pressure.

_____ 13. In a displaced fracture, the bone breaks through the skin.

_____ 14. Fractured bones must be set using a process called reduction.

_____ 15. When caring for a resident with a cast, you must make sure the cast does not get wet.

Identifying Types of Fractures

Identify each type of fracture.

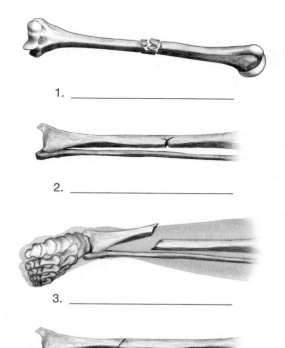

1. _____

2. _____

3. _____

4. _____

© Body Scientific International

Name: _____ Date: _____

Diseases of the Muscular System
Complete the following sentences.

1. _____ is a group of diseases that cause progressive weakness and loss of muscle mass due to atrophy.
2. In MD, abnormal _____ interfere with the production of proteins needed to maintain healthy muscle tissue.
3. Each type of MD is caused by a unique genetic _____, which is usually inherited.
4. The main sign of MD is progressive _____ weakness.
5. About one-half of MD cases are _____, which typically affects young boys.
6. Residents with MD may require the use of a(n) _____, which is a machine that forces air in and out of the lungs.
7. MD can reduce the efficiency of the heart muscle and cause difficulty swallowing, or _____.
8. _____ lateral sclerosis is a disease characterized by the gradual decline and deterioration of motor neurons in the brain and spinal cord, causing loss of the ability to speak, eat, move, and breathe.
9. As the spinal cord degenerates, _____ causes hardening of the muscles.
10. ALS may cause the muscles to waste away, or _____.

Care Consideration for Muscular Diseases
List the nine areas of care a holistic nursing assistant must consider when caring for residents with muscular diseases. Give an example of a care consideration in each area.

1. _____

   Example: _____

2. _____

   Example: _____

3. _____

   Example: _____

4. _____

   Example: _____

5. _____

   Example: _____

6. _____

   Example: _____

7. _____

   Example: _____

8. _____

   Example: _____

9. _____

   Example: _____

Matching Section 9.1 Key Terms, Part B
Match each definition with the key term.

A. abscess
B. anesthetic
C. aneurysm
D. aphasia
E. arrhythmias
F. arteriosclerosis
G. atherosclerosis
H. benign
I. biopsy
J. catheter
K. coma
L. dialysis
M. edema
N. fistula
O. hemiplegia
P. hypertension
Q. ischemia
R. malignant
S. metastasis
T. nodules
U. predisposition

_____ 1. paralysis on one side of the body
_____ 2. not cancerous
_____ 3. a condition in which a person cannot understand or use words
_____ 4. high blood pressure
_____ 5. a flexible tube that is inserted through a narrow opening into a body cavity
_____ 6. the process of removing waste products and excess fluid from the body
_____ 7. a condition in which arteries narrow due to plaque buildup
_____ 8. a medication that produces a loss of sensation
_____ 9. abnormal heart rhythms
_____ 10. an insufficient supply of blood to a tissue or organ
_____ 11. the removal of a small piece of tissue from a tumor using a special needle
_____ 12. cancerous
_____ 13. a distended and weak area in the wall of an artery supplying blood to the brain

60 The Nursing Assistant

Copyright Goodheart-Willcox Co., Inc.
May not be reproduced or posted to a publicly accessible website.

_____ 14. an abnormal and permanent opening between an organ and the exterior of the body

_____ 15. a tendency to suffer from a particular condition

_____ 16. an enclosed collection of pus in any part of the body

_____ 17. a state of deep and prolonged unconsciousness

_____ 18. the spread of cancer cells to other locations in the body

_____ 19. a condition in which arteries thicken, harden, and lose elasticity

_____ 20. retention of fluid

_____ 21. small, round, or knotlike collections of body tissue

Multiple Sclerosis (MS)

Identify whether each statement is true or false.

_____ 1. Common nervous system diseases include multiple sclerosis (MS), Parkinson's disease, and peripheral neuropathy.

_____ 2. Cardiologists specialize in caring for patients with neurological diseases.

_____ 3. Multiple sclerosis (MS) is a condition in which the immune system attacks myelin, the protective material that surrounds nerve fibers and muscles.

_____ 4. There is no cure when damaged nerve signals are slow or blocked.

_____ 5. Relapsing-remitting MS is the most common type, in which a person experiences a relapse followed by a remission.

_____ 6. Secondary progressive MS develops from relapsing-remitting MS after 10–20 years and does not include relapses or remissions.

_____ 7. Primary progressive MS is the most common type of MS.

_____ 8. In progressive relapsing MS, symptoms worsen between relapses.

_____ 9. Physical examinations and MRIs are typically used to diagnose MS.

_____ 10. Treatment for MS may consist of medications to ease symptoms and manage stress.

Parkinson's Disease

Select the *best* answer.

_____ 1. Parkinson's disease
   A. initially causes improved ability to think, which is related to the overproduction of neurons
   B. progresses gradually and causes neurons in the brain to break down or die
   C. causes neurons in the brain to produce more dopamine
   D. is easily diagnosed and prevented with blood tests

_____ 2. Which of the following is true of dopamine?
   A. It is not a vital chemical messenger.
   B. It causes abnormal brain activity when levels decrease.
   C. It is unrelated to the signs and symptoms of Parkinson's disease.
   D. It is the brain scan used to detect Parkinson's disease.

_____ 3. Risk factors for Parkinson's disease include
   A. gender, as men are less likely than women to get Parkinson's disease
   B. age, as Parkinson's disease often begins toward the middle or end of a person's life
   C. heredity, but not the environment
   D. the presence of cardiovascular disease

_____ 4. Symptoms of Parkinson's disease
   A. usually begin on one side of the body and may include pill rolling and tremors
   B. include fast movement, called bradykinesia
   C. rarely include balance problems and stiff muscles
   D. include loud, monotone outbursts

_____ 5. A treatment plan of care for Parkinson's disease
   A. does not often include attention to lifestyle issues such as exercise and diet
   B. always includes surgery to regulate certain parts of the brain
   C. would not include integrative medicine such as massage; tai chi; yoga; and music, art, or pet therapy
   D. may include prescription medications, physical therapy, speech-language therapy, IM, or surgery

Neuropathy

Complete the following sentences.

1. Sensory, motor, and autonomic nerves can be affected by a disease called _____.

2. If neuropathy affects _____ nerves, the signs and symptoms include tingling, pain, and numbness.

3. If neuropathy affects _____ nerves, there is weakness in the feet and hands.

4. If neuropathy affects _____ nerves, there may be problems with internal organs, which can increase heart rate and lower blood pressure.

5. If neuropathy involves a single nerve, it is called _____.

6. If neuropathy affects many nerves, it is called _____.

7. About one-third of all neuropathies are _____, which means the cause is unknown.

8. _____ neuropathy is a type of common neuropathy in which nerves carrying messages to the body are damaged or diseased.

9. Topical _____ that produce a loss of sensation may be used to treat neuropathy.

Sensory System Diseases and Conditions

Complete the following sentences.

1. Diseases and conditions of the sense organs are usually treated by healthcare providers such as _____, optometrists, and otolaryngologists.

2. A cataract is a condition in which a slow buildup of _____ on the lens of the eye causes clouding.

3. _____ is an incurable condition in which the optic nerve is damaged, possibly resulting in vision loss or blindness.

4. _____ glaucoma is the most common type of glaucoma and occurs when fluid builds up where the cornea and iris meet, creating pressure in the eye.

5. In _____ glaucoma, fluid at the front of the eye cannot drain through the angle and is blocked, creating severe pressure that constitutes a medical emergency.

6. _____ degeneration is an incurable eye disease caused by the deterioration of the macula, the central portion of the retina.

7. _____ macular degeneration is the more common form and is characterized by yellow deposits called *drusen*.

8. _____ are composed of lipids, or fatty proteins, that form when the eye fails to dispose of waste products.

9. _____ macular degeneration is caused by the growth of abnormal blood vessels underneath the macula.

10. The biggest risk factor for macular degeneration is _____, although other risk factors include genetics, race, smoking, and cardiovascular disease.

Otitis Media and Ménière's Disease

Select the *best* answer.

_____ 1. Which of the following is true of otitis media?
   A. It is commonly called an *ear infection*.
   B. It most commonly affects adults.
   C. It does not cause an earache.
   D. It does not affect a person's hearing.

_____ 2. Otitis media is characterized by
   A. ear pain and nasal discharge
   B. a slow onset of symptoms
   C. a red, bulging eardrum
   D. a ringing in the ears

_____ 3. Ménière's disease affects the
   A. outer ear
   B. eardrum
   C. ossicles
   D. inner ear

_____ 4. Ménière's disease is characterized by
   A. the early appearance of symptoms, usually between the ages of two and five
   B. spontaneous episodes of spinning called *vertigo*
   C. frequent bacterial infections
   D. periods of excessive fluid drainage from the inner ear

_____ 5. Ménière's disease may be treated with
   A. surgery, which will cure the disease
   B. over-the-counter allergy medications
   C. rehabilitation to improve balance and hearing aids
   D. prescription medications to reduce migraines

Diabetes Mellitus

Complete the following sentences.

1. Diabetes mellitus is a disease in which the body's ability to produce or respond to the hormone _____ is damaged.

2. Diabetes mellitus causes abnormal _____ of carbohydrates and elevates glucose levels in the blood and urine.

3. _____ diabetes occurs during pregnancy and often goes away after the baby is born.

4. In type _____ diabetes, the immune system destroys insulin-producing cells in the pancreas, leaving little or no insulin to be transported throughout the body.

5. Type _____ diabetes develops when cells become resistant to insulin and the pancreas is unable to produce sufficient amounts of insulin.

6. Another term for high blood glucose levels is _____.

7. Diabetes is often diagnosed using a blood test called _____ hemoglobin.

8. A(n) _____ or a continuous glucose monitor may be used to check blood glucose levels.

9. Type 1 diabetes requires that the hormone _____ be replaced, either via injection or a pump.

10. An insulin pump is attached to the body by a(n) _____.

11. _____ and exercise are particularly important for managing diabetes.

12. A side effect of diabetes, diabetic _____ is characterized by a buildup of ketones in the urine.

13. Blood glucose levels that drop too low may cause a condition called _____.

14. _____ care is particularly important for residents with diabetes and may not be part of a nursing assistant's scope of practice.

15. _____ can prevent insulin from working and cause blood glucose levels to rise.

Thyroid Disease

Identify whether each statement is true or false.

_____ 1. Hyperthyroidism and hypothyroidism are the two types of thyroid disease you will most commonly encounter when working as a holistic nursing assistant.

_____ 2. Women are more likely to experience thyroid disease than men.

_____ 3. Thyroid disease is unrelated to iodine deficiency.

_____ 4. Hypothyroidism refers to excess production of the thyroid hormone.

_____ 5. Hyperthyroidism may be caused by nodules developing in the thyroid gland.

_____ 6. Graves' disease occurs when the hypothalamus attacks the thyroid gland, causing it to produce too much thyroid hormone.

_____ 7. Hyperthyroidism does not cause any symptoms related to the cardiovascular system.

_____ 8. When the thyroid gland enlarges, it may create a growth called a nodule.

_____ 9. Hyperthyroidism occurs when the thyroid gland does not produce enough thyroid hormone.

_____ 10. Hypothyroidism may cause sluggishness, mental fog, a bloated feeling, and weight gain.

Identifying Diseases of the Cardiovascular System

Complete the following sentences.

1. _____ disease occurs when there is damage, injury, or disease in the inner layers of the coronary arteries.

2. When plaque and other waste products build up to narrow the arteries, this results in a condition called _____.

3. As the surfaces of arteries become clogged with _____, a person will experience angina and shortness of breath.

4. If the arteries become completely blocked, this causes a(n) _____ infarction, or *heart attack*.

5. Caused by reduced blood flow to the heart, _____ is described as a sensation of squeezing, pressure, heaviness, or tightness in the center of the chest.

6. _____ angina is caused by physical activity that makes the heart work harder, usually lasts for a few minutes, and then disappears with rest or prescription medication.

7. Myocardial infarction occurs when a completely blocked coronary artery causes _____, or lack of blood flow to the heart.

8. _____ heart failure is a condition in which the heart does not have the oxygen and nutrients it needs to pump blood effectively and has weakened pumping power.

9. Congestive heart failure can affect the kidneys and cause _____, or fluid buildup, in the arms, legs, ankles, feet, and lungs as the body becomes congested.

10. Coronary artery disease may also cause _____, or abnormal heart rhythms.

11. _____ accident is another term for *stroke*.

12. A(n) _____ stroke occurs when blocked arteries prevent blood from nourishing the brain.

13. _____ stroke occurs when an artery in the brain leaks blood or ruptures due to an aneurysm.

14. A transient ischemic attack (TIA) is also called a(n) _____.

15. Also called *peripheral artery disease*, peripheral _____ disease occurs when there is damage to blood vessels that supply blood to areas of the body other than the brain or heart.

Coronary Artery Disease

Select the *best* answer.

_____ 1. Coronary artery disease is diagnosed
   A. by a doctor who collects medical history, performs a physical examination, and orders special blood tests to check for enzymes that signal damage to the heart
   B. solely by a chest X-ray to see if the heart is enlarged
   C. by a nurse using an electrocardiogram (EKG or ECG) or echocardiogram
   D. by computerized tomography (CT) during a hospice visit

_____ 2. Coronary artery disease may be treated with
   A. medications to further narrow the arteries and reduce blood flow
   B. prescription medications to elevate blood pressure and cholesterol
   C. anti-inflammatory medications
   D. doctor-prescribed medications such as aspirin to reduce blood clotting

_____ 3. Percutaneous coronary intervention (PCI)
   A. is not typically used for coronary artery stenosis
   B. is a procedure in which a catheter with a tiny balloon at the tip is inserted into the narrowed artery and inflated
   C. uses a balloon to inflate an artery that is not blocked by plaque
   D. inserts a stint that inflates to keep the artery open

_____ 4. Coronary artery bypass surgery
   A. is used when an artery has been repaired with a stent
   B. is performed by a surgeon who inserts a vein or artery from the brain
   C. uses a graft to bypass a blocked coronary artery, allowing blood to flow around it
   D. is most appropriate for people who have only a single narrowed artery

_____ 5. When caring for residents with coronary artery disease, holistic nursing assistants should
   A. encourage the consumption of fruits, vegetables, and increased amounts of saturated fat
   B. encourage strenuous exercise routines
   C. encourage residents to eat large meals
   D. assist with smoking cessation plans, if the resident smokes

Cerebrovascular Accidents (CVAs)
Complete the following sentences.

1. A cerebrovascular accident (CVA), or *stroke*, occurs when a blood vessel in the brain becomes blocked due to atherosclerosis or _____.

2. A CVA may occur as the result of bleeding due to a ruptured _____, which is a distended or weak area in a blood vessel.

3. There are three types of strokes: ischemic stroke, hemorrhagic stroke, and _____ ischemic attack.

4. _____ strokes are the most common type of CVA.

5. A(n) _____ stroke occurs when an artery in the brain leaks blood or ruptures due to an aneurysm.

6. Hemorrhagic strokes may be either _____ or subarachnoid.

7. _____ hemorrhagic strokes are the most common and occur when an artery bursts and bleeds into surrounding brain tissue.

8. In a(n) _____ hemorrhagic stroke, bleeding occurs between the brain and its tissue covering.

9. High blood pressure, or _____, is a risk factor for hemorrhagic stroke.

10. It is not uncommon for a person to have a transient ischemic attack, or _____, and not know because it lasts for only a short amount of time.

Symptoms of a CVA
Read the scenario and complete the sentences that follow.

   Mrs. Jones is driving to town on a rural country road to get a few groceries. She experiences a sudden, severe headache in her left temple and swerves to the side of the road, jamming the car into park. Her right hand tingles, loses grip on the steering wheel, and falls to her lap. She squints to make sense of her reflection in the rearview mirror and is terrified to see her drooping mouth. She reaches for her purse in the backseat, but the right side of her body refuses to respond. She is able to retrieve her cellphone, but has difficulty dialing 9-1-1. She cannot understand the operator who answers and responds with slurred speech.

1. The loss of movement on one side of Mrs. Jones' body is called _____.

2. Mrs. Jones' slurred speech and inability to understand and use words is called _____.

Peripheral Vascular Disease (PVD)
Identify whether each statement is true or false.

_____ 1. Peripheral vascular disease occurs when there is damage to blood vessels that supply blood to areas of the body other than the brain and heart.

_____ 2. A family history of PVD may increase a person's chances of developing the disease.

_____ 3. Women over 60 years of age are more likely to develop PVD than men.

_____ 4. PVD symptoms begin quickly due to inadequate blood supply to the leg muscles.

_____ 5. If PVD is left untreated, gangrene can develop in the affected limb, and tissues may die and decay.

_____ 6. Treatment for PVD may include angioplasty, a procedure used to narrow obstructed arteries or veins.

The Respiratory System and Disease
Complete the following sentences.

1. The _____ is a viral infection of the respiratory system and affects the nose and throat.

2. A(n) _____ is a healthcare provider who specializes in diseases of the respiratory system.

3. _____ is a chronic lung disease in which the airways become inflamed, swell, and narrow.

4. Asthma may cause _____, a high-pitched, whistling sound during expiration.

5. Asthma symptoms may be mild or get worse, and a person may experience attacks or sudden intensifications called _____.

6. A(n) _____ may be used to diagnose asthma by measuring how much and how fast air is inhaled and exhaled.

7. A(n) _____ provides a score, or peak expiration flow rate (PEFR), to indicate how well a person's lungs are functioning.

8. A(n) _____ test measures the amount of air left in the lungs after a person takes a deep breath and exhales fully.

9. Using an inhaler or _____, people can manage asthma by breathing medication directly into the lungs.

10. Residents who use an inhaler are at risk for developing _____, a fungus that builds up on the lining of the mouth.

11. COPD is characterized by inflamed airways filled with _____, which reduces the amount of airflow into the body.

12. COPD usually includes two conditions, chronic bronchitis and _____.

13. Bronchitis is a prolonged condition in which the _____ passages become inflamed, causing membranes to swell and narrow the airways to the lungs.

14. Bronchitis can be _____ (lasting one to three weeks) or chronic (lasting three months or longer).

15. _____ is a condition that causes damage to the walls of air sacs in the lungs, trapping carbon dioxide during exhalation and leaving no room for fresh oxygen.

16. Rapid heart rate, or _____, may be associated with severe COPD.

17. _____ are inhaled medications that relax muscles around the airways, helping to improve breathing.

18. Residents with severe COPD may need _____ therapy delivered by nasal cannulas.

Diseases of the Immune and Lymphatic Systems

Identify whether each statement is true or false.

_____ 1. The primary function of the respiratory system is to defend the body against infection through natural immunity and acquired immunity.

_____ 2. Natural immunity is specific to bacteria or viruses and gives the body the ability to protect itself.

_____ 3. Acquired immunity is immunity people have at birth.

_____ 4. In an autoimmune disorder, the body produces antibodies that attack the body's own tissues instead of fighting infection.

_____ 5. Autoimmune disorders cannot be cured.

_____ 6. HIV weakens the immune system and causes people to become sick with infections that would not normally affect them.

_____ 7. HIV is transmitted via blood, semen, vaginal fluid, and saliva.

_____ 8. Acquired immunodeficiency syndrome (AIDS) is considered the most advanced stage of HIV with multiple symptoms affecting the entire body.

_____ 9. PreP medications may be prescribed if a person has been infected with HIV.

_____ 10. HIV/AIDS can be avoided by abstaining from sex, using condoms if engaging in sexual intercourse, and avoiding sharing needles.

Identifying Diseases and Conditions of the Immune System

Complete the table by identifying the missing diseases and conditions.

Diseases and Conditions of the Immune System		
Disease or Condition	Cause	Example
1. _____	Being born with a weak immune system	5. _____
2. _____	A disease that weakens the immune system	6. _____
3. _____	An overly active immune system	7. _____
4. _____	Immune system attacks itself	8. _____

GERD and Peptic Ulcers

Complete the following sentences.

1. The _____ system uses its essential functions of ingestion, digestion, absorption, and elimination to transform foods eaten into energy.

2. Common gastrointestinal system diseases and conditions are gastroesophageal reflux disease (GERD), _____ ulcers, gallbladder disease, and diverticulitis.

3. A(n) _____ is a specialist in diagnosing and treating gastrointestinal diseases and conditions.

4. _____ reflux disease is commonly called *acid reflux* and is characterized by the flow of acidic stomach contents back into the esophagus.

5. The cause of GERD is sometimes a(n) _____, or the bulging of the stomach into the chest through the diaphragmatic hiatus.

6. The key symptom of GERD is _____, or indigestion.

7. A serious complication of GERD is _____, or damaging inflammation in the esophagus that may lead to esophageal bleeding and ulcers.

8. People can find relief from GERD by controlling portions, eating at least two to three hours before going to bed, and taking over-the-counter _____ to neutralize acid.

9. To diagnose GERD, a doctor may order a(n) _____, in which the esophagus, stomach, and upper part of the small intestine are viewed using a special X-ray procedure.

10. _____ are sores or sometimes holes in the lining of the GI tract.

11. A gastric ulcer forms in the _____.

12. A(n) _____ ulcer forms in the small intestine.

13. _____ ulcers are rare and can form as a result of medications or alcohol.

14. Risk factors for developing a peptic ulcer include a family history of ulcers, stress, diet, long-term use or abuse of over-the-counter _____, and smoking.

15. A bacterial infection caused by _____ is present in most people who have duodenal and gastric ulcers and may be the primary cause of ulcers.

16. One treatment option for *H. pylori* is _____ given to kill the bacteria.

Gallbladder Disease

Select the *best* answer.

_____ 1. Gallbladder disease
A. results from the presence of gallstones in the kidneys
B. occurs when gallstones cause blockage so the gallbladder cannot empty normally
C. occurs when people who are at risk for gallstones do not have symptoms
D. is a disease that affects the urinary bladder

_____ 2. Gallbladder disease symptoms
A. may cause mild pain in the lower right part of the abdomen
B. cause pain that spreads to the lower back and shoots down the leg
C. can be steady or come and go and often improves when a person eats
D. may include yellowing of the skin and the whites of the eyes

_____ 3. To diagnose gallbladder disease,
A. the healthcare team will use modern diagnostic technology and disregard the resident's expression of pain
B. a doctor may order a diagnostic ultrasound of the abdomen to detect gallstones
C. a nursing assistant will assess the resident's abdomen for pain
D. the resident will undergo a cholecystectomy to determine the presence of gallstones

_____ 4. Care considerations of gallbladder disease include
A. a healthy diet, healthy weight, and prescription medications
B. the surgical fixation of the gallbladder
C. the surgical removal of the pancreas
D. incontinence care related to diarrhea

Diverticulitis

Identify whether each statement is true or false.

_____ 1. Diverticulitis occurs when pouches in the wall of the colon, called *diversions*, become inflamed or infected.

_____ 2. Risk factors for diverticulitis include aging, a diet high in animal fat and low in fiber, lack of exercise, obesity, smoking, and certain medications.

_____ 3. Signs and symptoms of diverticulitis include mild pain in the lower left abdomen that improves during activity, fever and chills, bloating and gas, and nausea.

_____ 4. The nursing assistant is responsible for conducting a medical history, physical examination, blood tests, and an X-ray or CT scan to diagnose diverticulitis.

_____ 5. Measures can be taken to prevent diverticula from becoming inflamed or infected.

_____ 6. When caring for residents with diverticulitis, nursing assistants should follow the plan of care and encourage a high-fiber diet, fluids, exercise, and relaxation.

_____ 7. If diverticulitis improves, solid food will be replaced with liquids to allow the intestine to heal.

_____ 8. Severe diverticulitis attacks may require discontinuing antibiotics.

_____ 9. If diverticulitis complications such as a perforation, abscess, or fistula occur, bowel resection surgery may be the next step.

_____ 10. During bowel resection surgery, diseased parts of the intestine are removed, and healthy portions of the intestine are reconnected.

_____ 11. A surgical opening in the abdomen for passing waste into an external bag is called a *colostomy*.

Urinary Tract Infections (UTIs)

Complete the following sentences.

1. A(n) _____ infection is an infection in which pathogens enter the body through the urethra and begin to grow.

2. A UTI that occurs in the kidneys is called _____.

3. The term *cystitis* refers to a UTI that occurs in the _____.

4. The term _____ refers to a UTI that occurs in the urethra.

5. Three common causes of UTIs are the transfer of bacteria from the _____, sexual activity, and the presence of a urinary catheter.

6. Compared to males, females are at _____ risk for UTIs.

7. Some signs and symptoms of a UTI include a strong and persistent urge to _____, a burning sensation, cloudy urine, and a foul smell.

8. Left untreated, UTIs may lead to urethral narrowing, called _____, and kidney damage.

9. Tests for diagnosing a UTI usually include a urine sample for laboratory analysis and a(n) _____, in which a small amount of urine is tested to identify the specific bacteria present.

10. To investigate frequent UTIs, a doctor may perform a(n) _____, which involves inserting a long, thin catheter with a lens into the urethra and urinary bladder to view the lining.

11. UTIs are usually treated with antibiotics and pain medications called _____.

12. To help prevent a UTI, nursing assistants should provide excellent perineal hygiene to ensure cleanliness after _____.

The Kidneys and Disease

Identify whether each statement is true or false.

_____ 1. Urologists are doctors who specialize in diagnosing and treating diseases and conditions of the urinary system.

_____ 2. In renal lithiasis, small, hard deposits composed of minerals and acid salts form in the gallbladder.

_____ 3. Kidney stones often form when the urine becomes more dilute and contains fewer crystal-forming substances.

_____ 4. Common causes of kidney stones include dehydration; diets high in protein, salt, and sugar; obesity; and family or personal history.

_____ 5. Kidney stones usually cause pain on the front of the body above the ribs, accompanied by pink, red, or brown urine that is foul smelling; urinary urgency; fever; nausea; and vomiting.

_____ 6. Treatment for kidney stones varies, but focuses on passing the kidney stone with large volumes of water until urine is clear.

_____ 7. Larger kidney stones may require the use of light waves to break up the kidney stones.

_____ 8. Nursing assistants can help residents with kidney stones by encouraging them not to drink fluids and straining all urine for evidence of passing a stone.

_____ 9. Renal failure occurs when the kidneys filter waste products from the blood too efficiently, disrupting the body's chemical composition.

_____ 10. Acute renal failure is a condition that usually resolves on its own with time.

_____ 11. Chronic renal failure is the gradual loss of kidney function and is usually caused by another disease.

_____ 12. Decreased urine output, edema, shortness of breath, chest pain, muscle weakness, drowsiness and fatigue, confusion, and nausea are all signs and symptoms of renal failure.

_____ 13. Advanced stages of renal failure or end-stage renal disease (ESRD) can lead to seizures or a state of deep and prolonged consciousness called *coma*.

_____ 14. To diagnose renal failure, a doctor may order a urinalysis to examine the chemical composition of urine.

_____ 15. To help diagnose renal failure, a nursing assistant may order blood tests to determine the level of kidney function, an ultrasound, a CT scan, or a biopsy to test kidney tissue.

_____ 16. People with renal failure are often prescribed a special diet with increased amounts of protein, phosphorus, calcium, sodium, and potassium.

_____ 17. End-stage renal disease (ESRD) occurs when the kidneys are so damaged they cannot function and have nearly or completely failed.

_____ 18. In hemodialysis, a machine is used to filter the blood of waste products.

_____ 19. In peritoneal dialysis, a catheter is inserted into the abdominal cavity to deliver a solution that absorbs waste and excess fluids.

_____ 20. When the kidneys are no longer able to remove waste products, a kidney transplant may be appropriate.

Common Reproductive System Diseases Among Males

Select the *best* answer.

_____ 1. Which of the following is a common reproductive system disease among males?
   A. uterine prolapse of the epididymis
   B. vaginitis of the prostate
   C. benign prostatic hypertrophy (BPH)
   D. diverticulitis

_____ 2. Benign prostatic hypertrophy (BPH)
   A. is also called *benign prostatic hyperplasia*
   B. is an enlarged pituitary gland
   C. is caused by hormonal changes and cell growth during puberty
   D. is normal aging that blocks the urethra, causing no symptoms

_____ 3. Which of the following are signs and symptoms of BPH?
   A. trouble starting the urine stream, but no difficulty stopping it
   B. a strong urine stream and the feeling that the bladder is completely empty after urination
   C. ease of urination
   D. urinary retention, infections, and kidney damage

_____ 4. Which of the following is true of BPH?
   A. It is cancerous, but does not interfere with the ability to achieve an erection.
   B. It is diagnosed by nursing assistants through a physical examination.
   C. It is diagnosed by nurses through a digital rectal exam.
   D. It is not cancerous, but a doctor may order a PSA test to rule out prostate cancer.

_____ 5. Care considerations for BPH include
   A. medications to eliminate urination
   B. helping the resident relax, maintaining good body hygiene, and assisting with special briefs if there is dribbling
   C. surgery to remove the testes and prostate gland
   D. encouraging the consumption of coffee and beer

Vaginitis

Identify whether each statement is true or false.

_____ 1. Vaginitis is never caused by bacteria, viruses, or a yeast infection.

_____ 2. Vaginitis may result from sexual contact, poor hygiene, lower levels of hormones causing vaginal dryness, and allergic reactions to environmental substances.

_____ 3. The signs and symptoms of vaginitis include changes in the color, smell, or texture of vaginal discharge; irritation; itching; and burning during urination.

_____ 4. A diagnosis is not necessary to prescribe medications for vaginitis.

_____ 5. To prevent vaginitis, nursing assistants should encourage residents to maintain good hygiene, avoid irritating substances, and wear restrictive clothing.

Uterine Prolapse

Apply the appropriate callouts to the image.
A. Rectum
B. Vagina
C. Bladder
D. Labia
E. Severely prolapsed uterus

© Body Scientific International

Understanding Cancer

Complete the following sentences.

1. _____ is a disease in which cells grow abnormally and out of control, crowding out normal cells.

2. When _____ occurs, cells from the original site of cancer spread to other parts of the body.

3. In many cancers, a lump called a(n) _____ will form.

4. When a tumor is _____, it is cancerous.

5. If a tumor is _____, it does not contain cancer cells.

6. A(n) _____ is a tumor consisting of fat cells that is usually benign.

7. The stages of cancer describe how far a cancer has _____.

8. Stage 1 indicates that cancer has not likely spread from its original site, and _____ is the most advanced stage of cancer.

9. Treatments for later stages of cancer may require a combination of surgery to remove the tumor and edges of healthy tissue, chemotherapy to shrink or eradicate cancer cells, and _____ to kill or slow the growth of cancer cells.

10. Factors that reduce the risk of developing cancer include living a healthy lifestyle, not smoking, and avoiding _____ substances.

11. Risk factors for cancer include age, family history, and exposure to toxic substances and _____ without protection.

12. General signs and symptoms of cancer may include weight loss, fatigue, fever, pain, changes in the skin, lumps, sores that do not _____, and changes in elimination.

13. Methods of diagnosing cancer include X-rays, blood tests, or a(n) _____.

14. _____ surgery is the removal of an organ before its cells become cancerous.

15. To provide _____ support, nursing assistants can be sensitive to and aware of a resident's feelings about and approaches to cancer diagnosis and treatment.

16. When caring for residents who have undergone radiation, nursing assistants should be gentle with _____ care and use mild soap and lukewarm water.

End-of-Life Care

Identify whether each statement is true or false.

_____ 1. For some people, poor quality of life and the spread of cancer lead to a decision to end treatment.

_____ 2. End-of-life care can be received at home or in long-term care settings, but not through hospice services.

_____ 3. Prescription medications are often used to relieve pain, anxiety, shortness of breath, nausea, and constipation.

_____ 4. Excellent holistic care continues through the end of life and even after death.

_____ 5. While some residents may desire alone time at the end of life, others prefer to communicate their worries with family members and those around them.

Matching Section 9.2 Key Terms

Match each definition with the key term.

A. acute pain
B. chronic pain
C. nonpharmacological
D. pain scales
E. stoic

_____ 1. devices used to measure the perception of the severity of pain

_____ 2. without the use of medication

_____ 3. an intense discomfort, often the result of trauma, that goes away within six months

_____ 4. a persistent, uncomfortable feeling that does not go away over time

_____ 5. detached from emotion or feeling

Understanding Pain

Complete the following sentences.

1. _____ can be mild, moderate, or severe and is described as a dull, aching, throbbing, stabbing, stinging, sharp, or crushing feeling.

2. Pain's _____, or source, and other factors such as cultural influences and the length of time pain is experienced influence the development and severity of pain.

3. Pain is felt, or _____, when pain receptors in the nervous system are stimulated.

4. Pain _____ send a signal that travels through nerves to the spinal cord, which responds to pain by causing a reflex action.

5. The _____ carries pain messages to the brain, where the messages are received by the thalamus and interpreted in the cerebral cortex.

6. Pain messages may be sent to multiple parts of the brain to cause particular reactions, such as increased _____ or sweating.

7. _____ pain is sudden and goes away relatively quickly with treatment.

8. _____ pain persists over time.

9. A repeating _____ of pain can lead to decreased activity, low interest in daily living, and diminished feelings of happiness and joy.

10. Some people are _____, or detached from feeling, and feel they can withstand pain without the help of medication.

Observing Pain

Complete the following sentences.

1. The responsibility of the holistic nursing assistant is to determine the level and intensity of a resident's pain and _____ it properly to the licensed nursing staff.

2. Knowledge of pain can help holistic nursing assistants take _____ actions that are not medication based according to the plan of care.

3. To assist in pain _____, holistic nursing assistants can be sensitive to pain responses, help the resident relax using deep breathing, provide comfortable positioning, and encourage calmness through music.

4. _____ can help a nursing assistant verbally describe the intensity of pain for the resident using numbers from 0, no pain, to 10, severe pain.

5. A pain scale that uses expressive _____ to illustrate different levels of pain can be helpful when working with young patients or residents who cannot communicate verbally.

Name: _____   Date: _____

Matching Chapter 10 Key Terms, Part A

Match each definition with the key term.

A. active listening
B. body language
C. clarification
D. closed-ended question
E. communication barriers
F. congruent communication
G. defense mechanisms
H. health literacy
I. interpreter
J. jargon
K. labeling
L. open-ended question

_____ 1. the process of restating what you believe was said to make sure you heard the message correctly

_____ 2. words, phrases, and language used by a specific group of people or culture

_____ 3. a question that requires only a one-word answer, such as *yes* or *no*

_____ 4. unconscious behaviors that enable people to ignore or forget situations or thoughts that cause fear, anxiety, and stress

_____ 5. a person who translates written or spoken words into another language

_____ 6. the process of showing interest in what a person is saying; includes paying attention, making eye contact, clarifying, and summarizing what a person has said

_____ 7. a question that requires more than a one-word answer

_____ 8. negatively describing someone using a specific word or phrase

_____ 9. a type of communication in which the sender's speech, facial expressions, and body language all send the same message

_____ 10. gestures and movements that communicate a person's thoughts and feelings

_____ 11. a person's ability to fully understand and use information about health, diseases, conditions, or treatments

_____ 12. any actions, behaviors, or situations that block or interfere with a person's ability to successfully send and receive messages

Holistic Communication

Complete the following sentences.

1. Even before people began to speak and write, they used cave paintings, rock carvings, and rock paintings to _____.

2. _____ is the way people exchange information with one another.

3. People send and receive messages both _____ (with words) and _____ (without words).

4. When communication is _____, it considers all aspects of a resident's body, mind, and spirit.

5. Holistic communication involves being fully _____ and focused on an exchange with another person.

6. Holistic communication promotes _____ and well-being.

7. Holistic communication keeps lines of communication _____ to achieve a caring environment.

8. Successful holistic communicators are accurate, honest, timely, and _____.

9. Holistic communication helps nursing assistants and residents develop trusting, respectful _____.

Understanding Communication

Identify whether each statement is true or false.

_____ 1. A holistic nursing assistant effectively communicates with residents, residents' families, and members of the healthcare team to deliver safe, quality care.

_____ 2. The four basic components of effective communication are the sender, mode of communication, recipient, and flashback.

_____ 3. In communication, the sender initiates communication, determines the content of the message, and evaluates the best way to deliver the message clearly.

_____ 4. The sender chooses the *mode of communication*, or the way the message will be sent.

_____ 5. The four modes of communication for sending a message are speaking, listening, using body language, and writing.

_____ 6. The mode of communication chosen rarely depends on the situation.

_____ 7. Clarity is important for ensuring the intended message is received accurately.

_____ 8. Crosscurrent communication occurs when verbal and nonverbal communication match.

_____ 9. Once a message is sent, the recipient receives the message by carefully listening to the spoken words and by observing the tone and pitch of the sender's voice and the sender's body language.

_____ 10. Feedback is a response from the recipient that confirms the sender and the recipient have the same, or a similar, perception of the message.

Identifying Components of Communication

Apply the appropriate labels to the image.

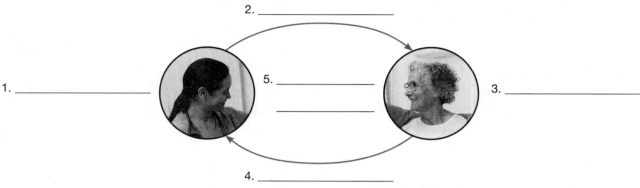

2. _____

1. _____

5. _____
   _____

3. _____

4. _____

ESB Professional/Shutterstock.com

Types of Communication

Select the *best* answer.

_____ 1. Which of the following is true of verbal communication?
   A. It occurs when people use spoken words to express themselves.
   B. It accounts for about 75 percent of all human communication.
   C. It is 90 percent nonverbal.
   D. It involves making facial expressions and body gestures.

_____ 2. Examples of nonverbal communication include
   A. pointing your finger, shaking your head, making facial expressions, or using body gestures
   B. telling a resident how you feel
   C. slumping your shoulders to convey confidence
   D. using a thumbs-down gesture to reflect a positive feeling

_____ 3. Body language is
   A. a type of nonverbal communication that uses gestures and body movements
   B. always direct and straightforward
   C. not as powerful as verbal language
   D. always interpreted by others the way it was intended

_____ 4. Which of the following is an example of positive nonverbal communication?
   A. shouting at a resident across the room
   B. invading personal space without permission to get personal cares done
   C. standing over a resident to communicate authority
   D. making eye contact, moving the eyebrows and forehead, using touch, and navigating zones of personal space

_____ 5. Which of the following is true of how comfortable zones of personal space are expressed in the United States?
   A. Personal space (1.5–4 feet) is reserved for business associates.
   B. Intimate space (1.5 feet or less) might be shared with family, very close friends, and pets.
   C. Social space (4–12 feet) is shared with very close friends.
   D. Public space (12 feet or more) is reserved for significant others.

Making Observations

Complete the following sentences.

1. Using the _____ of sight, smell, touch, and hearing improves observations and makes interactions more meaningful.

2. _____ a resident's facial expressions can help you realize if the resident is in pain.

3. The sense of _____ may identify a foul odor, which can alert the nursing assistant to a possible new infection.

4. The sense of _____ helps a resident feel cared about, but also reveals changes in skin temperature.

5. _____ observations provide measurable facts without personal interpretation.

6. _____ observations are based on opinions and personal interpretation.

7. A useful subjective observation could be a(n) _____ account of his or her experience or level of pain.

Overcoming Communication Barriers

For each communication barrier, explain how the barrier impedes communication and how the barrier can be overcome.

1. Jargon

_____

_____

_____

2. Stereotypes and labels

_____

_____

_____

3. Advice

_____

_____

_____

4. Cultural barriers

_____

_____

_____

5. Hearing impairments

_____

_____

_____

6. Vision impairments

_____

_____

_____

7. Speech impairments

_____

_____

_____

8. Cognitive disorders

_____

_____

_____

9. Defense mechanisms

_____

_____

_____

Recognizing Defense Mechanisms

Apply the appropriate labels to the table.

Defense Mechanisms	
Defense Mechanism	Description
1. _____	Rejecting the truth about one's feelings, experiences, or facts
2. _____	Refusing to remember a traumatic or painful situation
3. _____	Reverting back to childlike behaviors when fearful, anxious, or angry
4. _____	Transferring a bad or negative feeling, such as anger, away from the source and onto someone or something else
5. _____	Believing that others feel a certain way when, in fact, the feelings are yours
6. _____	Feeling one way inside, but outwardly expressing the feeling in an opposite way
7. _____	Focusing on facts, logic, and reasoning instead of a stressful feeling or uncomfortable emotion
8. _____	Using logic to excuse unacceptable behaviors and feelings

Accurate Communication

Using online resources, research how one of the best-known Superman actors died from a decubitus ulcer. Write down this information and then have the first person (who compiled the information) in a line privately read the information to the next person in line. The next person should verbally communicate (without reading, in private) the information to the third person, and so on until the last person is reached. Have the last person announce his or her understanding of the information to the entire group. Then, compare the original written information to the final verbal version. The objective of this activity is accurate reporting of the information without error, but this rarely happens. Errors usually happen in the retelling, illustrating the importance of accurate communication.

Ways to Improve Communication

Select the *best* answer.

_____ 1. If communication is difficult, it is best to
  A. use a communication strategy called passive listening
  B. be patient, listen carefully, and try to clarify and reflect what is being communicated
  C. initiate proper interrogation to help improve the communication barrier
  D. accept that active listening makes successful communication impossible

_____ 2. Which of the following describes active listening?
  A. showing interest in the person speaking and in what is being said by paying attention and providing good eye contact
  B. looking directly at the speaker with a stare
  C. using eye contact to help the speaker feel what he or she is saying is unimportant
  D. sitting down, leaning into the speaker's personal space, and nodding your head

_____ 3. Clarification involves
  A. saying, "I want to be sure I understand why you refuse to get along with me"
  B. saying, "What is your problem?"
  C. asking another person to clarify a message by saying, "I want to be sure you understood me; are you deaf?"
  D. restating what you believe was said to make sure you heard the message correctly

_____ 4. What is reflection?
  A. a technique in which the resident looks in a mirror and tells the nursing assistant how he or she feels
  B. a method of identifying a resident's feelings so they can be directly reported to the doctor
  C. a technique in which one listens, identifies the feelings expressed nonverbally, and asks questions to bring out those feelings
  D. a feeling of tension and frustration that the resident must release

_____ 5. The most effective questions
  A. are *why* questions that make people feel defensive and express their angry feelings
  B. result in one-word answers such as *yes* or *no*
  C. are open-ended questions that lead to more than a one-word answer
  D. will retrieve details that the resident may be trying to hide from his or her family

Health Literacy

Complete the following sentences.

1. _____ is the degree to which people fully understand and use information about their health, diseases, conditions, or treatments to manage their health, make appropriate health decisions, find necessary healthcare resources, share personal information, adopt healthy behaviors, and engage in self-care.

2. Poor health literacy can result when people ignore communication, misinterpret messages, or _____ the information or understanding to follow instructions or report abnormal symptoms.

3. A person's level of health literacy is influenced by reading and writing skills, ability to understand and calculate simple math, _____ about wellness and illness, and depth of knowledge about healthcare topics and systems.

4. Older adults, people from specific cultures, nonnative English speakers, and people with low incomes and educational levels are _____ likely to have below-average health literacy.

5. The extent of a person's health literacy is influenced by _____, knowledge and skills, situation, and ability to communicate.

6. The Patient Protection and Affordable Care Act includes a National Action Plan to Improve _____, which seeks to help individuals make informed decisions about their healthcare.

7. The responsibility for improving health literacy lies with _____.

8. To promote health literacy, nursing assistants can use all forms of communication available, choose words and examples that make the information understandable, offer simple instructions for better understanding, speak plainly, request an interpreter so the resident's primary language is used, speak slowly, and _____ listen.

Matching Chapter 10 Key Terms, Part B

Match each definition with the key term.

A. anger
B. assertive
C. caring
D. collaboration
E. compromise
F. conflict
G. fear
H. giving of self
I. interpersonal relationships
J. intimate relationships
K. phobias

_____ 1. providing assistance and comfort to positively affect the health and well-being of a resident

_____ 2. the process by which people work together to resolve conflict in a way that satisfies everyone

_____ 3. a disagreement between two or more people

_____ 4. bold and clear

_____ 5. relationships between two or more people who share similar interests or goals; meet physical or emotional needs

_____ 6. unsupported, exaggerated fears that sometimes interfere with daily life

_____ 7. an unpleasant feeling or emotion resulting from the threat or presence of danger

_____ 8. the process by which two sides of a conflict make concessions to find the best resolution

_____ 9. relationships between two people who have romantic feelings of love for each other

_____ 10. a strong feeling or emotion that develops from frustration, displeasure, or a threat

_____ 11. the quality of putting a resident's health and wellness needs before one's own needs as a caregiver

Interpersonal Relationships

Complete the following sentences.

1. There are four types of _____ relationships: family relationships, friendships, intimate relationships, and professional relationships.

2. _____ relationships are based on interactions between parents, siblings, and extended family members.

3. Families' patterns of communication are based on _____, habit, and familiarity.

4. Relationships called _____ are built on similar likes, dislikes, plans, goals, and desires.

5. _____ relationships develop from romantic feelings and love.

6. Nursing assistants develop _____ relationships with coworkers, residents, and residents' family members.

Building and Maintaining Professional Relationships

Complete the following strategies for building and maintaining professional relationships.

1. Be _____, be responsive, and focus on others.

2. _____ others' views and opinions.

3. Be _____ by ensuring residents have the assistance they need.

4. Be _____ by avoiding stereotypes and labels.

5. Be trustworthy and _____ so others can count on you.

6. Be appreciative, _____, and optimistic.

7. Be a(n) _____ player.

8. Manage _____ and conflict appropriately.

Feelings in Professional Relationships

Identify whether each statement is true or false.

_____ 1. Feelings have no place in a professional relationship.

_____ 2. It is not possible for a nursing assistant to transfer negative feelings onto a resident.

_____ 3. Transference can negatively affect relationships with residents and the nursing assistant's ability to provide holistic care.

_____ 4. Residents may also unconsciously transfer feelings about another person onto a nursing assistant.

_____ 5. To handle feelings well, the nursing assistant should focus on effective communication skills and the best way to deliver care.

Name: _____ Date: _____

Caring Skills

Apply the appropriate labels to the table.

Caring Skills	
Skill	**Description**
1. _____	Quality of making one's self available and open to others and putting residents' needs first
2. _____	Understanding for another person's feelings and emotions
3. _____	Willingness to wait and understand
4. _____	Knowledge of responsibility and commitment never to take shortcuts
5. _____	Pursuit of information about residents
6. _____	Ability to think and act quickly to overcome challenges and solve problems

Understanding Anxiety, Fear, and Anger

Complete the following sentences.

1. Residents may deal with _____ by crying, expressing anger, or shutting down emotionally.

2. Anxiety disorders include _____ (unsupported, exaggerated fears), panic, post-traumatic stress disorder (PTSD), and obsessive-compulsive disorder (OCD).

3. To identify anxiety, nursing assistants can _____ for heavy, short breaths; complaints about heart palpitations or chest pain; dizziness; sweating; muscle aches; dry mouth; and fluctuations in behavior or mood.

4. As caregivers, nursing assistants must recognize their own _____ of anxiety to be aware of and manage them.

5. To alleviate anxiety, caregivers can take slow, deep _____ and talk through feelings of anxiety with a coworker.

6. _____ is a feeling of being scared, emotionally out of control, and overwhelmed.

7. Fear is an unpleasant emotion that occurs in response to an identified _____ or the presence of danger.

8. Positive fear can serve as a healthy _____ and motivate the resident to change for the better.

9. Fear has physical effects due to the actions of the sympathetic nervous system (SNS), which causes the _____ response.

10. Fear cannot be overcome unless a person commits to _____ or eliminating his or her fear.

11. _____ is a powerful feeling that develops from frustration, displeasure, or a threat.

12. _____ is a mild form of anger; rage is an extreme form.

13. Instead of demonstrating anger outwardly, some people turn anger inward, which can cause serious physical symptoms and _____.

14. Often, residents' anger comes from residents feeling they have lost _____ over their own lives, leading to frustration or feelings of helplessness.

15. It is _____ for nursing assistants to exhibit anger or gossip about people with whom they are angry.

Conflict Management: Managing Feelings

Complete the three steps for managing feelings in the face of conflict.

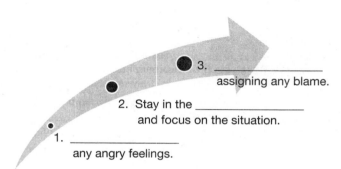

3. _____ assigning any blame.

2. Stay in the _____ and focus on the situation.

1. _____ any angry feelings.

Conflict Management: Problem Solving

List the six steps for using problem solving to manage
a conflict.

1. _____

   _____

   _____

2. _____

   _____

   _____

3. _____

   _____

   _____

4. _____

   _____

   _____

5. _____

   _____

   _____

6. _____

   _____

   _____

Name: _____   Date: _____

Matching Chapter 11 Key Terms

Match the definition with the key term
A. beliefs
B. cross-cultural communication
C. cultural humility
D. customs
E. diversity
F. ethnicity
G. ethnocentrism
H. kinship
I. prejudice
J. race
K. racism
L. rituals
M. traditions
N. trait

_____ 1. ideas that a person or group of people accept to be true

_____ 2. established practices and beliefs that are followed by a group of people over multiple generations

_____ 3. a feeling of being close or of having an association or connection

_____ 4. an opinion or feeling that is formed without facts and that often leads to unfair feelings of dislike for a person or group because of race, sex, or religion

_____ 5. a distinctive physical quality or characteristic

_____ 6. the presence of differences among people

_____ 7. awareness and understanding of one's own culture, as well as the cultures of others; includes knowledge of personal limitations, barriers, and gaps in knowledge and provides the openness needed to be sensitive to and respectful of other cultures

_____ 8. the use of practices and approaches that promote and improve relationships with people from different cultures

_____ 9. actions that are always done in the same way, often for religious purposes or as part of a ceremony

_____ 10. a group's identification with common social, cultural, and traditional practices that are shared within the group

_____ 11. intolerance, discrimination, or prejudice based on race

_____ 12. an outlook in which one judges another culture based on the beliefs and standards of one's own culture

_____ 13. a set of inherited physical characteristics, including skin, eye, and hair color

_____ 14. behaviors or practices that have special meanings or symbolism and that are handed down from one generation to another

Racial and Ethnic Diversity

Complete the following sentences.

1. Differences among people include racial diversity, ethnic diversity, family diversity, religious diversity, geographic diversity, generational diversity, and _____ diversity.

2. _____ is linked to a person's genetic makeup and cannot be changed.

3. Race can be identified using a person's distinctive physical characteristics, or _____, like skin, hair, or eye color.

4. _____ is a group's identification with shared social, cultural, and traditional practices.

5. _____ is a set of learned behaviors and is passed down through generations.

6. People of the same culture have shared _____, or behaviors that have special meanings, beliefs, and languages.

7. People of the same culture also have shared _____, or actions always done in the same way.

8. People of the same culture may have shared _____, which are established practices and beliefs.

Family Diversity

Identify whether each statement is true or false.

_____ 1. The traditional family includes a mother, a father, and a child or children.

_____ 2. When divorced parents marry other people and have children from both marriages, this forms a blended family.

_____ 3. Some families have two parents of the same sex.

_____ 4. Blended families are families with adopted or foster children.

_____ 5. An interstitial family is one in which several generations live in the same house.

_____ 6. Interracial families have family members from different races.

Religious Diversity

Complete the following sentences.

1. A(n) _____ is defined by a specific set of spiritual beliefs about supreme beings, a particular philosophy of life, a code of ethics, and a set of rituals.

2. In some religions, a(n) _____ being is seen as being responsible for all healing.

3. The religion most commonly represented in the United States is _____.

4. Nearly 6 percent of people in the United States follow other religions, such as Judaism, Buddhism, and _____.

5. The final 23 percent of people in the United States are unaffiliated with a religion. These people may consider themselves _____ (people who deny or disbelieve the existence of a supreme being) or agnostics (people who believe they cannot know if any supreme being exists).

Geographic Diversity

Identify whether each statement is true or false.

_____ 1. The places where people live are not an important consideration of diversity.

_____ 2. Different regions of the United States often have diverse cultural practices.

_____ 3. In the United States, regional accents vary, people have familiarity with different types of food, and people call items such as clothing or furniture by different names.

_____ 4. People may be accustomed to different types of transportation because of their geographic locations.

_____ 5. People who live in the city often utilize public transportation, while people in more rural areas may rely exclusively on personal vehicles.

Generational Diversity

Identify whether each statement is true or false.

_____ 1. In today's society, there are five diverse generations: the silent generation, baby boomers, generation X, millennials, and generation Z.

_____ 2. Stereotypes are helpful for understanding and interacting with different generations.

_____ 3. Nursing assistants should recognize generational diversity and value the qualities of only their own generation.

_____ 4. The better nursing assistants understand the differences between generations, the harder it will be for them to understand members of these generations.

_____ 5. Nursing assistants can build rapport with diverse generations through effective communication.

Sexual Diversity

Select the *best* answer.

_____ 1. Sexual orientation
   A. describes a person's emotional, romantic, and sexual attraction to males or females
   B. includes heterosexuality (attraction to members of the same sex)
   C. includes homosexuality (attraction to members of the opposite sex)
   D. includes asexuality (attraction to members of both sexes) and bisexuality (lacking sexual attraction for other people)

_____ 2. What is gender identity?
   A. a mental illness
   B. a feeling that a person's assigned sex (male or female) is the same as his or her gender identity
   C. a feeling that one's assigned sex is incorrect
   D. a person's sense of being a man or a woman and the expression of that sense

_____ 3. People born with a difference in sexual development (DSD)
   A. have a mixture of XYZ chromosomes
   B. have variations in their sexual anatomy and are not entirely in alignment with female or male anatomy
   C. may have male anatomy on the outside, have male anatomy on the inside, and identify as male
   D. are not identified until puberty

_____ 4. Other types of diversity
   A. do not include varied political beliefs
   B. exclude differences in levels of education
   C. include diversity in mental and physical abilities
   D. include political diversity, but not different levels of education

_____ 5. A holistic nursing assistant
   A. will likely care for many diverse cultures and groups
   B. will care only for a limited group of people unless he or she moves
   C. cares for the mind, body, and spirit of his or her favorite residents
   D. recognizes that not all residents deserve safe, quality care

Name: ____________________ Date: ____________

Challenges to Appreciating Diversity

Apply the appropriate labels to the table.

Challenges to Appreciating Diversity	
Challenge	**Description**
1. ____________	Judging another culture based on the beliefs and standards of one's own culture
2. ____________	An unfair belief that some people, objects, or situations are better than others
3. ____________	An opinion formed without facts that leads to unfair feelings of dislike for a person or group based on race, sex, or religion
4. ____________	A form of prejudice in which one believes one's own race is superior
5. ____________	An oversimplified, generalized, usually unfavorable opinion about a group of people

Cultural Humility

Complete the following sentences.

1. Cultural ____________ recognizes that there are differences among all people and acknowledges that it is impossible to learn everything about another person's culture.
2. Cultural humility focuses on the importance of ____________ one's own culture to understand its limitations, barriers, and gaps in knowledge.
3. Cultural humility attempts to achieve a sense of ____________ by encouraging people to be respectful of one another, be open to new ideas, and understand that each person should be treated as an individual.
4. A person who practices cultural humility is positively ____________ about how other people see the world and live.
5. ____________ dynamics in some cultures place a strong emphasis on older adults as decision makers with wisdom.
6. ____________ is a feeling of closeness between members of an extended family or community.
7. In some cultures, ____________ is valued to the extent that people are unwilling to acknowledge strong emotions or pain.
8. A resident's respect for ____________ figures may lead healthcare staff members to assume that everything is all right with the resident, when not everything is.
9. People's diets are often influenced by their ____________ or religious practices.
10. A holistic nursing assistant must be aware of any medical and religious ____________ restrictions a resident has and assist with accommodating any special requests by following the plan of care and reporting to the licensed nursing staff.
11. Residents' ____________ beliefs may prevent them from taking certain medications, receiving blood transfusions, and donating or receiving organs.
12. Cultural practices or religious beliefs may dictate ____________, which involves regard for decency of behavior, dress, and exposure of body parts to others.

Cross-Cultural Communication

Identify whether each statement is true or false.

_____ 1. Cross-cultural communication uses practices and approaches that promote and improve relationships with people from different cultures.

_____ 2. Successful cross-cultural communication does not take into account a culture's values, traditions, and customs.

_____ 3. Understanding how members of a culture communicate both verbally and nonverbally is not important for cross-cultural communication.

_____ 4. To ensure successful cross-cultural communication, nursing assistants should pay attention to residents' body language and be mindful of using gestures.

_____ 5. Using jargon is a good skill for cross-cultural communication.

_____ 6. When using cross-cultural communication, nursing assistants should never ask residents to repeat back what they heard.

_____ 7. Asking respectful questions to understand traditions is an important cross-cultural communication skill.

Diversity Awareness

With a partner, conduct a diversity awareness interview. Your partner should pretend to be a resident, and you should take the role of a nursing assistant. Create seven open-ended, diversity-related questions to ask your partner to better understand his or her cultural background and traditions. Then, trade places and answer your partner's questions. After both interviews, indicate whether you agree or disagree with the statements that follow and explain why.

1. Question: _____

_____

    Answer: _____

_____

2. Question: _____

_____

    Answer: _____

_____

3. Question: _____

_____

    Answer: _____

_____

4. Question: _____

_____

    Answer: _____

_____

5. Question: _____

_____

    Answer: _____

_____

6. Question: _____

_____

    Answer: _____

_____

7. Question: _____

_____

    Answer: _____

_____

8. Race is linked to a person's genetic makeup and cannot be changed. Do you agree or disagree?

_____

_____

9. Ethnicity is a group's identification with shared social, cultural, and traditional practices. Do you agree or disagree?

_____

_____

10. Some diverse family structures include traditional families, families with single parents, blended families, and intergenerational families. Do you agree or disagree?

_____

_____

11. A religion is defined by a specific set of spiritual beliefs about supreme beings, a particular philosophy of life, a code of ethics, and a set of rituals. Do you agree or disagree?

_____

_____

12. The places where people live, or people's geographic locations, are an important consideration of diversity. Do you agree or disagree?

_____

_____

13. It is important not to believe stereotypes about particular generations. Do you agree or disagree?

_____

_____

14. Gender identity refers to a person's sense of being a man or a woman and the expression of that sense. Do you agree or disagree?

_____

_____

Name: _____ Date: _____

Matching Chapter 12 Key Terms

Match each definition with the key term.

A. care conferences
B. change-of-shift report
C. critical observation
D. deformity
E. memory
F. numbness
G. nursing orders
H. objective observations
I. rationale
J. rounds
K. subjective observations
L. tingling

_____ 1. descriptions based on feelings or opinions

_____ 2. the appropriate use of both objective and subjective observation

_____ 3. routinely scheduled meetings that bring together all members of the healthcare staff who deliver care to a particular resident; during the meeting, the resident's plan of care is discussed

_____ 4. instructions outlining the actions that should be taken to achieve stated goals of care; are written by the RN

_____ 5. a sensation that feels like sharp points digging into the skin due to changes in nerve function

_____ 6. distortion of a body part

_____ 7. a verbal report that transfers essential information about residents from one shift to the next

_____ 8. an inability to feel anything due to changes in nerve function

_____ 9. descriptions based on facts

_____ 10. opportunities to monitor and discuss the status of a resident's condition or disease; are conducted inside or right outside the resident's room

_____ 11. the storage and remembrance of past experiences

_____ 12. the research- and science-based reasoning behind a specific nursing action

The Plan of Care

Complete the following sentences.

1. A written _____ is based on a comprehensive nursing assessment performed by the licensed nursing staff and provides guidance for delivering individualized, consistent care for each resident.

2. Plans of care are evaluated and _____ both routinely and when any resident changes occur.

3. Updates or changes in care are documented by the _____ nursing staff and are communicated to staff members across all shifts.

4. The communication of changes by the licensed nursing staff establishes _____ of care across shifts and among members of the nursing staff.

5. Plans of care are useful for determining _____ coverage because they detail the types of treatments needed, schedules for reporting and observing residents, and the amount and type of assistance staff will be required to provide.

6. Plans of care use the steps of the _____ process and other important components like doctors' orders.

7. _____, which are instructions for achieving care goals, are included in a plan of care.

8. A(n) _____ is different from a nursing diagnosis in that it identifies a disease or medical condition.

9. A registered nurse makes a(n) _____, diagnosis which is the identification of a health problem that can be improved through nursing care.

10. A(n) _____ is the desired change or outcome in a resident's condition and also might be called a *critical* or *clinical pathway*.

Nursing Orders

Nursing orders are instructions that outline the actions nursing staff members must take to help residents achieve desired goals. Complete the items that are usually included in nursing orders.

Nursing Orders

1. The _____ of the order

↓

2. The _____ to be taken

↓

3. The _____ (reasoning) for the actions

↓

4. The _____ of the action

↓

5. The _____ of the licensed nursing staff member who wrote the order

Plan of Care Evaluation

Identify whether each statement is true or false.

_____ 1. Evaluation of the plan of care is ongoing and is used to track and update progress toward achieving a goal.

_____ 2. Nursing assistants determine if nursing actions should be stopped, continued, or adjusted.

_____ 3. Evaluation is used to assess the overall effectiveness of the nursing plan of care.

_____ 4. Once updated, a written plan of care will be available to the nursing staff for reference.

_____ 5. A plan of care may be in the form of a Kardex or part of an EMR and may identify the most important treatments, medications, allergies, special diets, and care considerations to meet activities of daily living.

_____ 6. Nursing assistants share important observations and information that affect the plan of care.

Care Conferences

List the agenda items that are typically included in a care conference.

1. _____

_____

2. _____

_____

3. _____

_____

4. _____

_____

5. _____

_____

Rounds

Complete the following sentences.

1. _____ are opportunities to physically monitor and discuss the status of a resident's condition or disease.

2. Nursing rounds are typically conducted in the resident's _____ for privacy.

3. _____ rounds usually occur in hospitals and are led by doctors to teach medical students, not just to monitor and discuss a particular patient's disease or condition.

4. _____ rounds are conducted by the licensed nursing staff, typically occur in a resident's room, and check on a resident's condition and any special needs.

5. Rounds are used to provide staff members with information about their assigned _____.

6. Rounds may be performed hourly or at the end of a(n) _____.

7. _____ rounds have been shown to improve safety, encourage more effective delivery of care, and improve satisfaction.

8. Frequent and consistent monitoring helps _____ harmful events, such as possible falls or the formation of decubitus ulcers due to immobility.

Reports and Assignment Sheets

Identify whether each statement is true or false.

_____ 1. The change-of-shift report is a verbal report that transfers optional information about patients or residents.

_____ 2. When a change-of-shift report is shared, nursing staff members share accurate information about resident status, and plans for future care are discussed based on reports from the outgoing nursing staff.

_____ 3. It is critical that nursing staff members share any safety concerns and information about changes in a resident's condition or disease.

_____ 4. During the change-of-shift report, nursing assistants should listen carefully, ask pertinent questions, and take notes about information related to the residents in their care.

_____ 5. Assignment sheets never include noncare assignments, such as cleaning the supply room or checking inventory.

_____ 6. Nursing assistants should review their assignment sheets with the doctor, especially if caring for unfamiliar residents.

_____ 7. The assignment sheet is used to plan one's shift and delegate time-consuming tasks.

Organizing the Assignment Sheet

With a partner, review the sample assignment sheet shown in Figure 12.4 in the text. Then, review the tasks a nursing assistant completes for residents during a typical p.m. shift. Discuss and develop your own assignment sheet to organize the tasks for a p.m. shift.

Typical Tasks During a P.M. Shift

Obtain information about residents' names, code status, VS and pain, allergies, cognitive status, assistive devices, diet, dentures, thickened liquids, I&O, elimination needs, mobility, bathing, and bed strip schedule.

(1430) Attend staff change-of-shift report, review plan of care and assignment sheet, ask questions, understand plan of care, organize plan for shift with other staff, and check supper menu.

(1500) Meet residents and always complete one procedure before starting another.

Offer H_2O q2h, if no restrictions; complete head-to-toe observation (in private); check mental status; check skin for baseline; organize self and equipment for shift; perform environmental safety check; change resident position q2h; perform nail care and ROM exercises; check VS, pain, and ht./wt.; help with coughing and deep breathing hourly; assist with toileting q2h; assist with ambulation; check rooms; set out clothing; change linens; give partial bath or shower, as indicated; clean residents' faces, hands, and clothing; freshen hairdo; place eyeglasses and hearing aids; shave prn; answer call lights; tag team with partner for short bathroom and hydration breaks.

(1630) Assist residents to meal.

(1700) Assist with meal; document I&O, when complete; assist residents back to rooms or elsewhere and place call lights.

(1800) CNA meal break.

(1830) Perform oral care; assist with toileting q2h; give bath or shower, as indicated; assist resident out to bed; perform perineal care; apply topical treatments prn; give back rub; position resident on side and float heels; measure I&O; freshen H_2O prn and prior to leaving; take all trash and laundry out of halls at shift end; pass snacks; assist other staff.

(2130) Do bed checks every half-hour (or according to plan of care) and prior to leaving any resident.

(2330) Attend change-of-shift report.

Observation

Complete the following sentences.

1. Holistic nursing assistants must be sensitive to and aware of _____ in a resident's daily routine, behavior, communication, appearance, general mood, and physical health.

2. It is a good idea to observe residents during _____ care to identify changes.

3. It is particularly important to practice _____ when the charge nurse has asked the nursing assistant to observe for specific changes, such as a change in breathing patterns or wound drainage.

4. A holistic nursing assistant who is observing a resident looks for physical changes, expressions of emotion, responses to _____, and the progression or improvement of a resident's disease or condition.

Objective and Subjective Observations

Select the *best* answer.

_____ 1. Objective observations are
A. based on facts
B. not an important responsibility of a holistic nursing assistant
C. less measurable than subjective observations
D. ideas, thoughts, or opinions

_____ 2. Subjective observations
A. are based on feelings or opinions
B. have the primary purpose of eliminating bias and personal opinions
C. are more factual than objective observations
D. are based on the senses of sight, hearing, touch, and smell

_____ 3. Which of the following is true of observation challenges?
   A. They occur when the resident is visually impaired.
   B. They occur when an observation is not reported or recorded soon after it occurs.
   C. They occur when two staff members disagree about how to observe a resident.
   D. They do not affect holistic resident care.

_____ 4. Memory is
   A. the ability to recall details of the future
   B. the storage and remembrance of past experiences
   C. always reconstructive, in that people recreate what they think they saw
   D. reliable, so documentation can occur at the end of a shift

_____ 5. Critical observation
   A. is knowing when you should hide your observations
   B. can always wait until the change-of-shift report
   C. occurs when both objective and subjective observations are used appropriately
   D. must be reported to the charge nurse immediately, even if routine

Reporting Changes

Complete the following list of changes that should be reported to the licensed nursing staff.

1. changes in the resident's ability to _____
2. changes in _____, or ability to move
3. complaints of sudden, severe _____
4. a sore or reddened area on the _____ or swelling
5. complaints of a sudden change in _____
6. complaints of pain or difficulty _____
7. abnormal _____
8. complaints of pain or difficulty _____
9. _____
10. _____
11. vital signs outside the _____
12. joint pain, tenderness, or _____
13. complaints of _____ (lack of feeling) or tingling
14. lightheadedness or _____

Steps for Reporting

Complete the following steps for reporting information to the licensed nursing staff.

1. Give the resident's _____, room number, and bed number.
2. Include the _____ of the observation or the time of the specific care given.
3. Provide _____ observations about what was seen, heard, felt, or detected through the sense of smell.
4. Provide only subjective observations communicated by the _____, such as feelings of pain.
5. Identify any anticipated or requested resident _____.

Name: _____   Date: _____

Matching Chapter 13 Key Terms

Match each definition with the key term.

A. 12-hour clock
B. 24-hour clock
C. addendum
D. amendments
E. consultations
F. electronic health record (EHR)
G. electronic medical record (EMR)
H. manually
I. payroll
J. software applications

_____ 1. a type of amendment in which an item is added to a health record to correct an error

_____ 2. a method of indicating time that splits each day into two 12-hour periods: the 12 hours from midnight to noon (called *a.m. hours*) and the 12 hours from noon to midnight (called *p.m. hours*)

_____ 3. the amount of money an organization pays its staff

_____ 4. an electronic record that includes information about a resident's entire medical history and all healthcare experiences

_____ 5. corrections to a health record

_____ 6. a method of indicating time that divides the day into 24 hours, from midnight to midnight and numbered from 0 to 24

_____ 7. meetings with a healthcare expert in which the expert gives advice or information

_____ 8. a component of an EHR that includes administrative and clinical information about a single stay in a healthcare facility

_____ 9. software programs with different uses; also called *apps*

_____ 10. by hand

Types of Records

Complete the following sentences.

1. Healthcare _____ relate directly to care or aid the organization and daily function of the healthcare facility.

2. Some records are physical forms and must be completed _____, or by hand.

3. There are two primary types of records used in healthcare facilities: records that support and document _____ and records that ensure all functions in a facility operate smoothly and efficiently.

4. Records are often digital, but manual recordkeeping may still document vital signs and fluid intake or output at the resident's _____.

5. When residents are discharged or expire, their records are sent to a(n) _____ that stores and maintains the facility's health records.

6. A holistic nursing assistant is responsible for viewing and adding careful, accurate _____ in the health record.

7. Records that support and _____ care include EHRs; EMRs; paper records; admission, transfer, and discharge records; MARs; and plans of care.

8. An electronic _____ record is a digital record that contains all of a person's health information, including medical history and healthcare experiences.

9. An EHR often includes doctors' visits, hospital stays, surgical or medical procedures, annual physical examinations, referrals, and _____ (meetings) with other doctors, social workers, or therapists.

10. The benefits of using an EHR include instant sharing across healthcare providers and facilities and _____ friendliness through elimination of the vast amounts of paper used in manual recordkeeping.

11. The universal _____ of the EHR enables more coordinated, patient-centered care; eliminates duplication; and allows a smooth transition from one healthcare facility to another.

12. An electronic _____ record is a component of an EHR that includes information about a patient's single stay in a facility.

13. An EMR contains _____ information about a patient, including age, gender, insurance coverage, and other data such as religious preference.

14. The _____ information in an EMR includes all medical and health information, such as history, diagnosis, progress, laboratory test results, and consultations with specialists.

15. EMRs track information over _____, identify due dates for screenings or checkups, provide trends in treatment progress, and help monitor the quality of care given.

16. A(n) _____, sometimes called a *paper chart*, is a physical document that includes administrative and clinical information about a patient or resident.

17. A paper record stored in one facility is more challenging to share with other healthcare providers because it is not _____.

18. Admission, transfer, and discharge records provide information needed during admission to, transfer within, and discharge from a(n) _____ facility.

19. A medication _____ record is a part of an EMR that records the drugs or medications administered by the licensed nursing staff during a stay at a healthcare facility.

20. A(n) _____ is based on a comprehensive assessment of the resident, provides guidance for delivering individualized care, and may be recorded in the EMR.

Facility Operation Records

Identify whether each statement is true or false.

_____ 1. Some records in a healthcare facility ensure the facility operates smoothly.

_____ 2. Employment forms are completed during the process of hiring and are destroyed shortly after in the Human Resources department.

_____ 3. The Human Resources department in a healthcare facility keeps records related to employment, payroll, and required health information like drug screenings and immunizations.

_____ 4. Policies and procedures provide guidance and instructions for delivering care and working in a healthcare facility.

_____ 5. Order forms are used to ensure there are sufficient supplies available in a healthcare facility at all times.

_____ 6. An order form is only completed once every year.

_____ 7. Incident reports are completed when there has been an error or accident in a healthcare facility.

The Life Span of a Record

Select the *best* answer.

_____ 1. Which of the following is *not* part of a healthcare record's life span?
   A. mitigation
   B. creation
   C. maintenance
   D. destruction

_____ 2. Which of the following is true of healthcare records?
   A. They are not legal documents.
   B. They are not regulated by laws.
   C. They are affected by the needs of ongoing medical research and education.
   D. They are never destroyed.

_____ 3. All healthcare facilities have policies and procedures regarding
   A. ways to conceal harmful information in records
   B. the retention of records that are never destroyed
   C. which record-related laws to follow
   D. the maintenance, retention, and destruction of records

Advantages of Electronic Records

Identify whether each statement is true or false.

_____ 1. Using electronic medical records reduces the chance of medical errors.

_____ 2. The Centers for Medicare & Medicaid Services (CMS) has instituted an EHR incentive program giving healthcare providers and facilities a financial incentive to adopt, implement, upgrade, or demonstrate certified EHR technology.

_____ 3. The use of EHRs makes information sharing more difficult.

_____ 4. Information documented in an EHR should concern only the resident receiving care, and confidentiality must be maintained.

_____ 5. The use of EHRs makes confidentiality more vulnerable.

Understanding Confidentiality

Select the *best* answer.

_____ 1. Confidentiality requires that healthcare providers consider any information communicated by a patient or resident to be
   A. public
   B. illegal
   C. private
   D. reported

_____ 2. Which of the following protects the rights of patients and residents regarding the confidentiality of health records?
   A. OBRA
   B. HIPAA
   C. EPA
   D. None of the above.

_____ 3. Health information is considered
     A. any paper, oral, or electronic record shared with a healthcare provider, insurer, or similar entity that can be used to identify a resident
     B. electronic records, but not paper records, that can identify a resident
     C. paper or electronic records, but not oral records, that are shared with a healthcare provider
     D. records that are shared with healthcare providers, but not with insurers

_____ 4. If healthcare providers share information inappropriately,
     A. there will be no legal consequences
     B. they will be rewarded
     C. information will no longer be considered confidential
     D. the act can be considered an invasion of privacy

_____ 5. In addition to confidentiality, HIPAA also provides
     A. the right for people to inspect, review, and receive copies of their health records
     B. the right for healthcare providers to make health information public
     C. the right for nursing assistants to disregard confidentiality
     D. freedom from legal consequences for violating confidentiality

_____ 6. Residents must complete a formal request to
     A. be entitled to confidentiality
     B. express a desire for confidentiality
     C. receive records physically, but not electronically
     D. review records and receive them physically or electronically

Maintaining Confidentiality

Complete the following guidelines for maintaining confidentiality.

1. Maintain _____ and confidentiality at all times.
2. Never take (a)n _____ or video of residents or their families using a personal device.
3. Do not _____ residents by name outside the unit and facility.
4. Do not post information _____ that may lead to resident identification.
5. Do not _____ records out of curiosity.
6. _____ of a computer once you are done using it.
7. Choose a strong _____ and do not share it with others.
8. Promptly _____ any identified breaches of confidentiality or privacy.

_____ 9. Abide by the facility's _____ regarding the use of employer-owned electronic devices and personal devices in the workplace.
_____ 10. Remember that any _____ of confidentiality and privacy is grounds for discipline.

Technology in Healthcare Facilities

Select the *best* answer.

_____ 1. Digital communication and devices
     A. are used by the licensed nursing staff, but not by nursing assistants
     B. include cell phones, landline telephones, desktop computers, laptop computers, and wireless devices such as tablets
     C. use technology that slows the process of resident care
     D. have completely replaced paper records and documentation in healthcare facilities

_____ 2. Computers on wheels are
     A. cow-shaped desks on wheels
     B. wheeled into a resident's room and used to input or complete necessary documentation
     C. carried by nursing assistants along with a wireless device
     D. used only to record vital signs

_____ 3. In healthcare facilities,
     A. urgent needs and information are only communicated using e-mail
     B. pagers are used for information unrelated to resident care
     C. e-mail might be used to communicate announcements, scheduling, or meeting invitations and reminders
     D. devices and digital communication methods are only used if the healthcare facility is a doctor's office

_____ 4. Software applications (apps)
     A. are used by healthcare staff members, residents, and nursing assistants to diagnose illnesses
     B. do not offer information regarding coding for insurance or prescription refills
     C. are never secure, so healthcare providers cannot share protected information with other providers
     D. offer information about diseases, drug and nutrition references, ranges of laboratory values, clinical research, and healthcare training

_____ 5. Apps that store or share protected health information
     A. must be HIPAA-compliant for information security
     B. cannot be accessed through secure, HIPAA-compliant websites called online portals
     C. can be accessed by a resident's family without the resident's permission
     D. are used only for medical purposes, not for tracking diets, daily exercise, or blood pressure

Telephone Communication

Complete the following sentences.

1. Telephones in healthcare facilities are more than just devices; they provide a way to share and gather _____.

2. _____ the telephone is an important part of a holistic nursing assistant's daily responsibilities.

3. Appropriately _____ and sharing information over the telephone contributes to the delivery of safe, quality care.

4. The same _____ requirements and confidentiality that affect face-to-face and written communication also affect information shared over the telephone.

5. If important information is shared over the telephone, the nursing assistant should write this information down and verify by _____ the information back to the caller.

6. If the information shared is outside the nursing assistant's legal _____, the nursing assistant should let the caller know and seek a member of the licensed nursing staff.

7. The nursing assistant may ask the caller to wait, but if that is not possible, should take the caller's _____ so the appropriate person can follow up on the call.

8. Examples of calls that are outside the scope of practice include conveying doctors' orders, receiving or giving _____, or releasing any resident information.

9. Nursing assistants should treat each telephone call as a vital part of _____.

10. When answering telephone calls, nursing assistants should always remember to follow facility _____.

Using the Telephone

With a partner, review the nine principles for proper nursing assistant telephone communication found in the text. Then, apart from your partner, write a fictional scenario involving a resident calling a nursing assistant on the telephone. Call your partner on the telephone and act out your scenario. When your partner calls you, practice following the nine principles of proper telephone communication during the call.

Documentation

Complete the following sentences.

1. The purpose of _____ is to provide a timely, ongoing record of care that includes accurate, concise information about the care provided.

2. Doctors, licensed nursing staff members, and other healthcare providers use documented information to make determinations regarding a resident's _____, progress, necessary changes in treatment, medications, and care.

3. In documentation, the primary responsibility of nursing assistants is to enter information into resident _____ and complete forms with specific information according to scope of practice.

4. Nursing assistants sometimes fill out facility forms, such as order forms or _____ reports, which document accidents.

5. Successful nursing assistants follow documentation guidelines and remember that the health record is a(n) _____ document.

6. The nursing assistant should never document something if it was not _____.

7. Nursing assistants should never document for _____, even if members of the licensed nursing staff ask.

8. Nursing assistants observe for physical changes, expressions of emotions, responses to treatment, or the _____ of a resident's disease or condition.

9. Information observed may be either _____ (based on facts) or subjective (based on feelings or opinions).

10. If care was not provided as assigned, the nursing assistant should document this and _____ why these changes were made.

11. Care that was not completed should be _____ to the licensed nursing staff.

12. Nursing assistants often document using _____ that indicate vital signs, food eaten, or the intake and output of fluids.

13. Facilities that use paper records typically use blue or black _____ to document care.

14. Successful nursing assistants write legibly on every line without skipping lines and draw a(n) _____ through any blank spaces so that additional information cannot be written on the record by someone else.

15. After documenting care, nursing assistants sign their full _____ and title.

16. Before writing new notes, nursing assistants should read _____ notes to ensure continuity of care.

17. The _____ clock splits each day into two 12-hour periods: the 12 hours from midnight to noon (called *a.m. hours*) and the 12 hours from noon to midnight (called *p.m. hours*).

18. The _____ clock divides the day into 24 hours, from midnight to midnight, numbered from 0 to 24.

19. In the 24-hour clock, noon would be 1200, and midnight would be _____.

20. Nursing assistants should use _____ marks to document subjective resident comments and should use simple, descriptive terms.

The 24-Hour Clock

Apply the appropriate labels to the image.

A. 0900/2100
B. 2400/1200
C. 0600/1800
D. 0300/1500
E. 1000/2200
F. 0700/1900
G. 0100/1300
H. 1100/2300
I. 0800/2000
J. 0500/1700
K. 0200/1400
L. 0400/1600

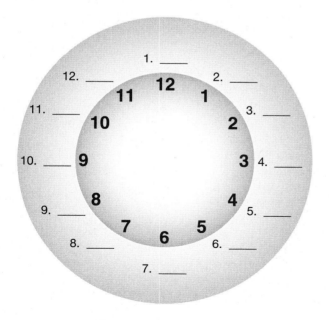

Correcting Errors

Identify whether each statement is true or false.

_____ 1. If errors occur during documentation, they must be corrected weekly.

_____ 2. The only person who can change, or amend, a record is the person who wrote the original entry.

_____ 3. Documentation corrections are legally called *commandments*.

_____ 4. Nursing assistants should always check facility guidelines for amending a health record.

_____ 5. If a documentation error is found, one should consult the person who entered the incorrect information and encourage him or her to amend the problem.

_____ 6. To correct a paper record, one should erase or use correction liquid or tape on the incorrect information, record the correct information, and initial or sign and date the correction.

_____ 7. To correct an electronic record, one should add an addendum that provides the corrected information without deleting the original information or rewriting it.

_____ 8. If information was forgotten during documentation, one should add a late entry with the missing information and details.

_____ 9. Once a correction or missing information is entered, it must be authenticated with a digital or manual signature that includes the date, time, and the person's full name and title.

_____ 10. Health records are not legal documents and do not need to be stored and accessible at all times.

Name: _____ Date: _____

Matching Chapter 14 Key Terms

Match each definition with the key term.

A. aerobic
B. anaerobic
C. antigens
D. antiseptics
E. autopsies
F. bacteria
G. bloodborne pathogens
H. chlorophyll
I. communicable diseases
J. culture
K. disinfectants
L. dormant
M. infection
N. lubricants
O. microorganisms
P. mucus
Q. noncommunicable diseases
R. phagocytosis
S. phenol
T. photosynthesis
U. saliva
V. toxins

_____ 1. an acid that can be used as a disinfectant in dilute form

_____ 2. needing oxygen to live

_____ 3. having slowed or stopped functions

_____ 4. substances foreign to the body that trigger the production of antibodies as part of the immune response

_____ 5. the process by which plants and other organisms convert light energy from the sun into chemical energy; allows the plant or organism to function

_____ 6. examinations conducted to determine cause of death

_____ 7. the process of cultivating living tissue cells in a substance favorable to their growth

_____ 8. a watery mixture found in the mouth that contains enzymes; lubricates the mouth and breaks down food

_____ 9. infectious microorganisms in the blood that can cause disease

_____ 10. diseases that are not contagious and cannot be transmitted by contact

_____ 11. able to live without oxygen

_____ 12. the invasion and growth of harmful, microscopic organisms in the body; leads to disease

_____ 13. a green substance found in plants that absorbs light and transfers it through the plant during photosynthesis

_____ 14. poisons

_____ 15. diseases that can be transmitted from one person, object, or animal to another; also called *contagious diseases*

_____ 16. fluids or substances that prevent the growth of microorganisms on the body

_____ 17. natural substances that reduce friction between surfaces

_____ 18. single-celled, microscopic organisms that can cause infection

_____ 19. living things, or organisms, that are so small they can only be seen through a microscope

_____ 20. a thick, slippery fluid that moistens and protects parts of the body

_____ 21. chemicals used to destroy or slow the growth of microorganisms to prevent them from spreading

_____ 22. the process by which a white blood cell engulfs and destroys foreign antigens

Body Defenses and Immunity

Complete the following sentences.

1. The body has biological armor that protects it from _____ (invasion by harmful, microscopic organisms) and disease.

2. The body's physical and chemical barriers that prevent disease-causing _____ from entering form the body's first line of defense.

3. The body is protected by a second, cellular line of defense called the _____ response.

4. The immune response describes the body's internal reaction to _____, which are disease-causing microorganisms.

5. _____ (redness and swelling), coughing, and sneezing help rid the body of infection or disease.

6. The _____ is the greatest first line of defense because it creates a physical barrier between the inner structures of the human body and the outside world.

7. The skin is only able to protect the body when it is healthy and _____.

8. Natural _____ secreted by the skin reduce friction and contain substances that prevent the growth of pathogens.

9. When the skin is cut, _____ are released to kill bacteria that may try to enter the body.

10. The nasal passages of the respiratory system are lined with mucous membranes that contain _____, a thick, slippery fluid that moistens and protects parts of the body.

11. Mucous membranes in the nasal passages contain tiny hairs called _____, which trap microorganisms that may cause infection or disease.

12. The eyes produce _____, which contain water, salt, antibodies, and enzymes that cleanse, lubricate, and stop bacterial growth on the eye's surface.

13. The _____ form a physical barrier that keeps foreign particles such as dust and dirt away from the eye.

14. The mouth secretes _____, a watery fluid that blocks the growth of pathogens.

15. The gastrointestinal (GI) tract is lined with _____ membranes that trap microorganisms.

16. The GI tract contains beneficial bacteria called *normal* _____ that change the chemical composition of the GI environment to prevent the growth of harmful bacteria.

17. _____ acid inside the stomach destroys potentially harmful microorganisms that may be found in ingested food.

18. The vagina is lined with mucous membranes and has a(n) _____ environment that helps prevent the growth of pathogens.

19. The _____ rinses pathogens out of the urinary tract and has mucous membranes for protection.

20. In the immune _____, the body distinguishes between its own tissues and cells and outside or foreign substances.

21. Foreign substances are known as antigens and may include _____ (poisons).

22. Cells with foreign antigens and toxins are identified by blood proteins called _____ as part of the immune response.

23. White blood cells engulf and destroy antigens through a process called _____.

24. Each time a new antigen enters the body, a new set of antibodies unique to that antigen develops, often causing permanent _____ to the disease.

25. Immunity can be acquired through _____, in which a mixture containing a very mild form of a disease triggers the body to build antibodies against the disease.

Phagocytosis

Apply the appropriate callouts to the image.

A. Enzymes start to destroy antigen
B. Antigen
C. Indigestible fragments are discharged
D. White blood cell engulfing antigen (bacteria, dead cells)
E. Antigen breaks down into small fragments

1. ____

2. ____

3. ____

4. ____

5. ____

© *Body Scientific International*

Vaccines

Identify whether each statement is true or false.

_____ 1. Vaccines are used to cure diseases.

_____ 2. Vaccines are developed in response to disease epidemics that can be fatal or cause disabilities (for example, smallpox, polio, measles, and whooping cough).

_____ 3. Some vaccinations require subsequent doses, called *boosters*.

_____ 4. When a person visits another country, he or she has not been exposed to the common diseases of that area and may require vaccination.

_____ 5. Vaccinations for travel to the United States include typhoid or yellow fever.

_____ 6. Annual vaccinations are available for diseases such as influenza or pneumonia.

_____ 7. Most vaccinations are given by injection, though some are given orally (such as those for polio or rotavirus) or through the nose.

_____ 8. In the United States, the Centers for Disease Control and Prevention (CDC) provides an immunization schedule for children ages 0–18 that includes vaccinations for varicella, inactivated poliovirus, measles, mumps, and rubella.

_____ 9. The CDC provides a schedule for adult vaccinations that includes diseases such as human papillomavirus (HPV) and Ebola.

_____ 10. Vaccinating a large majority of the population against a disease helps control the spread of disease by creating a type of mass immunity called *community unity*.

_____ 11. In the United States, vaccinations are typically required for school-age children, though some states make exceptions for parents who object for religious or other reasons.

_____ 12. Vaccinations are not required for people who work in healthcare.

The Inflammatory Response

Complete the following sentences.

1. The _____ response is characterized by redness and swelling in response to irritation, injury, or infection.

2. In the inflammatory response, body tissues secrete chemicals that cause blood vessels around the damaged area to _____.

3. Inflammation can make the affected area warm to the touch and cause a person to run a(n) _____, which destroys antigens or toxins.

4. The inflammatory response signals _____ blood cells and other cells to travel to the injured area of the body and attack toxins.

5. Often found at the site of injury, _____ contains tissue, dead antigens, and white blood cells.

6. Often, pressure from _____ and the increased body heat associated with inflammation cause pain.

Infection Risk

Identify whether each statement is true or false.

_____ 1. Infants and young children have overdeveloped immune systems, causing them and older adults to have more resistance to infection.

_____ 2. People in poor health have unlimited resistance to colds and the flu and often experience less severe symptoms than the general public.

_____ 3. People with autoimmune disorders or human immunodeficiency virus (HIV) often experience chronic conditions that lower immunity.

_____ 4. People who have been hospitalized, have been in a healthcare facility for a long time, have an artificial joint, or are on kidney dialysis are at increased risk for infection.

_____ 5. Residents in long-term care facilities are less susceptible to infection, particularly if they have urinary catheters or continuous central line intravenous (IV) catheters.

_____ 6. Urinary catheters and IV catheters increase risk for infection because they are foreign objects placed inside the body.

_____ 7. Increased susceptibility to infection is a major problem in healthcare facilities.

_____ 8. Infections acquired within healthcare facilities are called *healthcare-associated infections (HAIs)*.

Microorganisms and Pathogens

Select the *best* answer.

_____ 1. Microorganisms, also called *microbes*,
A. are large organisms that live around and within a person
B. are so small they are only visible through binoculars
C. can be found in the air, water, and soil and on plants, animals, and people
D. are useful and do not cause disease

_____ 2. Normal flora
A. live in the gastrointestinal tract and help with digestion
B. never cause problems when they travel to new locations
C. cannot move away from their places of origin
D. are disease-causing organisms

_____ 3. What are pathogens?
A. a punishment for evil
B. an imbalance of internal forces in the body
C. new treatments discovered by notable doctors and scientists
D. disease-causing microorganisms

_____ 4. Which of the following is true of disinfectants?
A. They were consumed during the 1800s by the French.
B. They eliminate offensive odors, but do not affect the growth of microorganisms.
C. They are chemicals used to destroy or slow the growth of microorganisms.
D. They are the same as antiseptics.

_____ 5. Hungarian doctor Ignaz Semmelweis
A. noticed a high mortality rate among men following childbirth in a hospital
B. noticed that women who gave birth in a hospital were treated by doctors
C. completed autopsies on women prior to childbirth
D. hypothesized that doctors were carrying pathogens on their hands and suggested hand washing as a solution

_____ 6. An English doctor, John Snow,
A. proved that microorganisms did not cause disease
B. traced a cholera epidemic in London to contaminated water
C. worsened a cholera epidemic by closing the water supply
D. caused a cholera epidemic in London by contaminating the water

_____ 7. French chemist Louis Pasteur
A. discovered that heating beer and wine to a certain temperature killed bacteria
B. caused liquids to spoil to create beer
C. used pasteurization to liquefy foods
D. was a microbiologist who studied the effects of pasteurization on animals

_____ 8. German doctor Robert Koch
    A. spread disease through infected animals
    B. showed that the bacterium *Bacillus anthracis* was unrelated to anthrax in cattle and sheep
    C. was infected by an agent isolated from an infected animal
    D. influenced the discovery of *Staphylococcus*, *Streptococcus*, and the microorganisms that cause cholera, typhoid fever, diphtheria, pneumonia, tetanus, meningitis, and gonorrhea

_____ 9. English doctor Joseph Lister
    A. applied discoveries about microorganisms to spread infection throughout England
    B. spread disease in his work during surgery
    C. soaked surgical bandages in phenol to prevent postoperative infections
    D. listed the types of organisms that caused phenol

_____ 10. Which of the following is true of germ theory?
    A. It holds that many diseases are caused by macroorganisms.
    B. It was made possible by the development of the microscope.
    C. It involves seeing tiny microorganisms visible to the naked eye.
    D. It is unrelated to epidemiology.

Bacteria

Complete the following sentences.

1. There are four types of microorganisms: _____, viruses, fungi, and parasites.

2. _____ are single-celled microorganisms that are often harmless, but can also cause infections in any part of the body.

3. Bacteria may be *aerobic* (needing oxygen) or _____ (not needing oxygen) and can only be seen under a microscope.

4. Bacteria are classified and named according to their sizes and _____.

5. There are three basic shapes of bacteria: _____ bacteria (*cocci*), rod-shaped bacteria (*bacilli*), and spiral bacteria.

6. _____ bacteria may be shaped like a comma (*vibrios*); may be shaped like a rigid corkscrew (*spirilla*); or may be long, thin, and flexible (*spirochetes*).

7. Bacteria group together and form _____.

8. Most bacteria that cause disease grow in a warm, dark, and moist environment and require _____ such as oxygen.

9. Bacteria can enter the body through the _____, nose, mouth, eyes, ears, lungs, urethra, and vagina.

10. Once bacteria gain entry, they _____ quickly, causing infection, destroying tissues and cells, and overwhelming the body.

Shapes of Bacteria

Apply the appropriate callouts to the image.

1. _____
2. _____
3. _____
4. _____
5. _____

Designua/Shutterstock.com

Bacterial Infections

Identify whether each statement is true or false.

_____ 1. Bacteria are the most common cause of infection in the body.

_____ 2. The type of bacterial infection does not change depending on the type of bacteria and location in the body.

_____ 3. Tuberculosis (TB) is caused by the bacterium *Mycobacterium tuberculosis* and is spread only through blood, semen, and vaginal secretions.

_____ 4. TB primarily attacks the lungs, but can also damage the kidneys, spine, and brain.

_____ 5. Risk factors for TB include a weakened immune system and travel to areas where TB is prevalent.

_____ 6. In latent TB, noncontagious bacteria are in the body, but no symptoms are present.

_____ 7. Latent TB is different from and cannot become active TB.

_____ 8. Patients with TB take antiviral medications for at least six to nine months and must take all of the medication prescribed.

_____ 9. Active TB is not contagious, so infection control precautions are not necessary.

_____ 10. Bacterial pneumonia is usually caused by *Streptococcus pneumoniae* and is an infection of the lungs that causes inflammation and fluid buildup.

_____ 11. Risk factors for bacterial pneumonia include an age under 65, asthma, a good diet, and abstinence from alcohol.

_____ 12. Common symptoms for bacterial pneumonia are high fever; chills; sweating; greenish, yellow, or bloody mucus; dyspnea; sharp, stabbing pain in the lungs; fatigue; loss of appetite; cyanosis in the lips and fingernails; and confusion.

_____ 13. Regular hand hygiene, good nutrition, exercise, sufficient sleep, isolation from those who are sick, and vaccines can help prevent pneumonia.

_____ 14. Effective treatments for pneumonia include antibiotics, medications for fever and pain, vigorous exercise, abstinence from fluids, and a dehumidifier to loosen mucus.

_____ 15. Acute appendicitis, diphtheria, conjunctivitis, tetanus, rheumatic fever, syphilis, pertussis, and Lyme disease are all examples of viral infections.

_____ 16. Antibiotics are the most common treatment for bacterial infections and are only available orally.

_____ 17. Penicillin, one of the first antibiotics, is no longer used to treat bacterial infections.

_____ 18. Antibiotic resistance develops when bacteria change to resist the effects of an antibiotic.

_____ 19. Bacteria that are resistant to more than one antibiotic are called *multidrug-resistant organisms (MDROs)*.

_____ 20. Examples of MDROs are methicillin-resistant *Staphylococcus aureus* (MRSA) and vancomycin-intermediate or vancomycin-resistant *Enterococcus* (VRE)

_____ 21. When a person has an infection that is antibiotic resistant, recovery time is typically very fast.

_____ 22. Good hygiene, cleanliness, and the cautious use of antibiotics can help prevent antibiotic resistance.

Viruses

Complete the following sentences.

1. _____ are small bundles of protein that cannot grow or multiply by themselves and take over host cells that are usually plant or animal cells.

2. After taking over a(n) _____ cell, a virus injects genetic material into the host and takes possession of its functions.

3. Host cells, once infected with a virus, reproduce the viral protein and _____ material, causing the virus to spread.

4. Some viruses spread through the _____ route, through water or food contaminated with feces.

5. Viral infections cannot be treated with antibiotics, but are treated with _____ prescription medications.

6. Rather than destroying a virus, antiviral medications _____ virus development.

7. _____ exist for viral pneumonia, the flu, polio, measles, mumps, rubella, and smallpox.

8. The common cold and influenza are separate viral infections that affect the _____ system and are contagious.

9. People over the age of _____, people with chronic medical conditions, pregnant women, and young children are at greatest risk for contracting the flu.

10. Symptoms of the _____ include fever, chills, cough, sore throat, runny or stuffy nose, muscle or body aches, headache, and fatigue.

11. Antiviral medications can lessen symptoms, shorten the time a person is sick, and prevent serious flu complications if taken within _____ day(s) of getting the flu.

12. Infection control precautions, rest, and increased _____ are important for recovery from the flu.

13. Other examples of _____ infections are chickenpox, measles, hepatitis, mononucleosis (mono), polio, rabies, shingles, HIV, and Ebola.

Fungi and Parasites

Identify whether each statement is true or false.

_____ 1. A fungus is an organism that lacks *chlorophyll*, a substance found in plants that absorbs and transfers light.

_____ 2. Fungi reproduce through spores, which are single-celled units capable of reproducing on their own.

_____ 3. Since they are capable of photosynthesis, fungi must digest food to live.

_____ 4. Types of fungi include mushrooms, molds, yeasts, and parasitic fungi.

_____ 5. A yeast infection occurs when the amount of yeast in the body becomes imbalanced, when people take antibiotics over a long period, or when bacteria that naturally keep yeast from growing become too suppressed.

_____ 6. Opportunistic fungi take advantage of opportunities to cause infection (for example, a weak immune system caused by HIV/AIDS).

_____ 7. Fungal infections cannot be treated using over-the-counter or prescription creams, ointments, or medications.

_____ 8. Examples of fungal infections include thrush, athlete's foot, vaginal yeast infections, ringworm, fungal eye infections, and pneumocystis pneumonia.

_____ 9. Parasites are organisms that live on or in hosts.

_____ 10. All parasites make the host organism sick.

_____ 11. Parasitic infections can be caused by three types of organisms: protozoa, helminths, and ectoparasites.

_____ 12. Protozoa like the *Plasmodium* parasite, which causes malaria, cannot live in drinking water.

_____ 13. Helminths, including tapeworms, ringworms, and hookworms, commonly live in the brain.

_____ 14. Ectoparasites like fleas and ticks live in or feed from human intestines.

_____ 15. Parasites can be spread through contaminated water, waste, fecal matter, blood, sexual contact, and mishandled or undercooked food.

_____ 16. Some parasitic infections are spread by insects, which carry the disease and transmit it while feeding off the host.

_____ 17. Lice are spread through direct contact, but not through contact with combs, brushes, hats, and other clothing.

_____ 18. Antibiotics and other medications such as lotions or creams can be helpful for treating some parasitic infections.

_____ 19. Treatment of a parasitic infection never includes removal of the infestation.

_____ 20. Examples of parasitic infections include bed bug bites, pinworm, foodborne diseases, head and body lice, malaria, and trichinosis.

How Infections Are Categorized

Select the *best* answer.

_____ 1. Local infections
  A. are confined to multiple areas of the body
  B. do not include boils
  C. include signs and symptoms of fever, redness, heat, pain, swelling, and pus or discharge that may be foul smelling
  D. are categorized as systemic

_____ 2. Which of the following is true of a systemic infection?
  A. It is widespread and travels throughout the body via the bloodstream.
  B. One example would be a boil.
  C. It has signs and symptoms of redness, heat, pain, swelling, and pus at the site.
  D. It always develops during a stay in a hospital.

_____ 3. Opportunistic infections (OIs)
  A. only develop under the circumstances of a strong immune system
  B. may develop when a person's immune system has been weakened by another infection
  C. do not infect the body
  D. create a second infection that fights the original infection

_____ 4. Healthcare-associated infections (HAIs)
  A. do not include central line-associated bloodstream infections (CLABSIs)
  B. are always acquired from catheters
  C. are unrelated to ventilator-associated pneumonia (VAP) and surgical site infections (SSTs)
  D. are acquired in a hospital or other healthcare facility

_____ 5. *Clostridium difficile* or *C. difficile*
  A. is an HAI that is only acquired by older adults and people with healthy immune systems
  B. is not related to the prolonged use of antibiotics
  C. develops when bacteria are transmitted by items contaminated with infected feces
  D. must be followed to prevent regulations

The Chain of Infection

Apply the appropriate labels to the image.

Chain of Infection

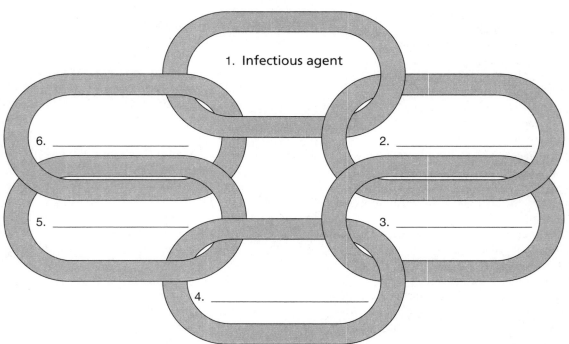

1. Infectious agent

6. _____

2. _____

5. _____

3. _____

4. _____

Name: _____ Date: _____

Disease Transmission

Complete the following sentences.

1. Diseases and infections are categorized by how they are _____, or spread.

2. Diseases that cannot be transmitted between people, objects, and animals are noncommunicable, or not _____.

3. Examples of _____ diseases include genetic diseases, cancers, mental disorders, autoimmune diseases, and heart disease.

4. _____ diseases are contagious and can be transmitted between people, objects, and animals.

5. Communicable diseases can spread through airborne transmission, contact transmission, vehicle or vector transmission, and bloodborne _____.

6. Communicable diseases can develop opportunistically or due to the reactivation of a(n) _____, or latent, organism with slowed or stopped functions.

7. _____, or droplet, transmission occurs when microscopic pathogens become suspended and move in the air or become trapped in dust.

8. If airborne pathogens are _____ by a host, they can cause illness.

9. Airborne _____ can occur when someone who is ill coughs, sneezes, talks, laughs, sings, or spits.

10. _____ transmission occurs when an infectious agent or reservoir housing a pathogen is exposed to a host through touch, sexual contact, blood, or body fluids.

11. In contact transmission, contact can be _____ through contaminated items such as soiled linen, clothing, a dressing soaked with drainage, or used specimen containers.

12. _____ transmission occurs when an infectious agent is ingested via contaminated food or water.

13. _____ transmission occurs when an infection is introduced into the skin or mucous membranes through an animal or insect bite.

14. Bloodborne pathogens are disease-causing microorganisms found in an infected person's _____.

15. Examples of bloodborne pathogens are hepatitis B virus (HBV), hepatitis C virus (HCV), and human _____ virus (HIV).

16. Bloodborne pathogens can be transmitted through exposure to human blood and other infectious body fluids, sharps-related injuries and _____ (punctures of the skin), and other injuries that break the skin.

Identification of an Infection

Identify whether each statement is true or false.

_____ 1. A person who suspects he or she has an infection should seek medical attention from a nursing assistant.

_____ 2. Observing related signs and symptoms can lead to the identification of an infection.

_____ 3. Infections cannot be identified using laboratory blood tests or X-rays.

_____ 4. A common blood test to identify infection is a white blood cell count because the body releases increased numbers of white blood cells into the bloodstream to fight the infection.

_____ 5. Blood or fungi cultures can help determine the type of microorganism causing the infection and the type of treatment.

_____ 6. A patient with an infection may be put into an isolation room to prevent the spread of infection until the results of a blood culture are available.

_____ 7. Urinary tract infections (UTIs) are tested using urine samples and cultures.

_____ 8. A doctor will often order an X-ray of the intestines and a fecal test to diagnose pneumonia.

_____ 9. The Mantoux tuberculin skin test (TST) is a lung function test used to identify TB.

_____ 10. In the Mantoux tuberculin skin test (TST), skin will react to the TB antigens if the person has TB.

CHAPTER 15 Infection Prevention and Control

Name: _____ Date: _____

Matching Chapter 15 Key Terms

Match each definition with the key term.

A. alcohol-based hand sanitizer
B. asepsis
C. contusions
D. dressing
E. excretions
F. exudate
G. friction
H. frostbite
I. isolation
J. lacerations
K. nonpenetrating wounds
L. penetrating wounds
M. personal protective equipment (PPE)
N. secretions
O. sharps
P. sterile
Q. sterile field
R. World Health Organization (WHO)
S. wound

_____ 1. free of living microorganisms
_____ 2. a protective material placed on a wound; sometimes called a *bandage*
_____ 3. a condition in which extreme cold temperatures cause freezing and damage to body tissues, such as the skin on the fingers, toes, nose, ears, cheeks, and chin
_____ 4. an area that is free from living pathogenic microorganisms
_____ 5. specialized clothing and accessories, such as gloves, gowns, masks, goggles, and other pieces of equipment, that are worn to protect against infection or injury
_____ 6. waste products expelled from the body
_____ 7. wounds that do not enter into or through the skin; are caused by rubbing or friction on the surface of the skin
_____ 8. the absence of infection or infectious material; also called *sterility*
_____ 9. a liquid that drains from a wound; is caused by tissue damage
_____ 10. the resistance between two objects or surfaces rubbing against each other
_____ 11. specific preventive measures that are used to limit or eliminate the spread of microorganisms from an infected person to others
_____ 12. an agency of the United Nations that focuses on international public health

_____ 13. a liquid, gel, or foam preparation containing alcohol; kills most bacteria and fungi and destroys some viruses found on the skin
_____ 14. wounds that tear body tissue and result in ragged edges
_____ 15. wounds that enter into or through the skin
_____ 16. an injury to body tissue that can be caused by a cut, blow, or other force; may be penetrating or nonpenetrating
_____ 17. substances produced and released by cells or organs
_____ 18. bruises caused by damaged or broken blood vessels; may cause swelling
_____ 19. objects such as needles, razors, broken glass, and scalpels that can penetrate the skin

Understanding Asepsis

Complete the following sentences.

1. Nursing assistants prevent infection by helping ensure _____, which is the absence of infections or infectious material.
2. Items that have come in contact with potential pathogens are considered _____, and items that have not been exposed to potential pathogens are considered *clean*.
3. Nursing assistants should touch _____ body parts or surfaces before touching those that are dirty or contaminated.
4. A nursing assistant must not touch his or her face, nose, or eyeglasses before touching a(n) _____.
5. Asepsis guidelines prevent touch _____, or the transfer of potential pathogens from a dirty to a clean surface or object.
6. Of the two types of asepsis, _____ asepsis is a clean technique used to reduce the number of microorganisms to control infection.
7. Medical asepsis procedures include hand hygiene, the use of personal protective _____, and isolation.
8. PPE includes specialized _____ and accessories such as gloves, gowns, masks, and goggles that protect against infection or injury.
9. The second type of asepsis, _____ asepsis, is a sterile technique used to completely eliminate microorganisms from the surface of an object.

Standard Precautions

Select the *best* answer.

_____ 1. Basic infection prevention and control practices used to prevent the spread of disease and deliver safe, quality care are called
A. transmission-based precautions
B. specific precautions
C. standard precautions
D. infection precautions

_____ 2. Practices that supplement standard precautions to prevent the spread of disease via direct contact with pathogens, droplets, and airborne pathogens are called
A. transmission-based precautions
B. droplet precautions
C. standard precautions
D. nonspecific precautions

_____ 3. In the United States, which organization guides standard and transmission-based precaution measures?
A. Environmental Protection Agency (EPA)
B. American Hospital Association (AHA)
C. American Academy of Pediatrics (AAP)
D. Centers for Disease Control and Prevention (CDC)

_____ 4. Which of the following is true of standard precautions?
A. They protect staff, patients, residents, family members, and visitors.
B. They only protect against bloodborne pathogens.
C. They do not protect against diseases spread through bodily fluids.
D. They protect the healthcare staff, but not visitors to a healthcare facility.

_____ 5. Standard precautions include
A. hand hygiene and recommendations against using PPE
B. cough etiquette, which involves coughing into one's hands
C. safe injection practices and the safe handling of sharps
D. lack of concern for potentially contaminated equipment and surfaces

_____ 6. Standard precautions should be used
A. on a case-by-case basis
B. appropriately and consistently with every patient or resident
C. only when there is enough time
D. only when there is an outbreak of a disease

Hand Hygiene

Identify whether each statement is true or false.

_____ 1. The role of hand washing in preventing the spread of infection was discovered in the nineteenth century and continues to be a critical infection control practice today.

_____ 2. Hand hygiene refers to hand washing, but does not include using alcohol-based hand sanitizer.

_____ 3. The CDC and the WHO are leaders in setting hand hygiene guidelines.

_____ 4. The WHO is an agency that focuses on public health administration in the United States.

_____ 5. Microorganisms can survive 30–180 seconds on the hands.

_____ 6. Hand hygiene should only be practiced when the hands are visibly soiled.

_____ 7. It is important to create friction when using alcohol-based hand sanitizers.

_____ 8. Wearing gloves is not a substitute for proper hand hygiene.

_____ 9. Effective hand hygiene is essential to infection prevention and control.

Hand Washing

Standard precautions require routine and proper hand washing to remove and prevent the spread of microorganisms. The following steps are part of the procedure for hand washing. For each set of steps, identify the proper order in which they should be completed by numbering them 1 through 7.

1. _____ Remove your hands from the water stream and apply soap. Work the soap into a thick lather over your hands, wrists, and the skin at least 1–2 inches above your wrists.

_____ Rub your palms together in a circular, counter-clockwise motion.

_____ Thoroughly wet your hands, wrists, and the skin 1–2 inches above your wrists.

_____ If your sleeves are long, use a clean, dry paper towel to push them up your arms.

_____ Locate a sink and supplies near the place care will be given.

_____ Using a clean, dry paper towel, turn on the faucet. Do not turn on the faucet with bare hands. Adjust the water temperature until warm and do not splash water on your scrubs.

_____ Remove or push up any watches with a clean paper towel. Remove rings or lather soap underneath them.

2. _____ Bend your fingers and interlock them and then rub from side to side. Clean under your fingernails by rubbing them against the other palm and forcing soap underneath them. Continue rubbing to clean around the tops of the nails. Reverse hands and repeat this step.

_____ Hold the fingers of the right hand together and place them in the middle of the left palm. Rub in a circular, counterclockwise motion.

_____ Push the fingers of the right hand between the fingers of the left hand and rub up and down.

_____ Hold the right thumb in the palm of the left hand. Rub in a circular, counterclockwise motion.

_____ With fingers interlaced, rub the palms together from side to side.

_____ Hold the left thumb in the palm of the right hand. Rub in a circular, counterclockwise motion.

_____ Push the fingers of the left hand between the fingers of the right hand and rub up and down.

3. _____ Discard the paper towel used to turn off the sink faucet into the waste container.

_____ Use a clean, dry paper towel to turn off the sink faucet. Your bare hand should not touch the sink faucet.

_____ Using a clean, dry paper towel, dry your hands and then your wrists, moving from the clean hand up toward the dirtier forearm.

_____ Drop the used paper towel into the waste container. If another paper towel is needed, use the same procedure. Never touch the waste container.

_____ Hold your hands under the running water with fingers pointing downward. Rinse your wrists and hands thoroughly.

_____ Wash your hands for a minimum of 20 seconds.

_____ Hold the fingers of the left hand together and place them in the middle of the right palm. Rub in a circular, counterclockwise motion.

Personal Protective Equipment (PPE)

Complete the following sentences.

1. Personal _____ equipment (PPE) is specialized clothing and accessories that protect the wearer from exposure to infectious materials.

2. PPE creates barriers that prevent microorganisms from making contact with the wearer's skin or _____ membranes.

3. PPE protects patients with compromised _____ systems from caregivers.

4. To be effective, PPE must be _____, or put on, and taken off according to procedure.

5. PPE includes gloves, gowns, masks, respirators, goggles, face shields, and in some cases, head covers and protective gear for the _____ (such as booties).

6. Gloves must be worn for touching blood, bodily fluids, mucous membranes, and _____, which are substances produced by cells or organs.

7. A nursing assistant should wear _____ if a resident has open or seeping sores or rashes, when handling soiled linens, and if the caregiver has scrapes, scratches, or chapped skin.

8. If a nonsterile _____ needs to be changed, nonsterile, disposable gloves are worn.

9. _____ gloves are completely free of living microorganisms and are worn for sterile procedures.

10. Some nursing assistants may need to use _____ gloves and other types of nonallergenic gloves.

11. _____ are required for completing certain procedures, particularly those that involve contact with blood, bodily fluids, secretions, and excretions.

12. Gowns are required for care given in a(n) _____ room to protect the skin and clothing from contamination.

13. A gown should be selected based on its resistance to _____ and may be disposable or reusable after proper cleaning.

14. _____ gowns are used when caring for residents in isolation, and sterile gowns may be necessary during an invasive procedure.

15. _____ protection is required if splashes or sprays of blood, bodily fluids, or secretions are anticipated or if a resident is in an isolation room.

16. _____ are the most reliable and practical eye protection against splashes, sprays, and respiratory droplets.

17. A(n) _____ protects the face from the chin to the forehead and sometimes over the top of the head.

18. A(n) _____ is worn to protect the nose and mouth from splashes or sprays of blood or bodily fluids and to prevent droplets from being transmitted by close contact.

19. Masks do not fit snugly on the face or provide a tight seal, so they are not reliable protection against _____ transmission.

20. A(n) _____ filters the air to prevent the inhalation of airborne microorganisms and must fit the wearer's face to provide a tight, effective seal.

Gloves

Identify whether each statement is true or false.

_____ 1. Standard and transmission-based precautions require the use of reusable, nonsterile gloves for a variety of procedures.

_____ 2. Before donning gloves, nursing assistants should select appropriately sized gloves and inspect them for cracks, holes, tears, or any discoloration.

_____ 3. It is acceptable for nursing assistants to wear rings underneath gloves.

_____ 4. The outside of a nonsterile glove is always considered contaminated, so gloved hands must be kept away from clothing and other clean areas.

_____ 5. Nursing assistants should wash their hands or use hand sanitizer prior to donning and after removing gloves.

Removing Disposable Gloves

The following steps are part of the procedure for removing disposable gloves. Identify the proper order in which they should be completed by numbering them 1 through 7.

_____ Slowly pull the second glove off, turning it inside out and drawing it over the first glove.

_____ Wash your hands to ensure infection control.

_____ Drop both gloves into the appropriate waste container.

_____ Pull the cuff of the first glove down, drawing it over your hand and turning it inside out.

_____ Use the gloved fingers of one hand to grasp the other, gloved hand. Grasp the gloved hand just below the cuff of the glove.

_____ Pull the first glove off your hand and hold it in the palm of the other, gloved hand.

_____ Insert the fingers of the ungloved hand under the cuff of the remaining glove on the other hand.

Gowns

Identify whether each statement is true or false.

_____ 1. Standard and transmission-based precautions require that healthcare staff members wear gowns during procedures in which they might be exposed to or transmit microorganisms.

_____ 2. A gown that is torn still creates an effective barrier that protects healthcare staff.

_____ 3. As often as possible, nursing assistants should carry out all procedures that require a gown at one time to avoid regowning.

_____ 4. A nursing assistant should always put on gloves after putting on a gown and should tuck the gloves under the cuffs of the gown sleeves.

_____ 5. It is acceptable to touch the outside of a gown as you remove it.

Removing a Gown

The following steps are part of the procedure for removing a gown. Identify the proper order in which they should be completed by numbering them 1 through 7.

_____ Repeat the last step to begin pulling the other arm out of its sleeve. Do not touch the outside of the gown as you pull the gown down off your shoulders and arms.

_____ Turn the gown inside out as you remove it. Hold the gown, turned inside out, away from your clothing and roll the gown so the contaminated outside faces inward.

_____ Wash your hands to ensure infection control.

_____ Dispose of the gown in the appropriate waste container before leaving the room.

_____ Reach behind the gown and untie both the neck and waist ties.

_____ Remove and discard your gloves. Be careful not to contaminate yourself.

_____ Slide your hands back into the sleeves of the gown. Using one hand (still inside the sleeve), hold the cuff of the opposite sleeve and begin pulling your arm out of that sleeve. Be careful not to touch the outside of the gown.

Applying a Mask or Respirator

The proper application of a mask or respirator provides a barrier that protects those who are giving and receiving care. The following steps are part of the procedure for applying a mask or respirator. Identify the proper order in which they should be completed by numbering them 1 through 7.

_____ Check that the mask or respirator fits properly and seals tightly on your face.

_____ Try to avoid coughing, sneezing, and unnecessary talking while wearing the mask or respirator. If the mask or respirator becomes moist, contaminated, or damaged, replace it. Do not let the mask or respirator hang around your neck when not in use.

_____ Adjust the mask or respirator over your nose, mouth, and chin by pinching the flexible portion over the bridge of the nose. The mask or respirator should fit snugly over the nose and under the chin. If you wear eyeglasses, the mask must also fit snugly under the bottom of your eyeglasses.

_____ Assemble the necessary equipment (the mask or respirator).

_____ Pick up the mask or respirator by its ties or elastic band. Place the mask or respirator over your nose, face, and chin.

_____ Secure the ties or elastic band of the mask or respirator behind your head and neck. Do not touch the portion of the mask or respirator that will cover your face. Only handle the ties or elastic band.

_____ Wash your hands or use hand sanitizer to ensure infection control.

Removing a Mask or Respirator

The following steps are part of the procedure for removing a mask or respirator. Identify the proper order in which they should be completed by numbering them 1 through 6.

_____ Wash your hands or use hand sanitizer to ensure infection control.

_____ If wearing gloves, remove and discard them. Be careful not to contaminate yourself.

_____ Untie the ties or remove the elastic band of the mask or respirator. Start with the ties or elastic band at the bottom of the mask or respirator and then untie or remove the ties or elastic band at the top.

_____ Use both hands to pull the mask or respirator away from your face.

_____ Grasp the mask or respirator by its ties or elastic band.

_____ Dispose of the contaminated mask or respirator according to facility policy.

Putting On and Removing Goggles or a Face Shield

Personal eyeglasses or contact lenses are not adequate eye protection. The following steps are part of the procedure for putting on and removing goggles or a face shield. Identify the proper order in which they should be completed by numbering them 1 through 7.

_____ Do not let the goggles or face shield hang around your neck when not in use.

_____ Wash your hands or use hand sanitizer to ensure infection control.

_____ Place the goggles or face shield on your face and eyes and adjust them so they protect the face and eyes.

_____ With ungloved, clean hands, remove your goggles or face shield by grasping the clean ear piece with both hands and lifting the goggles or face shield away from your face.

_____ Try to avoid coughing, sneezing, and unnecessary talking while wearing a face shield. If the goggles or face shield become moist, contaminated, or damaged, replace them.

_____ Discard the goggles or face shield in the designated receptacle according to facility policy. Do not reuse any disposable face protection. Wash your hands to ensure infection control.

_____ If wearing gloves, remove and discard them. The outside of the goggles or face shield is contaminated, so do not touch it with your bare hands.

Respiratory Hygiene and Cough Etiquette

Identify whether each statement is true or false.

_____ 1. Respiratory hygiene and cough etiquette are standard precautions that protect others from the spread of infection.

_____ 2. Actions related to respiratory hygiene and cough etiquette cause disease transmission and spread the respiratory secretions of residents.

_____ 3. Cough etiquette includes covering one's mouth and nose with a tissue when coughing or sneezing and using the nearest waste container to dispose of a tissue after its use.

_____ 4. Equipment and working surfaces must be cleaned and decontaminated yearly to reduce the number of microorganisms and prevent transmission.

_____ 5. During cleaning, foreign materials are removed from surfaces and equipment.

_____ 6. During disinfection, disinfectants prevent microorganisms from spreading and destroy many microorganisms depending on their strength.

_____ 7. Sterilization eliminates all forms of microorganisms using extreme physical or chemical processes, such as steam under pressure or liquid chemicals.

_____ 8. Gloves do not need to be worn during cleaning, disinfection, and sterilization procedures.

_____ 9. All disposable equipment can be reused once and then must be thrown away.

_____ 10. Contaminated equipment, clothing, and supplies are double-bagged in biohazard waste bags for proper handling and disposal.

Removal of Infectious Waste

Complete the following sentences.

1. The double-bagging procedure requires disposable gloves and two leak proof, plastic _____ waste bags.

2. Inside the isolation room, the nursing assistant holding the full bag of waste places the contaminated biohazard waste bag inside the _____ biohazard waste bag held by the nursing assistant outside the isolation room.

3. Before the contaminated biohazard waste bag is placed in the clean biohazard waste bag, the nursing assistant standing outside the isolation room should fold the top of the clean biohazard waste bag into a(n) _____.

4. The cuff at the top of the clean biohazard waste bag protects the nursing assistant's _____ from contamination.

5. The nursing assistant standing inside the isolation room should remove his or her PPE _____ leaving the room.

Transmission-Based Precautions

Select the *best* answer.

_____ 1. What are transmission-based precautions?
   A. contact precautions and droplet precautions, but not airborne precautions
   B. wearing goggles or face shields, but never gloves, during contact
   C. precautions used when splashes or sprays are not anticipated
   D. precautions used for residents who are known or suspected to be infected with specific pathogens

_____ 2. Cleaning a room properly after discharge
   A. removes soil and sterilizes microorganisms in the room
   B. is solely the job of housekeeping or environmental services
   C. includes the appropriate disposal of all linen, even clean linen
   D. involves the disposal of a resident's personal belongings

_____ 3. Contact precautions
   A. are used when microorganisms may be spread by direct or indirect contact
   B. require that gloves and a gown be worn upon entering the hallway
   C. require that gloves be worn in the dining room
   D. require that reusable items be discarded after use

_____ 4. Droplet precautions
   A. are used when an infection can be spread by respiratory droplets or contact with mucous membranes
   B. are used for influenza, but not for pertussis
   C. depend on respiratory droplets traveling fewer than 3–6 feet
   D. require that a face mask be put on after entering a room

_____ 5. Airborne precautions
   A. are required when a disease can be spread by contact
   B. are not used for airborne diseases such as measles and tuberculosis
   C. usually require the use of a respirator certified by the National Institute of Occupational Safety and Health (NIOSH)
   D. use HEPA filtration units to clean out infected wounds

_____ 6. Enteric precautions
   A. are the same as wound and skin precautions
   B. control diseases spread through direct or indirect oral contact with infected feces or contaminated articles
   C. encourage the spread of microorganisms that combat pathogens
   D. are used for heavy secretions from the respiratory system

_____ 7. The Occupational Safety and Health Administration (OSHA)
   A. sets safety standards related primarily to airborne pathogens
   B. protects residents in long-term care facilities from negligent caregivers
   C. developed research facilities for the study of the *Plasmodium* parasite and the Ebola virus
   D. sets standards that protect healthcare staff and others who are exposed to blood and other potentially infectious materials

_____ 8. OSHA safety standards
   A. prevent exposure to bloodborne pathogens and reduce the chance of infection if contact occurs
   B. require facilities to create, but not implement, exposure control plans
   C. prevent training for staff members who are exposed to blood
   D. are designed with the goal of protecting facilities from liability

_____ 9. Which of the following is true of isolation?
   A. It prevents all organisms from entering a room.
   B. It only protects residents from the healthcare staff.
   C. It involves wearing PPE, which may include masks, gowns, goggles, and gloves.
   D. It includes additional guidelines for reusing linens.

_____ 10. Strict isolation is
   A. followed by the nursing staff, but not by doctors or family members
   B. followed by the healthcare staff, but not by family members
   C. used to prevent noncommunicable diseases from spreading
   D. used to prevent the transmission of highly communicable diseases spread by contact or airborne routes

_____ 11. Respiratory isolation
   A. is used to prevent the transmission of bloodborne pathogens
   B. is used to prevent the transmission of microorganisms spread through sneezed or inhaled droplets
   C. never requires special ventilation and filtration systems
   D. is most effective when the resident shares the room with a roommate

_____ 12. Protective isolation is
   A. used to protect the nursing assistant from the pathogens of the resident
   B. used to protect those vulnerable to pathogenic microorganisms due to lowered immunity
   C. used for residents with healthy immune systems to prevent leukemia
   D. used for residents recovering from an abusive relationship

_____ 13. Which of the following is true of OSHA?
   A. It guarantees the right to a safe workplace for all staff.
   B. It provides a safe workplace that is contaminated with blood or bodily fluids.
   C. It requires healthcare facilities to provide costly training about exposure risk at the nursing assistant's expense.
   D. It requires healthcare facilities to remove workers who have had exposure incidents.

_____ 14. An exposure control plan
   A. includes free hepatitis B vaccines and immediate, confidential medical evaluation and follow-up
   B. provides free hepatitis B vaccines for residents, but not for caregivers
   C. prevents exposure to severe weather during resident outings
   D. is kept confidential at the administrative level of the facility to protect the facility from exposure

_____ 15. A written exposure control plan should include
   A. requirements for hepatitis B vaccination
   B. policies related to standard precautions, including hand hygiene practices and the use of PPE
   C. safe management and disposal of sharps
   D. All of the above.

Putting On and Removing Personal Protective Equipment (PPE)

In this activity, you will practice portions of the procedures for putting on and removing personal protective equipment (PPE). To prepare for this activity, review the procedural checklists for hand hygiene and putting on and removing gloves, goggles, gowns, and masks. Also have your FIRST CHECK procedural checklist nearby.

Form a group of three and assign each person a role. One person will be the nursing assistant, another a resident, and the third person will serve as the evaluator. Then complete each of the following steps:

1. Create a mock isolation room and choose a procedure that must be performed within the room. One way to create an isolation room is to draw a privacy curtain completely around a bed. Outside the room, set up an isolation cart or overbed table with the following items: hand sanitizer, a gown, a mask, goggles or protective eyewear, and gloves. Inside the room, place a waste container and hand sanitizer by the door.

2. Complete the FIRST, or Preparation, steps of the procedure, omitting any steps that are not applicable to the chosen procedure. Before entering the room, don PPE (gloves, a gown, a mask, and goggles or protective eyewear) using the proper procedure.

3. Did you have any difficulty applying the appropriate PPE? If so, what challenges did you face? Were any steps forgotten?

   _____

   _____

   _____

4. Perform the chosen procedure, being extra cautious not to contaminate yourself in the isolation room.

5. When the procedure is complete, remove gloves, goggles, the gown, and the mask following proper procedure. Perform hand hygiene before leaving the room and complete the remaining CHECK, or Follow-Up and Reporting and Documentation, steps of the procedure, omitting any steps that are not applicable.

6. Did you have any difficulty removing the appropriate PPE? If so, what challenges did you face? Were any steps forgotten?

   _____

   _____

   _____

7. Switch roles with your partners and then discuss any difficulties encountered while using PPE and performing the chosen procedure in isolation.

Understanding Wounds

Complete the following sentences.

1. A(n) _____ is an injury to body tissue caused by a cut, blow, or other force.

2. There are two major categories of wounds: _____ wounds and nonpenetrating wounds.

3. _____ wounds break through the skin and are often deep enough to cut through body tissues and organs.

4. _____ wounds are caused by rubbing or friction on the surface of the skin and do not break through the skin.

5. _____ are tear-like wounds that have ragged edges and may be caused by falling against a rough surface.

6. A bite or _____ from an insect or animal is another type of wound.

7. _____ wounds result from exposure to extreme temperatures.

8. _____ wounds result from inhalation or contact with chemical substances and can cause skin or lung damage.

9. _____ wounds are caused by high-voltage electrical currents entering the body and causing serious internal damage.

10. Nursing assistants observe, report, and document the condition of a wound, swelling, the color and amount of discharge, and odors that may indicate _____.

11. Drainage that is thin, watery, and slightly yellow or colorless is called *clear* or _____ *drainage* and is typically normal.

12. Drainage that is thin, watery, and slightly pink from blood is _____ and is typically normal.

13. Drainage of an abnormal color might be _____, or tinged with large amounts of blood, or be mostly blood.

14. _____ drainage is an abnormal type of drainage filled with pus; is typically gray, green, or yellow with a thick consistency; and usually signals an infection.

15. If wound drainage soaks a dressing, this needs to be _____ immediately.

16. _____ wounds may have a drain, or a small tube surgically inserted to drain fluid during the healing process.

Name: _____   Date: _____

Dressings

Identify whether each statement is true or false.

_____ 1. Dressings are used to protect wounds, prevent drainage, and promote comfort and healing.

_____ 2. Factors that help or hinder the wound healing process include the health and age of the person, nutritional and respiratory status, medications, cultural and socioeconomic factors, and other diseases.

_____ 3. People with diabetes often have slower healing processes due to poor blood circulation.

_____ 4. Gauze dressings are common, but dressings may also be made of other materials such as transparent adhesive film.

_____ 5. The dressing material used for a wound is selected based on what the nursing assistant is comfortable changing.

_____ 6. Some dressings are held in place by bandages.

_____ 7. Wet dressings are applied in several layers to absorb drainage, and dry dressings are saturated with a prescribed solution to promote healing.

_____ 8. A licensed nursing staff member will never ask a nursing assistant to assist with a nonsterile dressing change.

_____ 9. Sterile dressings are applied in a sterile field, which is an area with many living microorganisms.

_____ 10. Only supplies that have been sterilized can be placed or used in a sterile field.

_____ 11. Any area beyond the 1-inch margin, or space, around a sterile field is considered contaminated.

_____ 12. A sterile package that is open, torn, punctured, or wet is still considered sterile.

_____ 13. Airborne microorganisms can contaminate the sterile field, so drafts, coughing, sneezes, talking, and laughing must be prevented within the field.

CHAPTER 16 Maintaining a Safe Environment and Practice

Name: _____ Date: _____

Matching Chapter 16 Key Terms
Match each definition with the key term.

A. always events
B. Alzheimer's disease (AD)
C. clinically adverse events
D. commode
E. culture of safety
F. entrapment
G. fire triangle
H. flow meter
I. gait
J. gait belt
K. harm
L. hypothermia
M. incident report
N. nasal cannula
O. near misses
P. needlesticks
Q. never events
R. osteoporosis
S. RACE
T. range of motion (ROM)
U. restraint
V. safety data sheet (SDS)
W. transparency

_____ 1. an acronym for the process of responding to fire; stands for *rescue*, *activate alarm*, *confine the fire*, and *extinguish*

_____ 2. any physical equipment or chemical substance that prevents a resident from moving freely

_____ 3. the three elements (fuel, oxygen, and heat) needed to start a fire

_____ 4. routine activities and processes that are so important they must be performed reliably and consistently; result in effective admissions, transfers, discharges, and handoffs

_____ 5. the amount that a person can move a given joint voluntarily

_____ 6. a chair that contains a chamber pot; can be used as a toilet by people with mobility challenges

_____ 7. a narrow, flexible plastic tube used to deliver oxygen through the nostrils using nasal breathing

_____ 8. the shared commitment of a healthcare facility's leadership and staff to ensure a safe work environment

_____ 9. unplanned health outcomes that do not cause harm, even though they have the potential to; are considered *close calls*

_____ 10. a harmful event in which a resident falls between the bed and side rails

_____ 11. a device used to make sure a resident gets the prescribed amount of oxygen

_____ 12. a degenerative brain disease and the most common form of dementia; results in progressive memory loss, impaired thinking, disorientation, and changes in personality and mood; advanced cases lead to a decline in cognitive and physical functioning

_____ 13. a belt worn around a resident's waist that serves as a safety device when a resident stands and ambulates; sometimes called a *transfer belt*

_____ 14. a condition of abnormally low body temperature

_____ 15. medical errors

_____ 16. a form that records information about an unusual event, such as a resident injury; also called an *accident* or *occurrence report*

_____ 17. puncture wounds caused by needles

_____ 18. lack of secretive or hidden information; honesty

_____ 19. a manner of walking

_____ 20. actions or errors that result in harm, death, or significant disability; are usually preventable

_____ 21. unintended physical injury that requires additional monitoring, treatment, or hospitalization; may result in death

_____ 22. a condition of porous bones; characterized by low bone density

_____ 23. a document found in a facility safety plan that contains information about the potential hazards of a chemical product, use, storage, handling, and emergency procedures; also called a *material safety data sheet (MSDS)*

A Culture of Safety
Complete the following sentences.

1. If care given in a facility does not meet safety and quality standards, Medicare and some insurance companies may not reimburse the facility for the _____ of care.

2. The Centers for Medicare & _____ Services (CMS) monitors quality measures such as clinical care, patient outcomes, and recent hospital experiences.

Name: _____   Date: _____

3. Long-term care facilities are required to perform initial assessments on admission, conduct periodic assessments over a resident's stay, and develop _____ data sets (MDSs) that set a foundation for the assessment of all residents.

4. Assessment information is used to develop, review, and revise the resident's _____ with the goal of coordinating care and services to enable the best possible physical, mental, and psychosocial well-being.

5. A resident _____ instrument (RAI) is used to gather specific information and ensure resident care promotes quality of life.

6. Healthcare facilities must use safe practices to attain expected and required quality _____ and measures.

7. Effective healthcare staff members maintain safety standards and follow facility safety _____ to ensure their safety and the safety of patients, residents, family members, and others.

8. The World _____ Organization (WHO) defines *patient safety* as the prevention of errors and harmful effects to patients.

9. *Unsafe events* are processes or acts that result in hazardous healthcare conditions or _____ (unintended injury).

10. The Agency for Healthcare _____ and Quality (AHRQ) defines *patient safety* as freedom from accidental or preventable injuries resulting from medical care.

11. Care that improves patient safety _____ the occurrence of preventable, harmful outcomes.

12. The Institute of _____ (IOM) holds that people should not be harmed by care intended to help them.

13. Quality care should be based on sound scientific _____ and should respond to individual preferences, needs, and values.

14. Unnecessary waits and harmful delays should be reduced, and care should not be wasteful or _____ in quality due to patient diversity.

15. Healthcare facilities must demonstrate _____, or honesty, in reporting safety issues.

16. The National _____ Forum (NQF) states that safety practices are processes that provide evidence-based care, reduce the likelihood of harm, and maximize the likelihood of avoiding errors.

17. Safety guidelines include being mindful of safety at all times, always working to prevent errors or harm, learning from errors, and working to assure a culture of _____ for all healthcare staff members, facilities, patients, and residents.

18. The Centers for Disease Control and Prevention (CDC) defines a(n) _____ of safety as the shared commitment of a healthcare facility's leadership and staff to ensure a safe work environment.

19. A healthcare facility with a culture of safety has the necessary systems, procedures, and _____ to achieve safe, high-quality performance from the healthcare staff.

20. Healthcare facilities that enjoy a culture of safety promote the occurrence of _____, or routine activities and processes that must be performed reliably and consistently.

21. Always events result in effective admissions, transfers, discharges, and change-of-shift _____.

22. When errors occur in a culture of safety, the focus is on _____, not on who did it.

23. A culture of safety's approach to errors brings failures and issues out into the _____ immediately and deals with them in a blame-free, nonbiased, and nonthreatening way.

24. In a culture of safety, clinically _____ events (medical errors) and near misses (unplanned health outcomes that do not cause harm) can be reported without fear of punishment.

25. Holistic nursing assistants abide by all safety principles, policies, and procedures; pay attention to how personal, cultural, and ethnic differences impact safety; suggest solutions to problems; and report errors both informally to the charge nurse and formally through _____.

How Nursing Assistants Ensure Safety
Identify whether each statement is true or false.

_____ 1. Hazards for residents in long-term care facilities include falls; burns; decubitus ulcers; blood clots; medication errors; healthcare-associated infections (HAIs) such as *Staphylococcus* (staph), urinary tract infections, and pneumonia; and entrapment.

_____ 2. Holistic nursing assistants ensure resident safety by avoiding forever events, preventing accidents, conducting safety checks, preventing sharps-related injuries, and following facility safety plans.

_____ 3. Forever events are actions or errors that lead to serious resident harm, disability, or death.

_____ 4. Never events are serious, reportable events that can be grouped into seven categories: surgical events, product or device events, resident protection events, care management events, environmental events, radiologic events, and criminal events.

_____ 5. Preventing accidents requires personal awareness of safety hazards, safety promotion, safety policies and the facility's safety plan, risks, safety equipment, and infection prevention and control.

_____ 6. After providing care, nursing assistants should always check the resident's identification to be sure they provided care to the correct resident.

_____ 7. A nursing assistant needs one identifier (such as a name, identification number or bar code, date of birth, or photo) to verify a resident's identity.

_____ 8. To properly identify a resident, a nursing assistant could say the resident's name, ask the resident to state his or her full name, and compare the name with the identification bracelet.

_____ 9. In some healthcare facilities, residents prefer not to wear identification bracelets; these residents may be identified by at least one other identifier verification and their photo, which can be found in the EMR.

_____ 10. Nursing assistants should follow facility policy for the identification verification of residents who are unable to communicate.

Verifying a Resident's Identity

In this activity, you will practice verifying a resident's identity. To prepare for this activity, review the information about using two identifiers to verify a resident's identity. Also have your FIRST CHECK procedural checklist nearby.

Form a group of three and assign each person a role. One person will be the nursing assistant, another a resident, and the third person will serve as the evaluator. Then complete each of the following steps:

1. Complete the FIRST, or Preparation, steps for a procedure. Be sure to verify the resident's identity using two identifiers. The evaluator should make sure two identifiers were used.

2. What two identifiers did you use to verify the resident's identity? List at least two other identifiers you could have used.

_____

_____

_____

_____

_____

3. Complete the CHECK, or Follow-Up and Reporting and Documentation, steps for a procedure, omitting any steps that are not applicable.

4. Switch roles with your partners and then discuss what situations might make verifying a resident's identity challenging. List ways you could verify the identity of a resident who does not speak your language or is unable to communicate.

_____

_____

_____

_____

_____

Conducting a Safety Check

Complete the following sentences.

1. _____ checks play an important role in reducing risks and preventing accidents.

2. A nursing assistant should perform a safety check while giving care in a resident's room and before _____ the resident's room.

3. During a safety check, it is important to make sure the resident is _____ and comfortable in bed, in a chair, or in a wheelchair.

4. A bed or wheelchair must be in the _____ position so that it does not roll when the resident moves into or out of the bed or wheelchair.

5. If a bed's side rails are used, the resident must be situated to prevent _____, a harmful event in which the resident falls between the bed and side rails.

6. If side rails are not used, the bed must be placed in its _____ position so the resident does not fall.

7. After positioning a resident properly, a nursing assistant should check that any _____ from an IV or Foley catheter is attached properly and is not kinked.

8. It is important to place the _____ light in an accessible place for the resident.

9. During a safety check, pick up any items on the floor, _____ up any spills, and position any furniture or obstacles so they will not get in the resident's way.

Sharps-Related Injuries

Select the *best* answer.

_____ 1. Injuries caused by sharp objects such as razors, broken glass, or rough edges that break the skin are called
   A. abrasions
   B. contusions
   C. sharps-related injuries
   D. HAIs

_____ 2. What are needlesticks?
   A. sharp objects used to deliver medications
   B. punctures of the skin by needles
   C. sharps containers
   D. needles used in IV catheters

_____ 3. Puncture wounds from used needles
   A. can cause wounds, but do not transmit infections
   B. are harmless
   C. are a good reason to avoid giving care
   D. can transmit pathogens and cause infection

_____ 4. Sharps and needles must be disposed of
   A. in designated sharps containers
   B. in any facility waste container
   C. only at the end of the day
   D. only when there is risk for infection

Facility Safety Plans

Complete the following paragraph.

Facility (1.) _____
plans outline policies and procedures followed by all
healthcare staff that comply with federal, state, and
(2.) _____ laws and regulations related
to health and safety. Facility safety plans include regulations
and guidelines related to the following workplace safety
concerns: fire safety, biosafety, bodily fluids, radiation
and chemical safety, (3.) _____
waste and materials (HAZMAT) management and
emergency response, and accident investigation and
(4.) _____.

Work Hazards Affecting Nursing Assistants

Complete the following sentences.

1. The _____ Safety and Health
   Administration (OSHA) estimates that nursing and
   healthcare staff members are at risk for occupational
   exposure to bloodborne pathogens such as HIV, the
   hepatitis B virus (HBV), and the hepatitis C virus (HVC).

2. It is important that nursing assistants follow
   _____ pathogen precautions.

3. In addition to bloodborne pathogens, occupational
   safety hazards for nursing assistants include sharps-
   related injuries and _____
   disorders (MSDs).

4. Nursing staff members have reported high rates of MSDs,
   such as _____ and shoulder
   injuries caused by moving and repositioning residents.

5. Risk factors for developing MSDs include overexerting,
   performing multiple lifts, lifting a resident alone,
   lifting uncooperative or confused residents, lifting
   residents who cannot support their weight or who
   are heavy, and not being adequately trained in body
   _____.

6. Nursing assistants are _____
   for following safety principles and practices at all
   times, both during work and in everyday life.

Falls

Identify whether each statement is true or false.

_____ 1. Falls cannot cause serious injury.

_____ 2. Falls occur less frequently as a person ages, and
   those who fall once are likely to fall again.

_____ 3. Falls rarely result in hospital admission or
   admission to a long-term care facility.

_____ 4. Most falls occur in a resident's room between
   10:00 p.m. and 6:30 a.m. when there are fewer
   staff members and less activity in a resident's room.

_____ 5. At night, residents are more likely to leave their
   beds to go to the bathroom without asking for
   assistance, possibly leading to a fall.

_____ 6. Many people who fall suffer moderate-to-severe
   injuries such as dislocations, bruising, cuts to the
   skin, muscle tears, hip fractures, or head traumas.

_____ 7. Injuries are more likely to affect residents
   who have osteoporosis, and if a person with
   osteoporosis does fall, the injury is usually
   more severe.

_____ 8. Inadequate handrails, a slippery tub, an icy
   sidewalk, a pet, poor footwear, and insufficient
   lighting help prevent falls.

_____ 9. Health issues such as low blood pressure, sensory
   loss, stroke, dementia, medications, and nervous
   system disorders increase the risk of falling.

_____ 10. Immobility after a fall can cause complications
   such as dehydration, decubitus ulcers,
   hyperthermia, and pneumonia.

_____ 11. Older adults need to be particularly cautious
   about falls, as age alone is a significant risk factor.

_____ 12. Many older adults rely on assistive devices such
   as walkers and canes that increase the risk of
   falling if they fit poorly or are defective.

_____ 13. An older adult is less likely to fall if he or she
   has difficulty with balance, strength, perception,
   vision, range of motion, or coordination.

_____ 14. During ambulation, a nursing assistant must
   pay attention to a resident's balance and
   strength, potential loss of sensation or sensory
   impairment, level of vision and hearing, joint
   range of motion, and gait.

_____ 15. Balance, gait, muscle, or range–of-motion
   exercises can be very helpful for preventing falls
   in residents and building strength and balance
   to promote self-confidence.

ACT

Complete the following steps of the *ACT* acronym for
preventing resident falls.

1. **A:** _____

2. **C:** _____

3. **T:** _____

Fall Prevention

Complete the following sentences.

1. The first step in preventing falls is _____
   residents who are at risk for falls.

2. Usually, a doctor, licensed nursing staff
   member, or physical therapist will conduct
   a(n) _____ of a resident's
   medications, fall risk factors, and strategies to
   overcome risks.

3. The assessment of the doctor, licensed nursing staff
   member, or physical therapist forms the basis of the
   _____ risk program, which is
   developed as part of a resident's plan of care.

4. Healthcare facilities often use a visual
   _____, such as a sign, picture,
   or wristband, to indicate that a resident has an
   increased risk for falling.

5. Some facilities use resident seat monitors, bed and chair exit _____, and wrist or room motion monitors to alert the nursing staff that an at-risk resident is mobile without assistance.

6. To help prevent falls, a nursing assistant should work _____ and steadily when providing assistance with ADLs and ambulation.

7. Holistic nursing assistants frequently monitor and observe _____ and listen for calls of help, banging, alarms, or falling objects.

8. One fall-prevention strategy is to ensure a working _____ is always within each resident's reach.

9. Keeping a resident's _____ at the lowest possible level and placing mats around the bed can help prevent a fall.

10. Making sure a resident's room is well _____ and does not have glare is especially important for preventing falls for residents with poor eyesight.

11. Fall prevention involves keeping a resident's room _____, dry, and uncluttered; placing the resident's personal items within reach; and cleaning up small, nonhazardous spills immediately.

12. To help prevent falls, a nursing assistant can check that there are no wires, cords, or other tripping _____ in a resident's room.

13. Nursing assistants should encourage residents to use handrails or _____ bars and assist with shower chairs, if needed.

14. _____ that are stable and sturdy, are at a good height, and have armrests can assist in preventing falls.

15. To reduce the risk for a fall, nursing assistants should be aware of any _____ in a resident's medications and understand how changes may affect the resident.

16. Keeping a bedside _____ nearby can help prevent residents from falling while going to the toilet.

17. While walking down a hall in a healthcare facility, a nursing assistant should _____ all residents and their rooms to identify possible safety hazards.

18. Nursing assistants should use proper body _____ to pick up anything on the floor that should not be there and immediately clean up any spills.

19. _____ that provides good support and has closed backs, nonskid tread, and securely tied shoelaces can help prevent falls.

20. Nursing assistants can anticipate the _____ of residents (hunger, thirst, toileting, discomfort, boredom, or emotional needs) to help prevent ambulation without assistance.

21. It is important to remind residents and family members about a facility's _____ measures for preventing falls.

22. Nursing assistants should use caution when applying creams, bath oils, or powders to a resident's skin, as these substances can make surfaces _____.

23. If a resident wears eyeglasses, the eyeglasses should _____ properly and be nearby so the resident can reach them easily.

24. To help prevent falls, nursing assistants can discourage residents from wearing _____ gowns or robes.

25. Canes, walkers, and chair legs that have _____ tips can help prevent falls.

26. A nursing assistant should _____ the wheels on beds and wheelchairs whenever a resident is moving into or out of the bed or wheelchair.

27. When helping a resident ambulate, a nursing assistant can provide and use assistive devices, such as a(n) _____ belt.

Responding to a Fall

Identify whether each statement is true or false.

_____ 1. If a resident begins to fall while ambulating, it is best to ease him or her safely down to the floor.

_____ 2. Resident falls do not need to be reported.

_____ 3. If a resident falls, a nursing assistant should act quickly and leave the resident to find help.

_____ 4. A nursing assistant should stay with the charge nurse as he or she assesses the resident who has fallen to determine the next course of action.

_____ 5. After the assessment, it is important to observe the resident for unusual changes, such as changes in vital signs, drowsiness, dizziness, vomiting, or double vision.

_____ 6. An incident report is used to document the exact details of any injuries, falls, needlesticks, burns, errors in care, resident complaints, and faulty equipment.

_____ 7. Incident reports should be written several days after an incident to ensure that details are interpreted correctly.

Restraint Alternatives

Select the *best* answer.

_____ 1. What is Alzheimer's disease (AD)?
   A. a degenerative brain disease that leads to memory loss and impaired thinking
   B. a brain disease that causes disorientation, but not changes in personality
   C. a disease that affects the behavior of some residents, but rarely requires monitoring by a nursing assistant
   D. a common side effect of medications

_____ 2. A restraint is used
  A. when residents exhibit behaviors that staff members cannot tolerate
  B. when ordered by a doctor to keep residents from falling or harming themselves or others
  C. to inhibit the movements of a resident and make care easier for the nursing staff
  D. as ordered by the doctor, independent of facility policies and federal and state regulations

_____ 3. A chemical restraint
  A. is only used to treat medical conditions related to Alzheimer's disease
  B. must be used in a way that does not cause injury or emotional harm to the nursing assistant
  C. requires observation and monitoring every two hours by a nursing assistant
  D. is a medication that makes a resident drowsy or sleepy and unable to move freely

_____ 4. A physical restraint
  A. is the least restrictive type of restraint
  B. is ordered by a doctor, who will choose a restraint that keeps the resident safe and provides the greatest amount of freedom
  C. is used in healthcare facilities and is whatever keeps the resident safe (for example, a tucked sheet)
  D. can be avoided if the nursing assistant raises all side rails to keep the resident in bed

_____ 5. Risks of restraints
  A. decrease with the use of mobility rails, which prevent the resident from exiting the room
  B. increase with locking the bed wheels and lowering the bed close to the floor
  C. include bruises, choking, loss of muscle tone, decubitus ulcers, falls, and loss of dignity
  D. do not include the use of side rails to prevent entrapment

The Restraint-Free Environment

Identify whether each statement is true or false.

_____ 1. Medicare- and Medicaid-certified nursing homes cannot use restraints except to treat medical symptoms.

_____ 2. One key action that helps avoid the use of restraints is ignoring call lights, which prevents wandering, confusion, or getting out of bed.

_____ 3. Alternatives to restraints include call light placement and reminders, close observation of the resident, a bed in low position, and a bedside commode or urinal close to the bed.

_____ 4. Holistic nursing assistants can help prevent issues or challenges related to restraints by providing excellent care, monitoring, observing, and reporting and documenting any problems immediately.

_____ 5. Once the doctor has ordered a restraint and the informed consent document has been reviewed and signed, licensed nursing staff members have full responsibility for applying, monitoring, and removing restraints.

Fire Triangle

Apply the appropriate labels to the image.

1. _____   3. _____

2. _____

BALRedaan/Shutterstock.com

Fire Safety

Complete the following sentences.

1. Healthcare facilities face considerable risks during fire emergencies because of their large populations of nonambulatory residents and the difficulty of _____.

2. Nursing assistants and healthcare staff members must know how fires can start and how to _____ them.

3. For a fire to start, the three elements of the _____ must be present: fuel, oxygen, and heat.

4. _____ is any flammable solid, liquid, or gas.

5. Fires can be prevented by keeping heat away from _____ items.

6. If the facility fire alarm sounds, a nursing assistant should abide by the facility _____.

7. A facility code announcement will help a nursing assistant identify the _____ of the fire.

8. If on the floor of the fire, a nursing assistant should close the nearest resident, office, laboratory, and utility room _____ and clear the corridors.

9. A nursing assistant should not _____ residents unless specifically instructed to do so.

10. Nursing assistants should only attempt to extinguish a fire using a fire extinguisher after the _____, activate the alarm, and confine the fire steps are accomplished and the fire department is on its way.

11. There are several fire _____ types designed to extinguish different classes of fires.

12. For Class _____ fires (solid materials such as wood, paper, cloth, or trash), a water or multipurpose dry chemical extinguisher is used.

13. For Class _____ fires (gasoline, oil, paint, or other flammable liquids), a carbon dioxide or multipurpose dry chemical extinguisher is used.

14. For Class _____ fires (wiring, fuse boxes, computers, or other electrical sources), a dry chemical or multipurpose dry chemical extinguisher is used.

15. For Class _____ fires (powders, flakes, or shavings from metals), a class D extinguisher is used.

16. For Class _____ fires (combustible fluids, such as oils and fats), a dry or wet chemical extinguisher is used.

17. Fire extinguisher _____ should be performed on a regular basis by a designated person and should make sure extinguishers are fully charged and ready for use.

18. When using a fire extinguisher, remember the acronym _____.

19. Before using an extinguisher, a nursing assistant should identify a(n) _____ in case the fire extinguisher fails to operate properly or the fire cannot be completely extinguished.

RACE

Identify each step of the RACE system.

The RACE System	
Letter	**Step**
R	1. _____
A	2. _____
C	3. _____
E	4. _____

Using a Fire Extinguisher

Apply the appropriate labels to the image.

A. Aim nozzle at base of fire.
B. Squeeze the handles.
C. Sweep spray side to side.
D. Pull the lock pin.

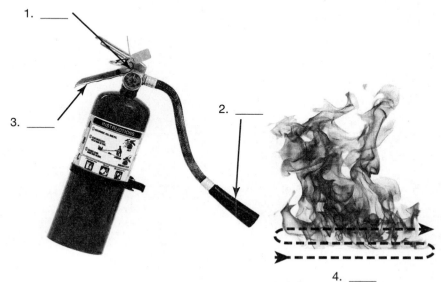

1. _____
2. _____
3. _____
4. _____

Thomas M Perkins/Shutterstock.com, Valeev/Shutterstock.com

Electrical and Chemical Safety

Identify whether each statement is true or false.

_____ 1. Electrical hazards can cause bodily shock, electrical fires, and explosions.

_____ 2. There are 14 main types of electrical injuries: electrocution, electrical shock, burns, and falls caused by contact with electricity.

_____ 3. Electrical hazards include electrical cords that are damaged or aging, faulty electrical equipment, and damaged electrical wall receptacles.

_____ 4. A facility safety plan provides directions regarding electrical safety, since many OSHA standards must be met.

_____ 5. Toxic exposure to hazardous chemicals can result from topical and spray medications; anesthetic gases; and chemicals used to clean, disinfect, and sterilize work surfaces and equipment.

_____ 6. OSHA hazard standards and facility-specific guidelines for chemical safety are outlined in the facility safety plan.

_____ 7. A bacterial safety data sheet (MSDS) contains information about potential hazards; the safe use, storage, and handling of chemical products; and emergency procedures.

_____ 8. Nursing assistants do not need to check that all hazardous chemicals are clearly labeled.

_____ 9. Nursing assistants should use appropriate PPE such as gloves, goggles, and gowns when handling hazardous detergents and chemicals.

_____ 10. If the eyes or body are exposed to hazardous chemicals, they should not be flushed with water.

Oxygen Safety

Complete the following sentences.

1. The need for oxygen therapy is determined by a doctor, who identifies the _____, or amount, of oxygen to be delivered.

2. In healthcare facilities, _____ nursing staff members are responsible for setting up oxygen equipment and tubing and adjusting the rate of oxygen.

3. A nursing assistant observes that the amount of oxygen delivered is _____ and that equipment and tubing are properly placed.

4. Any resident changes or problems in the delivery of oxygen should be _____ to the licensed nursing staff.

5. A(n) _____ ensures a resident gets the prescribed amount of oxygen.

6. A(n) _____ gauge shows the amount of oxygen being delivered.

7. Oxygen _____ is used to move oxygen from the tank, cylinder, or wall unit to the resident.

8. A(n) _____ cannula is commonly used to deliver oxygen and has two small prongs that deliver oxygen into the nose.

9. Oxygen _____ cover the nose and mouth and are used if a resident has difficulty breathing through the nose or needs a large amount of oxygen.

10. A(n) _____ adds moisture to oxygen and prevents the resident's nasal passages from drying.

11. Medical oxygen tanks and cylinders are labeled with a United States Pharmacopeia (USP) code and are marked with a colored diamond that reads _____.

12. Oxygen tanks and cylinders contain gas under high _____, and if they are not handled correctly, can cause serious damage, injury, or death.

13. Nursing assistants ensure that supplies and equipment involved in oxygen therapy are kept _____ and in good, working order according to facility policy.

14. Oxygen safety precautions are _____ outside any room or building in which oxygen is used or stored.

15. When oxygen is in use, it is important to prevent _____ electricity.

16. Oil-based face creams, hair dryers, or _____ razors should never be used while oxygen is in use.

17. Oxygen tanks and cylinders should be kept at least _____ feet away from open flames, space heaters, large windows, or any other source of heat.

18. It is important not to use cleaning solutions, paint thinners, or _____ spray cans near oxygen, as these can ignite a fire.

19. A holistic nursing assistant should observe and report _____ irritation, changes in breathing or vital signs, and changes in the operation of equipment to the licensed nursing staff.

20. Tucking _____ under the nasal cannula tubing can prevent the cheeks or skin behind the ears from becoming sore.

Name: _____   Date: _____

Matching Chapter 17 Key Terms
Match each definition with the key term.

A. ankylosis
B. atony
C. axilla
D. ballistic
E. body alignment
F. body mechanics
G. connective tissue
H. contracture
I. double pendulum
J. embolus
K. foot drop
L. joints
M. orthostatic hypotension
N. orthotic
O. posture
P. prosthetic
Q. restorative care
R. stroke
S. syncope
T. thrombus
U. trochanter rolls

_____ 1. the action of ambulation; the leg swings forward from the hip, and the heel touches and rolls forward to the toe

_____ 2. a condition of paralysis or weakness in the dorsiflexion muscles of the foot and ankle; results in the dragging of the foot and toes

_____ 3. a sudden blockage or rupture of a blood vessel in the brain; can cause a loss of consciousness, partial loss of movement, and speech impairment; also called a *cerebrovascular accident (CVA)*

_____ 4. the stiffening or immobility of a joint

_____ 5. a condition in which blood pressure falls when a person stands

_____ 6. actions that promote safe, efficient movement without straining any muscles or joints

_____ 7. a device that supports, aligns, or corrects a weakened, immobile, injured, or deformed part of the body

_____ 8. moving under one's own momentum against external forces of gravity and air resistance

_____ 9. a mass (most commonly a blood clot) that moves and can become lodged in a blood vessel and obstruct blood flow

_____ 10. the optimal placement of all body parts such that bones are in their proper places and muscles are used efficiently

_____ 11. the armpit

_____ 12. temporary unconsciousness; fainting

_____ 13. lack of sufficient muscular strength

_____ 14. a blood clot that forms within a blood vessel and does not move

_____ 15. a type of body tissue that connects or supports other body tissues, structures, and organs; is composed of collagen fibers that provide strength and elastic fibers that enable flexibility

_____ 16. an artificial device designed to replace a missing body part

_____ 17. the tightening or shortening of a body part (such as a muscle, a tendon, or the skin) due to lack of movement

_____ 18. the way in which a person holds his or her body; the manner in which the body remains upright against gravity when sitting down, lying down, or standing up

_____ 19. locations where two or more bones connect

_____ 20. soft rolls that are placed along the body and span from above the hip to above the knee; prevent external rotation of the hips; are usually premade or made from a towel or bath blanket and are usually 12–14 inches long

_____ 21. care that assists with any modifications and adjustments residents must make to live as independently as possible

Understanding Body Mechanics
Complete the following sentences.

1. Body _____ are actions that promote safe, efficient movement by using the correct muscles and movements to avoid straining muscles or joints.

2. _____, or the ability to move, enables people to walk, climb stairs, or drive a car.

3. Muscles contract and move bones with the help of _____ tissue, which joins muscles and bones together.

4. _____ refers to the way a person holds his or her body.

5. A stable center of gravity is established when a person keeps his or her back _____ and bends only at the knees and hips.

6. A line of gravity is established when a person keeps the back straight and lifts objects _____ to his or her body.

7. A wide base of support is established when the feet are kept _____-width apart (about 12 inches).

8. Proper body alignment when _____ involves tucking in the buttocks, pulling the abdomen in and up, keeping the back flat, holding the chest up and slightly forward, stretching the waist, centering the shoulders above the hips, holding the head up, tucking the chin in, leaning weight forward, and being supported on the outsides of the feet.

9. Good _____ aligns and reduces stress between bones and joints, reduces wear and tear on joints, strengthens the spine and muscles, and conserves energy.

10. Nursing assistants need to be _____ of body mechanics as they complete everyday activities.

Principles of Body Mechanics

Complete the following principles of body mechanics.

1. A stable _____ of gravity

2. A(n) _____ of gravity

3. A(n) _____ base of support

4. Proper body _____ when standing

Using Proper Body Mechanics

Complete the following sentences.

1. It is important to move in a smooth and _____ way, not in a jerky way.

2. Because _____ an object can be difficult, it is better to pull, push, or roll the object instead.

3. When possible, it is best to lift, move, or carry objects with _____ hand(s).

4. It can be helpful to use the strongest muscles of the hips and thighs instead of the _____ muscles.

5. When caring for a resident in bed, a nursing assistant should keep the work and supplies on the bedside table _____ to his or her body.

6. A nursing assistant can keep the supplies and steps in a procedure at a comfortable _____ by raising the bed.

7. Nursing assistants need to maintain good physical health to reduce the chance of _____ on the job.

8. Proper body mechanics apply to the _____ involved in standing, sitting, lifting, and reaching.

9. When _____, the buttocks should be at the back of the chair, the spine straight, and the feet flat on the floor.

10. When lifting, it is best to bend the knees, keep the back straight, and never _____ (bend at the waist with the legs straight).

11. Nursing assistants should avoid _____ or stretching the body when reaching for equipment or supplies.

12. Healthcare staff members may wear _____ to protect against back injuries during care.

Body Alignment and Positioning

Select the *best* answer.

_____ 1. Nursing assistants are responsible for
   A. preventing immobility
   B. monitoring, but not changing, resident positions
   C. monitoring and changing resident positions
   D. making residents ambulate

_____ 2. Which of the following is *not* the responsibility of a nursing assistant?
   A. determining how often a resident should be repositioned
   B. moving a resident up in bed
   C. turning a resident
   D. transferring a resident into a wheelchair

_____ 3. The optimal placement of all body parts such that bones and muscles are used efficiently is called
   A. repositioning
   B. body mechanics
   C. immobility
   D. body alignment

_____ 4. Proper body alignment describes how the head, shoulders, spine, hips, knees, and ankles
   A. become immobile
   B. bend and twist
   C. are moved through the range of motion
   D. line up with each other

_____ 5. Repositioning increases
   A. trouble sleeping
   B. comfort
   C. restlessness
   D. pressure and strain on the skin

_____ 6. Repositioning restores the functions of
   A. blood clots in the legs
   B. contractures
   C. respiratory and gastrointestinal systems
   D. foot drop

_____ 7. Repositioning helps prevent
   A. atrophy and ankylosis
   B. relaxation
   C. sleep
   D. respiratory function

_____ 8. How does repositioning affect the skin?
   A. It increases the risk of decubitus ulcers.
   B. It relieves pressure on the skin.
   C. It causes more strain on the skin.
   D. It causes the skin to become dirty.

Using Equipment and Devices

Identify whether each statement is true or false.

_____ 1. If uncertain about using a type of positioning equipment, nursing assistants should check with the licensed nursing staff.

_____ 2. Some equipment and devices can be interpreted as restraints, but using them will never violate resident rights or cause harm.

_____ 3. Pillows of various sizes can help protect the skin, prop up a limb, support the head, or support the back for comfort.

_____ 4. Rolled towels and blankets may be used to support a resident and maintain proper body alignment.

_____ 5. Trochanter rolls are made from rolled towels or blankets and span from the top of the pelvic bone to the mid thigh to prevent internal rotation of the hips.

_____ 6. A draw sheet can be folded in half, placed on the middle of the bed, and used by the nursing assistant to turn and position the resident.

_____ 7. A footboard is a flat panel placed on top of the feet at the end of the bed to prevent foot drop.

_____ 8. A hip abduction wedge, which is usually made of a stiff foam rubber material, keeps the hips closely adducted.

_____ 9. A bed board is a wide board placed over the mattress for additional support.

_____ 10. At a minimum, residents should be rotated through at least four body positions during a shift.

Body Positions

Complete the following sentences.

1. In Fowler's position, a resident is seated in bed, and the head of the bed is raised to a _____° angle.

2. When a resident is seated in bed, and the head of the bed is raised to a 30° angle, this is _____ position.

3. In _____ Fowler's position, the head of the bed is raised to a 60–90° angle.

4. In Fowler's position, a resident's _____ may be elevated with a pillow under the knees.

5. The resident's head should be supported with a(n) _____ in Fowler's position.

6. In semi-Fowler's position, a foot support may be needed to help prevent _____.

7. In _____ position, the resident lies flat on his or her back.

8. In supine position, the bed should be flat, and the resident's arms and legs should be _____.

9. A resident's _____ and hands should be supported with pillows in supine position.

10. In supine position, a small, rolled towel or blanket should be used to support the small of the resident's _____ and under the knees to relieve strain on the back.

11. A(n) _____ roll can be used to prevent a resident's hips from rotating outward in supine position.

12. In supine position, padding can be used to protect _____ points on the resident's elbows, knees, and tailbone.

13. _____ position is a special supine position often used for residents who need certain medical or surgical procedures.

14. In Trendelenburg position, a resident's extended or bent legs are raised above the _____.

15. In prone position, a resident lies facedown, flat on the _____.

16. A resident's legs are extended, and the _____ is turned to one side in prone position.

17. In prone position, a resident's _____ should be extended down at the sides or bent upward at the elbows.

18. Pillows may need to be placed under a resident's lower legs to reduce pressure on the _____ in prone position.

19. In _____ position, the resident lies on one side.

20. When placing a resident in lateral position, nursing assistants should support the resident's head with a pillow, flex the lower arm, and bend the upper knee and hip to relieve pressure on the _____.

21. In lateral position, _____ should support the resident's back to maintain the position.

22. In Sims' position, the resident lies partly _____ and partly lateral.

23. In Sims' position, the resident's left leg and arm should be _____, and the right leg and arm should be flexed.

24. A resident's left arm should rest _____ him or her in Sims' position.

Following Positioning Guidelines

Select the *best* answer.

_____ 1. Resident positioning and repositioning requires
A. a material safety data sheet of the different body positions
B. attention to the resident's genetics
C. notification of facility mechanics for assistance
D. assistance if the resident is frail, is overweight, or has drainage tubes or an IV catheter

_____ 2. Which of the following is a safe resident-handling technique?
  A. maintaining a wide, stable base of support
  B. positioning the bed at the lowest height when providing care
  C. positioning the resident's hips at the level of the nursing assistant
  D. rotating the nursing assistant's spine to reach the resident's pressure points

_____ 3. Residents should be moved
  A. onto bed linens that are clean, dry, and wrinkled
  B. carefully and smoothly to avoid shearing of the skin
  C. quickly to decrease complaints of dizziness, shortness of breath, and rapid heartbeat
  D. with or without resident permission

_____ 4. Which of the following is an example of safe preparation?
  A. observing the resident in advance to determine whether care will be given
  B. using a mechanical lift and gait belt for every resident
  C. following specific safety guidelines
  D. avoiding asking other busy staff members for help

_____ 5. It is important for a holistic nursing assistant to ask
  A. other staff members for help as needed
  B. a paralyzed resident to ambulate independently
  C. other staff members to give the care
  D. if the resident is in pain only after changing the resident's position

Positioning in Bed

Complete the following sentences.

1. Proper _____ in bed provides good body alignment, helps maintain skin integrity, prevents decubitus ulcer formation, and promotes comfort and relaxation.

2. If moving an immobile resident up in bed, a nursing assistant should place pillows under the head and against the _____ to protect the head.

3. To slide a supine resident up in bed, two nursing assistants should grasp each side of the draw sheet, and in unison on the count of _____, gently slide the resident.

4. When positioning residents, nursing assistants can use proper body _____ by standing straight and facing the bed with knees slightly bent and feet pivoted toward the head of the bed.

_____ 5. If moving a resident with some _____ up in bed, a nursing assistant can put one arm under the resident's shoulders and the other arm under the resident's hips and ask the resident to bend his or her knees, brace the feet and hands firmly against the mattress, and on the count of three, push toward the head of the bed.

Turning a Resident in Bed

Identify whether each statement is true or false.

_____ 1. When a resident must remain in bed, shearing can help prevent skin breakdown, promote comfort, and prepare residents for care procedures.

_____ 2. An immobile resident, whether in bed or seated in a chair, should be repositioned or turned at least every four hours.

_____ 3. To turn a resident, a nursing assistant should assist the resident to bend his or her knees and cross the arms over the chest, reach over the resident and grasp the lift sheet at the shoulder and hip, and safely turn the resident.

_____ 4. Using proper body mechanics, a nursing assistant should roll a resident as a unit, gently and smoothly toward him or her.

_____ 5. A nursing assistant can use pillows to make further body alignment adjustments in the center of the bed and should straighten out the resident's clothing, bed linens, and any tubes.

Logrolling

Complete the following sentences.

1. During _____, a resident's body and spine are kept in straight alignment without twisting.

2. One of the nursing assistant's responsibilities is to _____ any tubing, such as IV catheters or urinary drainage bags, from being dislodged during logrolling.

3. During logrolling, disposable _____ are worn only if required for infection prevention and control.

4. In logrolling, the resident's entire _____ is moved to the side of the bed nearest the lead nursing assistant.

5. During logrolling, the resident's arms are crossed over the chest, a pillow is placed lengthwise between the resident's _____, and on the count of three, two nursing assistants roll the resident in a single movement using a draw sheet.

Dangling

Identify whether each statement is true or false.

_____ 1. An important first step prior to a resident getting out of bed is *dangling*, or sitting at the edge of the bed.

_____ 2. Sitting before standing increases the risk of orthostatic hypotension, a condition in which blood pressure falls when a resident stands.

_____ 3. Orthostatic hypotension occurs when gravity causes blood to pool in the abdomen and legs, decreasing blood pressure as less blood circulates back to the heart.

_____ 4. Orthostatic hypotension is more common in adults ages 65 and older because special receptors that sense and regulate blood pressure slow down with age.

_____ 5. An older heart may not beat fast enough to make up for a drop in blood pressure, and certain medications may contribute to orthostatic hypotension.

_____ 6. If orthostatic hypotension occurs, a resident may feel lightheaded or dizzy after standing up, feel weak, experience syncope, and become a fall risk.

_____ 7. A nursing assistant should stand behind a seated resident in case of a fall forward.

_____ 8. It is the nursing assistant's responsibility to observe the resident and tell the resident if he or she is dizzy or lightheaded.

_____ 9. During dangling, nursing assistants should check vital signs, check for difficulty breathing, and note if the skin is pale or bluish in color.

_____ 10. If a resident has difficulty breathing, a nursing assistant should return the resident to a lying position and notify the charge nurse during the next shift change.

Transferring a Resident

Complete the following sentences.

1. _____ residents from their beds to a chair, wheelchair, or stretcher is a procedure that requires concentration and safety awareness.

2. Transfer sheets, slides, roll boards, and wooden or plastic slide or transfer boards are typically used for transfers between beds and _____.

3. A(n) _____, sometimes called a transfer belt, is a safety device that nursing assistants can use to help prevent falls in residents who are standing or ambulating.

4. Mechanical _____ may be used to move residents who are extremely overweight, cannot bend their bodies, or are unable to bear weight on their feet.

5. A plastic or wooden _____ board is placed between the bed and stretcher, extending from the resident's shoulder to hips, and a lift sheet is typically used to transfer the resident over the board.

Identifying the Parts of a Wheelchair

Apply the appropriate labels to the image.

A. Wheel and hand rim
B. Footplate
C. Side panel or skirt guard
D. Armrest
E. Handgrip (push handle)
F. Arm
G. Front rigging
H. Wheel
I. Brake (wheel lock)
J. Tipping lever

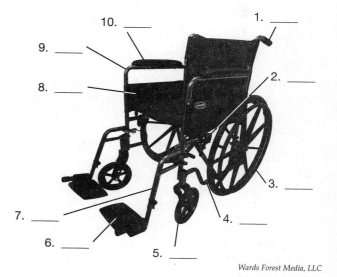

Wards Forest Media, LLC

Transferring from a Bed to a Chair or Wheelchair

Transferring a resident in one smooth or pivoting motion minimizes fatigue and promotes safety. The following steps are part of the procedure for transferring from a bed to a chair or wheelchair. For each set of steps, identify the proper order in which they should be completed by numbering them 1 through 5.

1. _____ Knock before entering the room.

   _____ Greet the resident and ask the resident to state his full name, if able. Then check the resident's identification bracelet.

   _____ Introduce yourself using your full name and title. Explain that you work with the licensed nursing staff and will be providing care.

   _____ Wash your hands or use hand sanitizer before entering the room.

   _____ Ask the licensed nursing staff how this procedure fits into the plan of care, if there are doctor's orders for the procedure, if there are any special instructions or precautions, and if the resident can be moved into the positions required for this procedure.

2. _____ Explain the procedure in simple terms, even if the resident is not able to communicate or is disoriented. Ask permission to perform the procedure.

_____ Provide privacy by closing the curtains, using a screen, or closing the door to the room.

_____ Lock the bed wheels and then lower the bed to its lowest position.

_____ Use Mr., Mrs., or Ms. and the resident's last name when conversing.

_____ Bring the necessary equipment into the room. Place the following items in an accessible location: a chair or wheelchair, a gait belt, a bath blanket, a robe and slippers, and a pillow.

3. _____ Apply a gait belt around the resident's waist over his clothing. The buckle of the gait belt should be in the front. Thread the belt through the teeth of the buckle and through the belt's two loops to lock it.

_____ Assist the resident to the edge of the bed and to a dangling position.

_____ Stabilize the chair for safety. If transferring the resident into a wheelchair, lock the wheels of the wheelchair and raise the footplates. Be sure the front swivel wheels of the wheelchair are facing forward.

_____ Position the chair or wheelchair next to the bed. If the resident has a weak side, position the chair or wheelchair so the resident can transfer using his stronger side.

_____ If there are side rails, raise and secure the rails on the opposite side of the bed from where you will be working. Lower the rail on the side you are working.

4. _____ Place one of your feet between the resident's feet and place your other foot outside one of the resident's feet. This will allow you to lock a sliding resident's knee with your knees.

_____ Place your feet so that you have room to pivot them toward the chair.

_____ Check that the gait belt is snug, but that there is still enough room to place your fingers under the belt.

_____ Stand in front of the resident with your feet about 12 inches apart.

_____ Face the resident and hold on to the gait belt using an underhand grasp for greater safety.

5. _____ Instruct the resident to hold on to your shoulders or arms, but not to put his arms around your neck.

_____ Once the resident is standing in front of the chair or wheelchair, ask if the resident feels the chair or wheelchair on the back of his legs.

_____ Continue to hold on to the gait belt while the resident gains his balance. Have the resident stand erect with his head up and back straight. Suggest the resident shift his weight from one foot to the other to become comfortable standing before starting the transfer.

_____ Using the gait belt, assist the resident into a standing position. Lift the resident using your arm and leg muscles. Bend your knees and keep your back straight. Do not twist your body.

_____ Face the chair or wheelchair and move your feet toward it as the resident follows, taking baby steps.

6. _____ Assist the resident into a seated position using proper body mechanics.

_____ Instruct the resident to put his hands on the armrests.

_____ Arrange the resident's robe and clothing and cover the resident's legs with a bath blanket. Make sure the bath blanket does not touch the floor or the wheels of the chair.

_____ Position the resident properly. The back and buttocks should be supported by the back of the chair or wheelchair. If there are footrests, place the resident's feet on them. There should be some space between the backs of the knees and calves and the edge of the seat. A small pillow behind the resident's lower back may provide support.

_____ Observe the resident for signs of discomfort or dizziness.

7. _____ Place the call light and personal items within reach.

_____ Conduct a safety check before leaving the room. The room should be clean and free from clutter or spills.

_____ Wash your hands or use hand sanitizer before leaving the room. Communicate any specific observations, complications, or unusual responses to the licensed nursing staff. Record this information, along with the care provided, in the chart or EMR.

_____ If transporting a resident using a wheelchair, push the wheelchair from behind and keep your body close to the chair. When entering an elevator, pull the wheelchair in backward. When leaving an elevator, wait until everyone leaves and then push the open button, turn the wheelchair around, and pull the wheelchair out of the elevator backward.

_____ Once the resident is back in his room, make sure his body is in alignment and he is safe and comfortable.

Transporting a Resident Using a Wheelchair

In this activity, you will practice transferring a resident from a bed to a wheelchair and manipulating, assembling, and disassembling wheelchair parts. To prepare for this activity, review the procedural checklist for Transferring a Resident from a Bed to a Wheelchair. Also have your FIRST CHECK procedural checklist nearby.

Form a group of three and assign each person a role. One person will be the nursing assistant, another a resident, and the third person will serve as the evaluator. Then complete each of the following steps:

1. Complete the FIRST, or Preparation, steps of the procedure, omitting any steps that are not applicable to the Transferring a Resident from a Bed to a Wheelchair procedure.

2. Did you omit any steps that are not applicable to the Transferring a Resident from a Bed to a Wheelchair procedure? If yes, explain which step(s) were omitted and why.

_____

_____

_____

_____

3. Lock the wheels of the wheelchair and swing the footrests outward. Remove the footrests and remove the armrest.

4. Assist the resident partner with putting on nonskid footwear and a gait belt.

5. Following the procedure for Transferring a Resident from a Bed to a Wheelchair, practice safe wheelchair transfer. Assist the resident into the wheelchair using the signal "on the count of three." The resident should not assist the nursing assistant. The nursing assistant must perform all the steps. The evaluator should assess how well the nursing assistant follows the procedure.

6. Reattach the wheelchair's armrest and footrests, being careful of the resident's lower extremities. Position the resident's feet on the footrests and remove the gait belt.

7. Instruct the resident to place his or her hands on his or her lap. Monitor the resident's hands throughout the entire procedure.

8. Take the resident for a wheelchair ride, being alert for safety at all times.

9. Upon returning, lock the wheels of the wheelchair, reapply the gait belt, and swing the footrests outward. Remove the footrests for practice and assist the resident back to bed.

10. Complete the CHECK, or Follow-Up and Reporting and Documentation, steps of the procedure, omitting any steps that are not applicable to the procedure.

11. Did you omit any steps that are not applicable to the procedure? If yes, explain which step(s) were omitted and why.

_____

_____

_____

_____

12. Switch roles with your partners so each partner has the opportunity to be the nursing assistant.

Transferring to a Chair or Wheelchair Using a Lift

Moving a weak or immobile resident with a mechanical lift promotes safety and comfort during the transfer process. The following steps are part of the procedure for transferring to a chair or wheelchair using a lift. For each set of steps, identify the proper order in which they should be completed by numbering them 1 through 5.

1. _____ Introduce yourself using your full name and title. Explain that you work with the licensed nursing staff and will be providing care.

_____ Ask the licensed nursing staff how this procedure fits into the plan of care, if there are doctor's orders for the procedure, if there are any special instructions or precautions, and if the resident can be moved into the positions required for this procedure.

_____ Knock before entering the room.

_____ Practice safety by asking for assistance from a coworker.

_____ Wash your hands or use hand sanitizer before entering the room.

2. _____ Explain the procedure in simple terms, even if the resident is not able to communicate or is disoriented. Ask permission to perform the procedure.

_____ Greet the resident and ask the resident to state his full name, if able. Then check the resident's identification bracelet.

_____ Provide privacy by closing the curtains, using a screen, or closing the door to the room.

_____ Bring the necessary equipment into the room. Place the following items in an accessible location: lift, the appropriate size and type of sling for the resident's weight and size, a chair or wheelchair, a robe and slippers, and a bath blanket.

_____ Use Mr., Mrs., or Ms. and the resident's last name when conversing.

3. _____ Roll the resident toward you and position the sling under him. You may need to roll the resident from side to side to maneuver the sling beneath him. The lower part of the sling should rest behind the resident's knees, and the upper part should rest beneath the resident's upper shoulders.

_____ If there are side rails, raise and secure the rails on the opposite side of the bed from where you will be working. Lower the rail on the side you are working.

_____ Position the lift bar and frame over the bed in an open position. Lock the lift's wheels.

_____ Lock the bed wheels and then lower the bed to the lowest position.

_____ Position the chair or wheelchair next to the bed and stabilize the chair for safety. If transferring the resident into a wheelchair, lock the wheels of the wheelchair and raise the footplates. Be sure the front swivel wheels of the wheelchair face forward.

4. _____ Attach the sling to the lift following the instructions in the manufacturer's handbook.

_____ Make sure the open ends of the lift's hooks that will attach to the sling face away from the resident.

_____ Ask the resident to fold his arms across his chest.

_____ When the lift holds the resident freely above the bed and is stable, move the resident away from the bed. Your coworker should support the resident's legs.

_____ Position the resident above the chair or wheelchair.

5. _____ Gently lower the resident as your coworker guides him into the chair or wheelchair. If the resident is being lowered into a chair, be sure the chair will not move.

_____ Make sure the resident's feet and hands are positioned comfortably in the chair.

_____ Cover the resident with a blanket. Make sure the blanket does not touch the floor.

_____ Follow your facility's policy to determine if the sling can be left beneath the resident.

_____ Lower the lift's bar so you can easily unhook the sling.

6. _____ Remove, clean, and store equipment in the proper location. Remove soiled linens and discard disposable equipment.

_____ Make sure the resident is comfortable and place the call light and personal items within reach.

_____ Wash your hands or use hand sanitizer before leaving the room. Communicate any specific observations, complications, or unusual responses to the licensed nursing staff. Record this information, along with the care provided, in the chart or EMR.

_____ Conduct a safety check before leaving the room. The room should be clean and free from clutter or spills.

_____ Wash your hands to ensure infection control.

Transferring from a Bed to a Stretcher

Select the *best* answer.

_____ 1. During transfer to a stretcher, the stretcher should be
   A. between the nursing assistant's and the resident's body
   B. behind the nursing assistant's body
   C. on the other side of the room
   D. beneath the resident in the bed

_____ 2. Which part of the resident's body is usually transferred to the stretcher first?
   A. right side
   B. left side
   C. upper part
   D. lower part

_____ 3. A stretcher should be pushed
   A. with the resident's head facing forward
   B. sideways
   C. with the resident's feet facing forward
   D. with the side rails down

Promoting Comfort

Identify whether each statement is true or false.

_____ 1. Holistic nursing assistants use a resident's preferred position for rest, if possible, and follow the plan of care.

_____ 2. Straightening linens, changing soiled linens and bedding, and covering the feet and legs all promote comfort.

_____ 3. A resident's position must be adjusted at least every six hours for maximum comfort, and pillows, blankets, or rolls can be used.

_____ 4. Nursing assistants should identify and disconnect any mechanical sources of discomfort, such as tubes, drains, syringe caps, or other equipment.

_____ 5. It is important to alert the licensed nursing staff if residents complain of discomfort related to tubes and drains.

Understanding Ambulation

Complete the following sentences.

1. _____, or walking around, is essential for achieving optimal well-being.

2. Ambulation improves circulation and muscle tone, preserves lung tissue and airway function, and helps promote muscle and joint _____.

3. Ambulation requires an action called a(n) _____ pendulum, in which the two legs coordinate so that one foot is always in contact with the ground.

4. When a person walks, the leg leaves the ground and swings forward from the hip; this is the _____ pendulum.

5. When the leg strikes the ground, the heel touches first and rolls through to the toe; this motion is the _____ pendulum.

6. During running, a(n) _____ phase occurs when both feet are off the ground at the same time and the body's momentum moves it forward.

Name: _____ Date: _____

The Stages of Ambulation
Complete each stage of ambulation in the illustration.

1. Assist the resident into a(n) _____ position.

2. Assist the resident in _____.

3. The resident begins _____.

Assisting with Ambulation
Identify whether each statement is true or false.

_____ 1. Before beginning ambulation, a nursing assistant should always ask if the resident is feeling any pain.

_____ 2. Depending on a resident's level of mobility, ambulation with a resident may require the use of a full-body lift, sit-to-stand lift, or gait belt.

_____ 3. The physical environment and equipment do not pose risks and do not need to be organized prior to ambulation.

_____ 4. Holistic nursing assistants include the resident in all actions of ambulation so the resident knows what to expect.

_____ 5. It is important to use good posture and proper body mechanics when assisting residents.

_____ 6. If a resident begins to collapse during ambulation, a nursing assistant should try to hold the resident up.

_____ 7. Significant others may assist with ambulation even if members of the licensed nursing staff have not given permission.

_____ 8. One responsibility of nursing assistants is encouraging and assisting with mobility for residents who are ill and want to stay in bed.

_____ 9. If the resident has a weak right side, the nursing assistant should stand behind and slightly to the right of the resident.

_____ 10. If the resident has a weak left side, the nursing assistant should stand behind and slightly to the left of the resident.

Abbreviations and Acronyms Related to Mobility
Identify the abbreviation for each meaning in the table.

Abbreviations and Acronyms Related to Resident Mobility	
Abbreviation or Acronym	Meaning
1. _____	ambulation
2. _____	bed rest
3. _____	bathroom privileges
4. _____	head of bed
5. _____	out of bed
6. _____	up as desired
7. _____	wheelchair

Assistive Devices Used During Ambulation
Select the *best* answer.

_____ 1. Which of the following is true of canes?
A. They are useful for residents who have had surgery and cannot ambulate.
B. They cannot improve balance or assist stability.
C. They help residents who have arthritis that results in restricted movement.
D. They are used by all older adults recovering from a stroke.

_____ 2. Crutches
A. are often used by residents who have short-term conditions
B. do not assist residents with amputations
C. cause disabilities due to insufficient support
D. require less upper body strength than a walker

_____ 3. A functional grip cane
A. is a type of single-shaft cane used for adolescents
B. has a straight handle for a steadier grip
C. provides support for residents who require a mechanical lift
D. has a slim, contoured handle that collapses with weight

Name: _____   Date: _____

_____ 4. The quad cane
    A. has a base with six, skid-resistant prongs
    B. should be held on the resident's weaker side
    C. offers more stability than a single-shaft cane and assists with balance
    D. should be in line with the resident's elbow crease when the elbow is slightly bent

_____ 5. Which of the following is true of walkers?
    A. They are helpful for residents who have had surgery on the upper limbs.
    B. They are carried by residents to break a fall.
    C. They are preferred to canes or crutches because they decrease strength.
    D. They let residents use their arms to take weight off the lower body.

_____ 6. A walker must fit
    A. the resident properly, with the handles even with the resident's wrist
    B. the resident properly as the resident stoops to ambulate
    C. the resident properly, with elbows straight holding on to the walker
    D. into the plan of care ordered by a nursing assistant

_____ 7. A standard, pickup walker
    A. provides a narrower base of support
    B. is used by residents who prefer a quad cane
    C. is used by residents who cannot pick up the walker while ambulating
    D. has four solid, rubber-tipped legs with a wide base

_____ 8. A rolling walker, or rollator, has
    A. motorized legs with wheels or casters that roll during ambulation
    B. four legs with wheels or casters that roll during ambulation and sometimes hand brakes
    C. four wheels on the front and six wheels on the back
    D. a platform to ride on like a scooter

_____ 9. Which of the following is true of ambulating with a walker?
    A. Residents may gradually be able to ambulate for longer periods of time using a walker.
    B. Residents will not become tired if properly ambulating with a walker.
    C. Residents should practice climbing stairs with a walker.
    D. Nursing assistants do not need to monitor a resident with a walker.

_____ 10. A walker should be placed
    A. so the resident can stand up and walk around the walker
    B. so the resident can grip it with one hand and use it to stand
    C. about one step ahead of the seated resident with the legs level on the ground
    D. so the resident can take the first step with the strongest leg

_____ 11. Standard underarm crutches
    A. can be adjusted for height, have padding, and are for short-term use
    B. have a U-shaped underarm support to distribute weight
    C. feature a horizontal, padded armrest and straps
    D. are slipped on and off through a forearm cuff

_____ 12. When providing assistance with crutches, nursing assistants should
    A. know that all healthcare facilities will allow them to ambulate a resident with crutches
    B. ignore special procedures, but follow basic training for ambulating residents with crutches
    C. help residents with splintered crutches ambulate
    D. always check facility policies and procedures before assisting

_____ 13. Which of the following statements about gait is true?
    A. A four-point gait is used when both legs have no weight-bearing ability.
    B. A two-point gait is used when both legs can bear some weight.
    C. A three-point gait is used when an affected, or injured, leg can bear all weight.
    D. A swing-through gait is used when the legs are paralyzed, but not in braces.

Abbreviations and Acronyms Related to Rehabilitation and Restorative Care

Identify the abbreviation for each meaning in the table.

Abbreviations and Acronyms Related to Rehabilitation and Restorative Care	
Abbreviation or Acronym	**Meaning**
1. _____	active-assistive range of motion
2. _____	abduction
3. _____	activity of daily living
4. _____	continuous passive motion
5. _____	range of motion

Rehabilitation and Restorative Care

Complete the following sentences.

1. Rehabilitation and restorative care are complementary services that work together to help residents regain lost abilities, maintain abilities, and _____ further loss of abilities because of illness, trauma, or disability.

126   The Nursing Assistant

2. The first goal of _____ care is to preserve and support improvements accomplished by rehabilitation.

3. The second goal of restorative care is to offer _____ and adjustments that enable residents to live as independently as possible.

4. Restorative care is intended to increase residents' _____ and to help residents achieve and maintain the highest possible physical, mental, and psychosocial function.

5. Older adults often require both rehabilitation and restorative care after a(n) _____, or a blockage of a blood vessel in the brain.

6. Rehabilitation and restorative care can be given in hospitals, outpatient clinics, long-term care facilities, residential care facilities, or an older adult's _____.

7. There are _____ requirements for the provision of specific rehabilitation and restorative services in nursing facilities.

8. Rehabilitative and restorative care may last only a few _____ or can occur over a long period of time due to the type or chronic nature of a disease or condition.

9. Rehabilitative care typically includes _____ therapy, occupational therapy, speech therapy, and activity or recreational therapy.

10. Once care has been ordered by the doctor, the healthcare team consults with the resident and often the _____ to determine a plan of care based on realistic goals.

11. A resident's positive _____, coping skills, willingness to participate, and family

support can make a difference with restorative care.

12. A(n) _____ therapist can provide range-of-motion exercises, muscle strengthening, and treatments such as heat and water therapy, electric nerve therapy, traction, and massage therapy.

13. _____ therapists provide support with ADLs, which include bathing, dressing, cooking, and eating to enhance independence.

14. _____ therapists help residents with communication and swallowing.

15. The _____ director or recreational therapist provides activities that promote socialization, encourage mobility, and improve self-esteem.

16. Nursing assistants help in restorative care by focusing on resident _____, providing encouragement, celebrating successes, observing resident progress, and providing ongoing documentation.

17. In rehabilitative care, regular exercise helps maintain joint mobility and prevent contractures, _____ (lack of strength), and atrophy of the muscles.

18. Regular exercise stimulates circulation to prevent the formation of a(n) _____, or an immobile blood clot.

19. Regular exercise can help prevent a dangerous _____, or mobile blood clot.

20. Nursing assistants assist residents with _____ (ROM) exercises to improve heart and lung function, increase flexibility, prevent decubitus ulcers, improve mood, and aid in meeting care goals.

Types of ROM Exercises

Identify the type of ROM exercise for each description in the table.

Types of ROM Exercises	
Type	**Description**
1. _____ _____	Uses the full range of motion of one or more body parts and does not require the physical help of healthcare staff
2. _____ _____	Is used when a resident needs help achieving the full range of motion in one or more body parts
3. _____ _____	Is used when a resident cannot move one or more body parts, requiring complete assistance from the healthcare staff

Assisting with ROM

Identify whether each statement is true or false.

_____ 1. ROM exercises are usually performed quickly and gently to avoid hurting the resident or harming the joints or bones.

_____ 2. If a resident is in pain, ROM exercises must continue, but the licensed nursing staff should be notified.

_____ 3. There are sometimes contraindications for ROM exercises, or situations in which ROM exercises should not be used.

_____ 4. A nursing assistant should discuss the schedule and importance of ROM exercises with the resident to encourage participation.

_____ 5. When performing ROM exercises, a nursing assistant should begin at the top of the body and work down, supporting each joint through its range of motion at least eight times.

Body Movements

Identify the body movement for each description in the table.

Body Movements	
Movement	**Description**
1. _____	The act of bending a joint
2. _____	The act of straightening a joint
3. _____	An exaggerated, or extreme, extension
4. _____	Lateral (sideways) movement away from the midline (an invisible line running vertically through the body)
5. _____	Lateral movement toward the midline of the body
6. _____	Turning of a body part around an axis, or fixed point
7. _____	Rotating a body part in a complete circle
8. _____	Rotating a body part away from the body
9. _____	Rotating a body part toward the body

Using Assistive Devices

Complete the following sentences.

1. _____ devices help people function safely and independently in healthcare facilities and at home.

2. A(n) _____ is an artificial device designed to replace a missing body part.

3. One example of a prosthetic is _____, which may replace all or some of a person's teeth and gums.

4. _____ eyes typically consist of glass or plastic prostheses made to look like eyes and placed in the eye sockets.

5. A(n) _____ is a device that supports, aligns, or corrects a weak, immobile, injured, or deformed body part.

Name: _____ Date: _____

Matching Chapter 18 Key Terms

Match each definition with the key term.

A. apical pulse
B. apnea
C. aural
D. axillary temperature
E. body mass index (BMI)
F. bradycardia
G. bradypnea
H. carotid pulse
I. Celsius (C)
J. diastolic blood pressure
K. dyspnea
L. Fahrenheit (F)
M. hyperventilation
N. hypotension
O. hypoventilation
P. hypoxia
Q. ideal body weight (IBW)
R. probe
S. radial pulse
T. stertorous breathing
U. stethoscope
V. systolic blood pressure
W. tachycardia
X. tachypnea
Y. temporal arteries
Z. tympanic temperature

_____ 1. the pressure of blood against the arteries when the heart muscle contracts

_____ 2. a calculation that uses height and weight to determine whether a person is a healthy weight, overweight, or underweight

_____ 3. slow, shallow breathing

_____ 4. unusually rapid breathing

_____ 5. the healthiest weight for an individual

_____ 6. pulse that is slower than 60 beats per minute

_____ 7. a period of absent breathing

_____ 8. the pressure of blood against the arteries when the heart muscle relaxes

_____ 9. deep, rapid breathing

_____ 10. blood pressure that is too low

_____ 11. a type of breathing that sounds like snoring

_____ 12. body temperature measured by placing a thermometer into the ear

_____ 13. related to the ear

_____ 14. temperature scale in which water freezes at 32° and boils at 212°

_____ 15. long, thin medical instrument used to measure temperature

_____ 16. a heart rate of more than 100 beats per minute

_____ 17. arteries located on each side of the head

_____ 18. unusually slow breathing

_____ 19. temperature scale in which water freezes at 0° and boils at 100°

_____ 20. heartbeat measured by listening to the apex of the heart with a stethoscope

_____ 21. body temperature measured by placing a thermometer under the armpit

_____ 22. heartbeat measured by feeling the carotid artery

_____ 23. difficult breathing

_____ 24. lack of adequate oxygen in the body

_____ 25. heartbeat measured by feeling the inside of the thumb side of the wrist

_____ 26. a medical device used to listen to body sounds such as breathing, heartbeat, and lung and bowel sounds

Understanding Vital Signs

Complete the following sentences.

1. _____ signs are the rates or values of a person's temperature, pulse, respirations, and blood pressure.

2. Vital signs are considered *vital* because they relate to essential body _____.

3. When vital signs are measured, a resident's height and _____ may also be measured and recorded.

4. Temperature is recorded in degrees and may be measured using either the Fahrenheit or _____ scale.

5. Temperatures can be oral, rectal, _____, tympanic, or temporal.

6. Tympanic thermometers measure the temperature of blood vessels in the _____.

7. The most commonly used pulse locations are the radial artery, apical artery, and _____ artery.

8. A high body temperature can signal that a resident has a(n) _____.

9. It is best to count _____ rate with no warning immediately after the pulse is taken.

10. To measure blood pressure, a nursing assistant will need a manual or electronic _____.

Measuring and Recording Vital Signs

Identify whether each statement is true or false.

_____ 1. The Celsius scale is most commonly used to measure body temperature in the United States.

_____ 2. Today, healthcare facilities only use digital thermometers.

_____ 3. A patient who is very ill in the hospital will only have vital signs taken during admission.

_____ 4. A stethoscope is used to help measure radial pulse.

_____ 5. Carotid pulse is normally taken when a resident is unconscious.

_____ 6. Individual facility guidelines do not impact how vital signs are recorded.

_____ 7. It is important that nursing assistants recognize when vital signs are not within normal range and report these findings immediately to the licensed nursing staff.

_____ 8. Measuring respiration rate helps determine a resident's level of blood oxygenation.

_____ 9. It is always best to alert residents before measuring their respiration rate.

_____ 10. Body temperature is regulated by the cerebellum.

Locations for Measuring Temperature

Consider the following scenarios and identify the *best* location for measuring the patient's or resident's body temperature.

1. A resident is receiving oxygen via a nasal cannula. She had a cerebrovascular accident (CVA), fell, and has a contusion on her forehead. She has an affected left side and an IV catheter in her upper right arm. She is experiencing bowel and bladder incontinence. Which location should the nursing assistant select to obtain her temperature?

_____

2. A patient is one year of age. He is vomiting and sweating. His father reports that he has been pulling at both ears. Which location should the nursing assistant select to obtain his temperature?

_____

3. A resident requires monthly, routine vital signs and is enjoying excellent health at 89 years of age. She has bilateral hearing aids, has a wig, and is oriented to person, place, and time. Which location should the nursing assistant select to obtain her temperature?

_____

4. A patient is attending his yearly physical examination at a medical office. Which common method is most likely used to obtain his temperature?

_____

5. A patient is unconscious and has head trauma related to a motor vehicle accident. His extremities are unaffected. Which location should the nursing assistant select to obtain his temperature?

_____

Identifying Average Body Temperature Ranges

Complete the table by identifying the missing Fahrenheit temperature ranges for individuals 12 years and older.

Average Ranges of Body Temperature	
Thermometer	**Twelve Years and Older**
Oral	1. _____ (36.4°C–37.5°C)
Rectal	2. _____ (37.0°C–38.1°C)
Tympanic	3. _____ (37.0°C–38.0°C)
Axillary	4. _____ (35.9°C–37.0°C)
Temporal Artery	5. _____ (36.2°C–37.8°C)

Identifying Pulse Locations

Apply the appropriate callouts to the image.

A. Dorsalis pedis pulse
B. Brachial pulse
C. Temporal pulse
D. Femoral pulse
E. Carotid pulse
F. Popliteal pulse
G. Apical pulse
H. Radial pulse

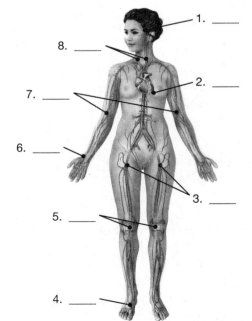

© Body Scientific International

The Stethoscope

Select the *best* answer.

_____ 1. The stethoscope is used to measure
A. an apical pulse
B. a radial pulse
C. urinary output
D. a resident's height

_____ 2. A stethoscope should be disinfected
A. after use
B. before use
C. every year
D. Both A and B.

_____ 3. If a nursing assistant cannot hear heartbeat clearly, he or she should
A. tell the resident that his or her heartbeat cannot be heard
B. rotate the diaphragm and try again
C. document that the heartbeat cannot be detected
D. report to the licensed nursing staff

_____ 4. The stethoscope is commonly used
A. to hear radial pulse
B. with an automatic vital signs machine
C. to measure manual blood pressure
D. to measure a resident's temperature

_____ 5. A stethoscope is composed of
A. a cuff and sphygmomanometer
B. two earpieces, rubber or plastic tubing, a brace, a diaphragm, and a bell
C. a light and electronic monitor
D. an oximeter and lead wire

Measuring Pulse Rates

Complete the following sentences.

1. Pulse rate is measured by _____ or hearing the pulse and counting the number of beats in one minute.

2. _____ pulse is taken when a resident is breathing normally and sitting.

3. Pulse rate is measured in _____.

4. The _____ of a pulse describes the pause between beats.

5. A pulse that is weak, or _____, is hard to feel.

6. A pulse that is slower than 60 beats per minute is called _____.

7. A fast pulse of 100 beats or more per minute is called _____.

8. Counting a(n) _____ pulse is the most common method of measuring heart rate and its quality.

Average Resting Pulse Rates Per Minute

Complete the table by identifying the missing resting pulse rates.

Average Resting Pulse Rates Per Minute	
Letter	**Step**
Adults	1. _____
Teenagers	2. _____
Children	3. _____
Infants	4. _____

Measuring a Radial Pulse

In this activity, you will practice portions of the procedure for measuring a radial pulse. To prepare for this activity, review the procedural checklist for Measuring a Radial Pulse. Also have your FIRST CHECK procedural checklist nearby.

Form a group of three and assign each person a role. One person will be the nursing assistant, another a resident, and the third person will serve as the evaluator. Then complete each of the following steps:

1. Complete the FIRST, or Preparation, steps of the procedure, omitting any steps that are not applicable to the Measuring a Radial Pulse procedure.

2. Did you omit any steps that are not applicable to the Measuring a Radial Pulse procedure? If yes, explain which step(s) were omitted and why.

_____

_____

_____

3. Ask the resident partner to sit in a chair. The evaluator should sit on one side of the resident, with the nursing assistant on the opposite side of the resident. The evaluator and nursing assistant will count the resident's radial pulse on either wrist. When ready to begin, the nursing assistant will note the time on the clock and tell the evaluator to start. Both the evaluator and nursing assistant will count the resident's pulse for a full minute.

4. Do not state the result at the end of the minute. Instead, the nursing assistant and evaluator should write down their results on separate pieces of paper. Show each other your results. The results must be within four beats of each other to pass. Keep practicing with new resident partners until you achieve this goal.

5. Once the nursing assistant and evaluator have achieved a radial pulse measurement within four beats of one another, the nursing assistant should complete the final five CHECK, or Follow-Up and Reporting and Documentation, steps of the procedure, omitting any steps that are not applicable to the procedure.

6. Did you omit any steps that are not applicable to the Measuring a Radial Pulse procedure? If yes, explain which step(s) were omitted and why.

_____

_____

_____

Respiration Facts

Identify whether each statement is true or false.

_____ 1. The rate of respiration is the measurement of a resident's cardiac cycle.

_____ 2. Respiration rate helps determine a resident's level of blood oxygenation.

_____ 3. A resident's respiration rate provides information about conditions such as asthma, heart disease, and even infections.

_____ 4. When measuring respiration rate, a nursing assistant should count each inhalation and exhalation separately.

_____ 5. It is best to count respiration rate with no warning immediately after pulse is taken.

_____ 6. A normal adult's respiration rate is 12–20 breaths per minute.

_____ 7. Hyperventilation is characterized by slow, shallow breathing.

_____ 8. Observing how well a resident is breathing is not as important as determining respiration rate.

_____ 9. A pulse oximeter is used to measure blood oxygenation.

_____ 10. Apnea occurs when there is a period of no breathing at all.

Counting Respirations

In this activity, you will practice portions of the procedure for counting respirations. To prepare for this activity, review the procedural checklist for Counting Respirations. Also have your FIRST CHECK procedural checklist nearby.

Form a group of three and assign each person a role. One person will be the nursing assistant, another a resident, and the third person will serve as the evaluator. Then complete each of the following steps:

1. Complete the FIRST, or Preparation, steps of the procedure, omitting any steps that are not applicable to the Counting Respirations procedure.

2. Did you omit any steps that are not applicable to the Counting Respirations procedure? If yes, explain which step(s) were omitted and why.

_____

_____

_____

3. Ask the resident partner to lie down on a bed. Both the evaluator and nursing assistant will count the resident's respiration rate. When ready to begin, the nursing assistant will note the time on the clock and tell the evaluator to start. Both the evaluator and nursing assistant will count the resident's respiration rate for a full minute.

4. Do not state the result at the end of the minute. Instead, the nursing assistant and evaluator should write down their results on separate pieces of paper. Show each other your results. The results must be within two breaths of each other to pass. Keep practicing with new resident partners until you achieve this goal.

5. Once the nursing assistant and evaluator have achieved a respiration rate measurement within two breaths of one another, the nursing assistant should complete the final five CHECK, or Follow-Up and Reporting and Documentation, steps of the procedure, omitting any steps that are not applicable to the procedure.

6. Did you omit any steps that are not applicable to the Counting Respirations procedure? If yes, explain which step(s) were omitted and why.

_____

_____

_____

Taking a Blood Pressure

When taking blood pressure, nursing assistants must follow the proper procedure to ensure the measurement is accurate. The following steps are part of the procedure for taking a manual blood pressure. For each set of steps, identify the proper order in which they should be completed by numbering them 1 through 5.

1. _____ Knock before entering the room.

_____ Introduce yourself using your full name and title. Explain that you work with the licensed nursing staff and will be providing care.

_____ Explain the procedure in simple terms. Ask permission to perform the procedure.

_____ Wash your hands or use hand sanitizer before entering the room.

_____ Greet the resident and ask the resident to state his full name, if able. Then check the resident's identification bracelet. Use Mr., Mrs., or Ms. and the last name when conversing.

2. _____ Clean the earpieces of the stethoscope with an antiseptic wipe and warm the diaphragm with your hands before cleaning it with antiseptic wipes.

_____ Squeeze the cuff to expel any remaining air.

_____ With your fingertips, locate the brachial artery at the inner aspect of the elbow.

_____ Unroll the blood pressure cuff and loosen the valve on the bulb of the sphygmomanometer by turning it counterclockwise.

_____ Position the resident's arm so it rests level with the heart with the palm turned upward.

3. ____ Close the valve on the bulb of the sphygmomanometer by turning it clockwise.

____ Place the center of the cuff, usually marked with an arrow, above the brachial artery.

____ Find the brachial pulse.

____ Wrap the cuff smoothly and snugly around the exposed arm about 1 inch above the elbow.

____ Place the earpieces of the stethoscope in your ears.

4. ____ Inflate the cuff to 180 mmHg.

____ Deflate the cuff by slowly turning the valve on the bulb of the sphygmomanometer counterclockwise at an even rate of 2–4 millimeters per second.

____ Place the warmed diaphragm of the stethoscope over the brachial artery. Hold the measuring scale level with your eyes.

____ Continue deflating the cuff slowly and evenly. Note the dial reading when the sound (beat) disappears. This is the diastolic blood pressure.

____ Listen carefully while the cuff is deflating. Note the dial reading when you hear the first sound (beat). This is the systolic blood pressure.

5. ____ Report abnormal results to the appropriate licensed nursing staff member immediately.

____ Return the stethoscope to its storage location.

____ Record the blood pressure on a pad, on a form, or in the electronic record.

____ Return the cuff to its case or wall mount.

____ Clean the earpieces and diaphragm of the stethoscope with antiseptic wipes.

Factors That Affect Blood Pressure

Explain how each of the factors listed here can affect blood pressure.

1. Diet: _____

_____

2. Weight: _____

_____

3. Exercise: _____

_____

4. Race: _____

_____

5. Time of day: _____

_____

6. Position: _____

_____

7. Cigarettes and alcohol: _____

_____

8. Drugs or medications: _____

_____

9. Stress, fear, or pain: _____

_____

Measuring Height and Weight of an Ambulatory Resident

In this activity, you will practice portions of the procedure for measuring the height and weight of an ambulatory resident. To prepare for this activity, review the procedural checklist for Measuring the Height and Weight of Ambulatory Residents. Also have your FIRST CHECK procedural checklist nearby.

Form a group of three and assign each person a role. One person will be the nursing assistant, another a resident, and the third person will serve as the evaluator. Then complete each of the following steps:

1. Complete the FIRST, or Preparation, steps of the procedure, omitting any steps that are not applicable to the Measuring the Height and Weight of Ambulatory Residents procedure.

2. Did you omit any steps that are not applicable to the Measuring the Height and Weight of Ambulatory Residents procedure? If yes, explain which step(s) were omitted and why.

_____

_____

_____

_____

3. Complete the procedure for measuring the resident's weight and height using a balance scale.

4. Complete the final five CHECK, or Follow-Up and Reporting and Documentation, steps of the procedure, omitting any steps that are not applicable to the procedure. Assume that the resident will be returning to bed after the procedure.

5. Did you omit any steps that are not applicable to the Measuring the Height and Weight of Ambulatory Residents procedure? If yes, explain which step(s) were omitted and why.

_____

_____

_____

_____

Measuring the Height and Weight
of Bedridden Residents

Select the *best* answer.

_____ 1. The height of a bedridden resident is typically
measured with
   A. a balance scale
   B. a bed scale
   C. a tape measure
   D. a hydraulic lift

_____ 2. Between which two points is the height of a
bedridden resident measured?
   A. top of the head to the bottom of the heel
   B. neck to the bottom of the heel
   C. top of the head to the ankle
   D. forehead to the top of the toes

_____ 3. While being weighed in a lift scale, bedridden
residents should hold
   A. their arms above their heads
   B. their arms out to either side
   C. their arms crossed over their chests
   D. their arms to their sides

_____ 4. The weights of a lift scale should be adjusted when
   A. the resident is lowered back to the bed
   B. the resident is lying in bed
   C. the resident is hanging freely in the sling
       over the bed
   D. the resident is holding on to the sling bar

Name: _____ Date: _____

Matching Chapter 19 Key Terms

Match each definition with the key term.

A. auscultation
B. glucometer
C. guaiac test
D. inspection
E. laryngeal mirror
F. occult blood
G. ophthalmoscope
H. otoscope
I. palpation
J. percussion
K. point-of-care testing (POCT)
L. specimens
M. speculum
N. sputum

_____ 1. a medical instrument used to examine the ears

_____ 2. a medical instrument used to examine the vagina or other body cavities

_____ 3. the act of placing one hand on the surface of the body and striking or tapping a finger on that hand with the index finger or middle finger of the other hand

_____ 4. the act of listening to the internal sounds of the body with a stethoscope

_____ 5. a medical instrument used to examine the mouth, tongue, and teeth

_____ 6. a diagnostic procedure used to detect fecal occult blood

_____ 7. a blend of saliva and mucus; also called *phlegm*

_____ 8. the act of using the hands to examine the body

_____ 9. a medical instrument that measures blood sugar levels

_____ 10. the presence of very small amounts of blood in the feces

_____ 11. specimen collection in the place where a resident is receiving care

_____ 12. a medical instrument used to examine the eyes

_____ 13. the visual examination of a body part

_____ 14. samples of a bodily substance

The Physical Exam

Complete the following sentences.

1. A physical _____ (PE) is typically performed in a medical facility, either annually or as needed, to determine the status or condition of a patient's body systems and functions.

2. The role of the nursing assistant is to _____ the room and resident for a physical examination.

3. Prior to a physical examination, patients provide _____ related to their health history, current medications, supplements, nutrition, exercise, sleep, pain, mental health, past surgeries, hospitalizations, and relevant family medical history.

4. Information shared by a patient is often documented by the nursing assistant, who enters the information into the patient's electronic _____.

5. A physical examination is performed by a doctor, _____ practitioner, or physician assistant who reviews the patient's health history and information before beginning the examination.

6. A patient's _____ signs are measured by a nursing assistant or medical assistant.

7. Health _____ tests may be ordered for checking cholesterol levels, testing for osteoporosis, conducting Pap smears for female patients, and conducting prostate cancer screenings for male patients.

8. In a(n) _____ physical exam, the healthcare provider examines each body system.

9. The healthcare provider starts at the patient's head and moves toward the feet in a(n) _____ examination.

10. _____ is the visual examination of a body part (for example, observing for bruises).

11. _____ is the use of the hands to feel an object such as a lump or mass in the body.

12. _____ is the method of placing one hand on the surface of the patient's body and then striking or tapping a finger on that hand with the index finger or middle finger of the opposite hand.

13. Percussion examines a patient's underlying body _____ for changes or fluid in the abdominal or chest cavities.

14. _____ is the method of listening to the internal sounds of the body (for example, using a stethoscope to listen to heartbeat).

Types of Physical Examinations

Identify whether each statement is true or false.

_____ 1. Some types of physical exams include comprehensive annual, pre-employment, travel, well-woman, well-man, and well-baby exams.

_____ 2. An annual physical examination is an opportunity to evaluate body system function and any diseases or conditions.

_____ 3. Early diagnosis of a disease or condition, such as type 2 diabetes or cancer, often leads to a more negative prognosis, particularly if treatment begins without delay.

_____ 4. An annual physical examination often includes an assessment of vital signs, routine laboratory tests; chest X-rays; electrocardiograms; and screenings for diabetes, colon or lung cancer, cardiovascular problems, bone mineral density, vision, hearing, and skin health.

_____ 5. Examples of X-rays include the annual flu shot and the pneumococcal, shingles, or herpes zoster vaccines.

Well-Woman Examinations

Identify whether each statement is true or false.

_____ 1. Sometimes a well-woman exam is performed by a gynecologist, primary care provider, or other appropriate licensed healthcare provider during an annual comprehensive physical examination.

_____ 2. The well-man examination usually includes a pelvic examination, Pap smear, and clinical breast exam.

_____ 3. After a woman reaches 70 years of age, a mammography is included as part of the well-woman exam.

_____ 4. Women younger than 25 years of age are usually screened for chlamydia and gonorrhea, and an annual pelvic examination is recommended for women 21 years of age and older.

_____ 5. A pelvic examination includes inspection of the external genitalia, the use of a medical instrument called a *frenulum* to examine the vagina and cervix, and the manual palpation of the uterus and ovaries.

_____ 6. Men over 40 years of age usually have a *rectovaginal examination*, which identifies signs of possible tumors behind the uterus, on the walls of the vagina, or in the rectum.

_____ 7. A Pap smear is performed as part of the pelvic examination and determines if there are abnormal cells that may lead to cancer in the cervix.

_____ 8. Clinical breast exams are recommended for women who are over age 40 or who have a family history of or risk factors for breast cancer.

_____ 9. Women younger than 40 years of age should observe their breasts for any changes and perform yearly breast self-examinations (BSEs) several days after menstruation.

_____ 10. Mammography is the process of x-raying the breasts for cancer.

Well-Man Examinations

Select the *best* answer.

_____ 1. A well-man examination
   A. is identical to the comprehensive physical examination for women
   B. is performed by a urologist, primary care provider, or other appropriate healthcare provider
   C. is never combined with an annual comprehensive physical examination
   D. is a separate exam for children

_____ 2. Which of the following is true of the well-man exam?
   A. It includes a prostate cancer screening and testicular, penis, and hernia exams.
   B. It doesn't include discussions about lifestyle behaviors.
   C. It focuses exclusively on testing for STIs.
   D. It does not include laboratory testing.

_____ 3. A prostate-specific antigen (PSA) serologic assay
   A. is completed by the doctor through auscultation of the prostate
   B. is usually combined with mammography
   C. is the most common test for diagnosing prostate cancer
   D. should not be performed for men over 50 years of age

_____ 4. Which of the following is true of digital rectal examination?
   A. It identifies any questionable areas of the cervix.
   B. It involves the insertion of a gloved finger into the rectum to feel the size of the prostate.
   C. It is not routinely performed for men over 50 years of age.
   D. It is not useful for men who have a high risk of prostate cancer.

_____ 5. An inguinal hernia
   A. is inspected for sores, rashes, swelling, or ulcers
   B. is palpated for lumps, changes in size, or breast tenderness
   C. is the presence of heart palpitations
   D. occurs when part of the intestine sticks out through a weak spot in the abdominal wall

Well-Baby Examinations

Complete the following sentences.

1. _____ exams begin one month after birth when the mother and infant visit a pediatrician, primary care provider, or other appropriate licensed healthcare provider.

2. A baby's _____ is an integral part of the exam and one of the most important measurements.

3. Weight is an indicator of adequate _____ and growth and is used to calculate medication dosages, if needed.

4. During a well-baby exam, nursing assistants practice _____ hygiene and provide privacy for the baby and mother.

5. A nursing assistant must check the baby's _____ before measuring weight.

6. A baby _____ is used to measure a baby's weight.

7. A baby scale must be adjusted to _____ before the baby is placed on it.

8. Before being weighed, a baby must be _____, the diaper must be removed, and the skin must be cleaned.

9. A baby should be placed on the _____ of a baby scale.

10. While weighing a baby, a nursing assistant should keep one hand over the baby to prevent the baby from _____.

11. When a baby is being weighed, the weight bar must be moved to the correct weight until the scale _____.

12. After being weighed, a baby should be placed on a safe _____, diapered, and dressed.

13. Once a baby is weighed, the baby should be given to the _____ or placed in a safe location.

Milestone Examinations

Match each milestone examination with the age at which it occurs.

A. One month
B. Two months
C. Four months
D. Six months
E. Nine months
F. One year

_____ 1. The ability to walk and feed self with hands is checked.

_____ 2. Head control and emerging teeth are checked.

_____ 3. The shape of the head, reflexes, and muscle tone are checked.

_____ 4. Response to sound, new teeth, and shape of head are checked.

_____ 5. A physical exam checks the head, heart, lungs, eyes, ears, mouth, body, abdomen (umbilical stump), genitals, and movement of limbs.

_____ 6. Response to sound and muscle control when sitting up are checked.

Physical Examination Equipment

Identify whether each statement is true or false.

_____ 1. A thermometer measures a resident's temperature.

_____ 2. A sphygmomanometer is used to measure blood pressure.

_____ 3. A stethoscope is used for palpating blood pressure, heart and lung sounds, and pulse.

_____ 4. Tongue depressors are used to examine the rectum.

_____ 5. An otoscope is an instrument that examines the eyes.

_____ 6. An ophthalmoscope is an instrument that examines the ears.

_____ 7. Flashlights are sometimes used to examine the pupils for dilation.

_____ 8. An eye chart is part of STI screening.

_____ 9. A laryngeal mirror is a device that examines the mouth, tongue, and teeth.

_____ 10. Tuning forks help test hearing.

_____ 11. A percussion or reflex hammer is used to tap body parts to test reflexes.

_____ 12. A speculum is used to examine the vagina and many parts of the male reproductive system.

_____ 13. The nasal speculum is used to inspect the reflex passages.

_____ 14. Sheets or drapes are used to cover a patient for the physical examination.

_____ 15. Soiled instruments, gloves, tissues, paper towels, and disposable coverings and drapes are disposed of in specific containers.

_____ 16. Disposable gloves can be reused between residents.

_____ 17. Lubricant is not typically used for a digital rectal exam.

_____ 18. Alcohol wipes may be needed to sanitize equipment during a procedure.

_____ 19. Cotton-tipped applicators are sometimes used for obtaining specimens.

_____ 20. Specimen containers do not need to be labeled with a resident's identification information.

Positions and Draping for Examination
Apply the appropriate labels to the images.

A. Knee-chest position
B. Dorsal recumbent position
C. Fowler's position
D. Lithotomy position
E. Supine position
F. Sims' position
G. Prone position

_____ 1.

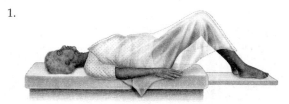

© Body Scientific International

_____ 2.

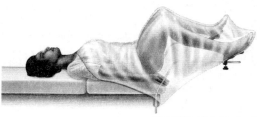

© Body Scientific International

_____ 3.

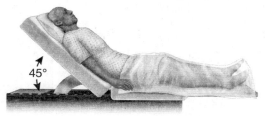

45°

© Body Scientific International

_____ 4.

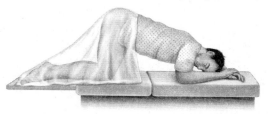

© Body Scientific International

_____ 5.

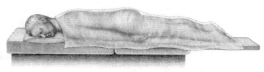

© Body Scientific International

_____ 6.

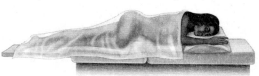

© Body Scientific International

_____ 7.

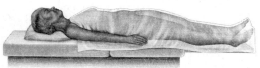

© Body Scientific International

Draping a Patient
Complete the following sentences.

1. _____ recumbent position is used to examine the vagina or rectum.

2. In dorsal recumbent position, the drape should cover the chest and _____ area.

3. Lithotomy position is used to examine the _____.

4. In lithotomy position, the drape should cover the body, but not the _____.

5. _____ position is often used to examine the legs and feet.

6. In Fowler's position, the drape should cover the _____.

7. _____ position is used to examine the rectum.

8. In knee-chest position, the drape should cover the _____ and legs.

9. _____ position is used to examine the spine and legs.

10. In prone position, the drape should cover the _____ and legs.

11. _____ position is a left side-lying position usually used to examine the rectum and sometimes the vagina.

12. In Sims' position, the drape should extend from the shoulders to the _____.

13. _____ position is used to examine the front of the body and the breasts.

14. In supine position, the drape should extend from under the _____ to the toes.

15. It is important to be respectful when positioning and draping and avoid needless _____ of the patient.

Specimens
Select the *best* answer.

_____ 1. Specimens are
   A. samples of a bodily substance that cannot cause disease
   B. collected for testing to provide information about a resident's mental health
   C. collected to provide critical information prior to a procedure or surgery
   D. taken every two hours during a physical examination

_____ 2. Which of the following is true of sputum?
   A. It is a blend of saliva and feces.
   B. It is analyzed for the presence of a specific pathogen.
   C. It is tested if a urinary tract infection (UTI) is suspected.
   D. It is an antibiotic used to destroy a pathogen.

_____ 3. What is point-of-care testing (POCT)?
A. collecting specimens in the place a resident is receiving care
B. using the sharp part of a glucometer to measure blood sugar
C. sending a resident via ambulance to a point of care
D. informing a resident of the important points in his or her care

_____ 4. Requisition forms (also called *laboratory slips*)
A. accompany labeled specimen containers delivered to the cafeteria
B. contain the resident's full name, sex, and marital status
C. never require a doctor's order
D. are completed by a licensed nursing staff member or the laboratory

_____ 5. The results from testing a specimen
A. do not relate to accurate specimen collection
B. should not be explained to a resident by a nursing assistant
C. are *positive* when they indicate no presence of infection or disease
D. are *negative* when they indicate results are not within normal range

_____ 6. A specimen in culture media
A. is coughed up from the lungs and sent to the laboratory
B. is placed in a dish containing special material to kill the natural flora
C. does not grow if the results are positive, indicating infection
D. grows if results are positive, necessitating further analysis to identify the pathogen

_____ 7. What is the collection method for a sputum sample?
A. urination
B. feces
C. coughing
D. clean catch

_____ 8. Which specimen is often used to detect the presence of medications and drugs?
A. sputum
B. urine
C. feces
D. skin

_____ 9. A stool sample is needed for
A. an occult blood test
B. a sputum culture
C. 24-hour urine specimen collection
D. a dipstick test

Sputum Specimens

Complete the following sentences.

1. Before taking a sputum specimen, a nursing assistant should ask the licensed nursing staff if _____ protective equipment should be worn during the procedure.

2. It is best to collect sputum specimens in the early _____, before the resident has had anything to eat or drink.

3. A resident should be positioned in _____ position or sit on the side of the bed to make it easier to cough.

4. It is important to instruct the resident not to touch the _____ of the specimen container or lid.

5. The resident should take _____ deep breath(s) and then cough deeply to bring up sputum from the lungs.

6. A nursing assistant should double-check that the specimen identified on the _____ matches the specimen collected and the requisition form.

7. The specimen container containing sputum should be placed in a(n) _____ transport bag.

8. After collecting the sputum specimen, the nursing assistant should offer the resident a glass of _____ and an emesis basin to cleanse the mouth.

9. Labeled sputum specimen containers should be sent or taken to the _____ or another assigned location with the requisition form.

Urine Specimens

Identify whether each statement is true or false.

_____ 1. Urine specimens are tested in three ways: observation of color, odor, and clarity; dipstick examination; and microscopic examination in a laboratory.

_____ 2. Healthy urine is usually cloudy, amber in color, and odorless.

_____ 3. The more hydrated a resident is, the darker the urine will be. Conversely, if a resident is dehydrated, urine will be light in color.

_____ 4. Most changes in urine color are permanent and are caused by food colors or medications.

_____ 5. Red urine usually indicates the presence of blood in the urine (called *hematuria*).

_____ 6. Cloudy urine with pus or mucus might signal a UTI.

_____ 7. A foul odor, such as a fishy smell, in the urine may be a sign of a bladder infection.

_____ 8. Observing and testing urine can detect the presence of sugar, glycosuria, ketones, and protein.

_____ 9. Nursing assistants can test a urine specimen using a dipstick reagent, which reacts to the presence of particular substances by changing color.

_____ 10. Urine specimens or cultures are viewed through a telescope to identify substances in the urine.

_____ 11. For microscopic examination, a urine specimen container should be 1/3 to 1/2 full.

_____ 12. Routine urine specimen analysis detects chemicals and medications in the urine, identifies the presence of infection, and can help diagnose diseases, such as diabetes.

_____ 13. Before the collection of a midstream urine specimen, the perineal area is cleansed. The specimen is collected midway through urination after a short stream of urine has exited the urethra.

_____ 14. For a 24-hour urine specimen, all of the urine expelled over a weeklong period is collected in a container to be analyzed by the laboratory.

_____ 15. Urine straining is done when kidney or bladder stones need to be retrieved for laboratory testing.

Routine Urine Specimen Collection

Nursing assistants follow instructions and facility policy for the proper collection of urine specimens to achieve accurate results. The following steps are part of the procedure for collecting a routine urine specimen. For each set of steps, identify the proper order in which they should be completed by numbering them 1 through 5.

1. _____ Place the following items in an accessible location in the room: urinary hat, bedpan or urinal and cover, disposable gloves, urine specimen container and lid label, urine graduate, completed laboratory requisition form, specimen transport bag with a biohazard label, a pen and form or digital device for recording the intake and output (I&O), and a paper towel.

   _____ Complete the label by printing the resident's name and room number, the time and date of the specimen collection, and the doctor's name. Place the label on the specimen container.

   _____ Provide privacy by closing the curtains, using a screen, or closing the door to the room.

   _____ Wash your hands or use hand sanitizer to ensure infection control.

   _____ Put on disposable gloves.

2. _____ Remove and discard your gloves. Wash your hands or use hand sanitizer to ensure infection control. Put on a new pair of gloves.

   _____ If the resident used a bedpan or urinal, cover it and take it into the bathroom. If measuring the resident's I&O, pour the urine from the bedpan or urinal into a clean graduate.

   _____ Ask the resident not to have a bowel movement or put toilet paper into the urine specimen. Provide a bag or waste container for the toilet paper.

   _____ Have the resident urinate into a urinary hat in the front half of a toilet, into a bedpan, or into a urinal.

   _____ Note the total urine output amount and record it on the paper or electronic intake and output form.

3. _____ Place the specimen container in a specimen transport bag. Use a biohazard bag or label, if needed. Do not let the specimen container touch the outside of the bag.

   _____ Empty the rest of the urine into the toilet. Remove, clean, and store equipment in the proper location. Remove soiled linens and discard disposable equipment. Remove and discard your gloves. Wash your hands or use hand sanitizer to ensure infection control.

   _____ Place a paper towel on a flat surface.

   _____ Put the lid on the specimen container. Double-check that the specimen identified on the label matches the specimen collected. Make sure the lid is tightly placed and attach the requisition form.

   _____ Remove the lid from the urine specimen container and place it, inside facing up, on the paper towel. Carefully pour about 120 mL of the urine directly from the graduate into the specimen container. Do not touch the inside of the specimen container or lid.

Collecting a Urine Specimen

For this activity, you will practice collecting a urine specimen without contamination. With a partner, gather and set up the needed supplies for collecting and measuring urinary output. Practice emptying liquid from a bedpan into a graduated cylinder. As you empty the liquid, identify clean and dirty surfaces and use paper towel barriers to avoid contaminating your hands and supplies. Your partner should observe and silently document every time your hands or supplies are contaminated and should provide feedback after the procedure is complete. Switch roles with your partner so you both have practice collecting the specimen.

Stool Specimens

Complete the following sentences.

1. _____ specimens help detect blood in the stool, identify possible infections, and screen for colon cancer.

2. Stool specimens can be examined for signs of colon cancer or the presence of noncancerous _____, or growths.

3. The fecal _____ blood, or guaiac, test detects blood in the stool.

4. A resident may need to _____ certain foods and medications three days prior to the guaiac test to prevent inaccurate results.

5. A Hemoccult kit contains a(n) _____ slide, which has front and back portions covered with a paper flap and a developer solution.

Fecal Occult Blood Test

Proper collection of a stool specimen is necessary to ensure an accurate fecal occult blood test. The following steps are part of the procedure for performing a fecal occult blood test. For each set of steps, identify the proper order in which they should be completed by numbering them 1 through 5.

1. _____ Place a paper towel on a flat surface. Open the front flap of the Hemoccult slide, exposing the guaiac paper.

   _____ Label the outside of the Hemoccult slide with the resident's name, the date, and the time the specimen was collected.

   _____ Secure a Hemoccult kit, paper towel, and wooden tongue blade. Open the Hemoccult kit.

   _____ Provide an explanation of the procedure you will be performing.

   _____ Practice hand hygiene and standard precautions. Ensure privacy and check the resident's identification.

2. _____ Close the front flap of the Hemoccult slide and turn the slide over to the reverse side.

   _____ Repeat the procedure using stool from a different part of the stool specimen. Smear the stool in Box B on the Hemoccult slide.

   _____ Open the back flap of the Hemoccult slide. Apply two drops of the developer solution to each box on the guaiac paper and wait 30–60 seconds before reading the results. If the slide turns blue, occult blood is present in the stool (considered *guaiac positive*). If the slide does not change color, there is no occult blood in the stool (considered *guaiac negative*). Complete the remainder of the procedure according to facility policy.

   _____ Using the wooden tongue blade, collect a small amount of stool from a fresh stool specimen.

   _____ Smear a small amount of stool in Box A on the Hemoccult slide.

Name: _____ Date: _____

Name: _____   Date: _____

Matching Chapter 20 Key Terms

Match each definition with the key term.

A. bath blanket
B. disposable protective pad
C. draw sheet
D. dysrhythmia
E. fatigue
F. hallucinations
G. sleep deprivation
H. traction
I. ward

_____ 1. a room in which several patients are given care in a healthcare facility

_____ 2. a small or regular-size flat sheet folded in half that is placed lengthwise over the middle of the bottom sheet of the bed and is used to help turn a resident in bed; also called a *pull sheet*, *turning sheet*, or *lift sheet*

_____ 3. visual, verbal, or physical perceptions of objects that are not real, but are mistaken for reality

_____ 4. weights, pulleys, and tape used to exert a slow, gentle pull; used to treat a muscular or skeletal disorder (such as a fracture) or to bring displaced bones back into place

_____ 5. a blanket, usually made from cotton or another absorbent material, that keeps a resident warm during a bed bath; may also be used as a protective covering to maintain resident modesty and warmth during procedures

_____ 6. a pad that is small, often multilayered, leak proof, and highly absorbent; can be placed under the buttocks of incontinent residents, used to absorb drainage, or used during procedures to prevent the bed from becoming soiled

_____ 7. an irregular or abnormal heart rhythm

_____ 8. a loss or deficiency of the recommended hours of sleep

_____ 9. a feeling of extreme tiredness or exhaustion

Healthcare Facility Rooms

Complete the following sentences.

1. Holistic nursing assistants who are familiar with the organization of residents' _____ will be best able to help residents feel comfortable and safe and promote a healing environment.

2. Long-term care facilities must comply with _____ requirements mandating that care and services enhance quality of life and that residents are treated with dignity and respect.

3. Historically, healthcare facilities did not offer private rooms. Instead, several patients received care in the same _____, or large room.

4. Modern rooms in a healthcare facility are either private with one resident or semiprivate with two residents and a shared _____ with safety modifications such as handrails.

5. Residents must be able to easily hang, store, and remove their _____ items.

6. Each room has a bed, which is sometimes called a(n) _____ bed due to its style and function.

7. A movable _____ table is used for personal care and meal trays, but should not be used for placing contaminated items without a barrier.

8. A(n) _____ stand usually holds personal items and has room on top for a telephone.

9. One or two _____ are normally located next to each bed to accommodate visitors.

10. A(n) _____ board opposite the bed may contain important information that is updated for each shift.

11. In some facilities, _____ equipment and blood pressure equipment are installed in the wall above or beside the bed.

12. Communication systems or _____ lights near or on the bed enable communication between the resident and healthcare staff.

13. Some residents may need _____ equipment (weights, pulleys, and tape that help treat muscular and skeletal disorders).

14. Privacy _____ enclose the area around the bed, and when there are no curtains, screens are used.

15. A room in a(n) _____ care facility may look like a typical bedroom in a home in which residents have the right to retain and use personal items and furnish as space permits.

Call Lights

Identify whether each statement is true or false.

_____ 1. Call lights are primarily used for communication between nursing assistants and the licensed nursing staff.

_____ 2. Answering a call light slowly helps prevent residents from wandering, becoming confused, getting out of bed, and falling.

_____ 3. A call light should always be within a resident's drawer.

_____ 4. Emergency call lights are typically found in residents' cars.

_____ 5. The call light communication system uses an alert and response cycle.

_____ 6. When a resident presses a call light, this activates a signal to a device that displays the room number at the nurses' station.

_____ 7. A call light may cause an alert light or sound, such as a ring or buzz, above or on the side of the door to a resident's room.

_____ 8. Healthcare staff members should answer call lights by intercom or phone call, respond to the page, or go to the room to see what is needed.

_____ 9. Once the staff member who answers the call light is in the room and able to assist, the call light should be turned on.

_____ 10. To orient residents to the call system, nursing assistants should show residents where call lights are located and how to use them.

_____ 11. If a resident cannot use a call light, a nursing assistant should check with the licensed nursing staff, the plan of care, and facility policy on how best to respond to the resident's needs.

_____ 12. A timely response to a call light increases a resident's dissatisfaction with care.

_____ 13. Frequent call light use by a resident may be the result of fear or anxiety, past experiences with long wait times, or boredom.

_____ 14. No matter how many times there is a call, a nursing assistant must never pass up an illuminated call light.

_____ 15. Rounding increases awareness of present or potential resident needs and can reduce unnecessary call light use.

Reducing Frequent Call Light Use

Complete the following guidelines for reducing frequent call light use.

1. Observe the resident's _____, ask if the resident is comfortable, and reposition the resident, if needed.

2. Make sure the _____ is accessible and is on the resident's stronger side.

3. Put the telephone, TV remote control, and bed light switch within the resident's _____.

4. Place the overbed _____ next to the bed.

5. Position the tissue box and drinking _____ so they can be easily reached.

6. Put the _____ container next to the bed.

7. Ask about the resident's _____ level and report any pain to the licensed nursing staff immediately.

8. Prior to leaving a room, ask the resident if there is anything else you can do before you go, be sincere with eye contact, and show interest in the resident's _____.

9. If appropriate, remind the resident that you or another member of the nursing staff will be back again to _____ on him or her during the shift.

Promoting a Healing Environment

Select the *best* answer.

_____ 1. A healing environment
   A. fosters the individual rights of residents and humanizes their experience
   B. involves understanding how rooms are arranged, eventually responding to call lights, and respecting personal items
   C. is not regulated by federal and state laws, regulations, and standards
   D. protects nursing assistants more than resident rights and outlines care requirements

_____ 2. To promote a safe, healing environment, nursing assistants should
   A. always accommodate resident preferences
   B. organize rooms to ensure resident safety
   C. maintain cleanliness and delegate procedures to the licensed nursing staff
   D. ensure proper temperature and ventilation of resident space heaters

_____ 3. Which of the following would help promote a healing environment?
   A. keeping room temperature between 81°F and 101°F
   B. waiting for older adults to report any room temperature outside the normal range
   C. opening a door or window to provide sufficient ventilation
   D. healing a resident in a warm environment

_____ 4. Resident rooms must
   A. have proper ventilation to help prevent odors
   B. achieve odor control using sterilization after elimination
   C. be ventilated during sterile dressing changes
   D. be cleared of garbage and soiled linens weekly

_____ 5. Personal space is
   A. the area around a person in which he or she feels most comfortable
   B. an unfamiliar person entering into a space
   C. frightening and draws residents into themselves
   D. meant to protect a resident's personal items

_____ 6. What can nursing assistants do to provide a healing environment?
   A. provide extension cords to ensure enough electrical outlets are available
   B. observe for sufficient lighting so residents can read easily and function even with impaired vision
   C. offer residents their personal phones to make phone calls in their rooms
   D. ensure that seating in the resident's room allows for easy transfer without a gait belt

_____ 7. Which of the following is true of safeguarding personal items?
   A. It involves taking all clothing and personal items.
   B. It is completed according to facility policy after the resident's discharge.
   C. It begins at admission and continues until transfer or discharge.
   D. It includes labeling the outsides of clothing or shoes.

_____ 8. Resident valuables
   A. may not be placed in the facility safe
   B. kept in the facility safe are auctioned off after discharge
   C. are discouraged for long-term care stays
   D. include clothing, jewelry, handbags, wallets, photos, books, and plants or gifts

_____ 9. Holistic nursing assistants
   A. pay for personal items that are special and irreplaceable to residents
   B. have the responsibility to keep a resident's personal items
   C. move personal items carefully so they never fall or break
   D. ask for permission before going through a resident's personal items in the bedside stand or closet

Completing an Inventory of Personal Effects

In this activity, you will practice completing an inventory of personal effects. To prepare for this activity, review the scenario that follows. Also have your FIRST CHECK procedural checklist nearby.

Scenario

When the nursing assistant meets Mrs. Carter, Mrs. Carter is sitting in a wheelchair fully dressed in a loose-fitting pantsuit with a coat, gloves, knitted hat, only one shoe on the left foot, and a loose sock on the right foot. Mrs. Carter is two days postoperative for a partial right knee replacement and has been admitted for physical and occupational therapy prior to returning home. She clutches her purse, sighs, and looks at her watch. She wears a beautiful ruby necklace and dabs her eyes with an embroidered handkerchief. There is a wheeled walker near the bed, and Mrs. Carter's husband is hanging a nightgown in a closet that is already full with clothing and three more left shoes. He states, "The surgeon says she'll be here six days, so I packed her suitcase with six more pantsuits and matching blouses and seven nightgowns, pairs of socks, and pieces of underwear. Her eyeglass and hearing aid cases are in the drawer. She can't hear very well, so be sure to take the batteries out tonight or her hearing aids won't work in the morning. I put her denture cup and brush on the bathroom sink. The lower partial is still in the cup, but she's wearing the full upper one. A bathrobe is hanging on the hook, and there are two more in the closet. I left her right shoes at home to save space and brought my radio to listen to the game. I can't get her to take her coat off. She says she isn't staying."

Form a group of three and assign each person a role. One person will be the nursing assistant, another Mrs. Carter, and the third person will serve as the evaluator. Then complete each of the following steps:

1. Complete the FIRST, or Preparation, steps, omitting any steps that are not applicable to the process.

2. Did you omit any steps that are not applicable to the process of completing an inventory of personal effects? If yes, explain which step(s) were omitted and why.

   _____

   _____

   _____

3. Print the inventory of personal effects form from the text and complete the document with the partner representing Mrs. Carter. The evaluator should also complete the inventory based on the scenario given. Compare inventories and keep working until the two inventories match. Then, the nursing assistant and resident partner should sign at the bottom of the inventory form.

4. Complete the CHECK, or Follow-Up and Reporting and Documentation, steps, omitting any steps that are not applicable to the process.

5. Did you omit any steps that are not applicable to the process of completing an inventory of personal effects? If yes, explain which step(s) were omitted and why.

_____

_____

_____

Beds and Bed Making

Complete the following sentences.

1. _____ beds can be raised, lowered, and repositioned using a controller.

2. The position of a(n) _____ bed can be changed using a crank mechanism at the end of the bed.

3. For safety reasons, the crank mechanism on a manual bed must be in the _____ position when not in use.

4. The wheels at each corner of a bed can be locked or unlocked using a(n) _____ lever by the wheels or a lever under the bed.

5. Beds in some long-term care facilities do not have side rails, but have an ambulatory _____ rail.

6. A bed that is _____ contains a resident.

7. _____ beds can be made closed or open.

8. If a bed will not be occupied for an extended period of time, it should be made _____ with the top linens pulled up.

9. _____ beds have the top linens pulled down because they will soon be occupied.

10. A(n) _____ bed has linens opened lengthwise so a patient can be transferred safely and comfortably from a stretcher to the bed after a surgery or procedure.

11. A(n) _____ sheet is placed lengthwise over the middle of the bottom sheet of a bed and is used to turn or move a resident in bed.

12. _____ blankets are used as protective coverings to maintain resident modesty and warmth during various procedures.

13. A disposable protective pad, sometimes called a(n) _____ pad, is made from washable cotton or a disposable, paperlike material.

14. Disposable _____ pads are used to promote the comfort of incontinent residents, absorb drainage, and prevent the bed from becoming soiled during procedures.

15. If a flat sheet is used for the bottom sheet of a bed, a nursing assistant can help maintain a resident's skin integrity by making the bed with _____ corners.

16. A(n) _____ is a breeding ground for pathogens and must be changed routinely and when it appears to be soiled.

17. If making an occupied bed containing an overweight resident, nursing assistants should always ask for _____.

18. If residents have dressings, tubes, or an IV catheter, nursing assistants should be sure not to _____ these devices when changing linens.

19. It is important to be mindful of fragile _____ as a resident is moved to prevent scrapes or bruises.

20. Creating a(n) _____ can ensure the bed linen is not too tight around and on top of the feet.

21. Once _____ are brought into a room, they cannot be used for another resident, not even a roommate.

22. Nursing assistants should wear disposable _____ when removing soiled linens for infection prevention and control.

23. _____ linens, whether they are clean or dirty, can spread pathogens and create static electricity.

24. When changing a pillowcase, a nursing assistant should help the resident move his head and keep the resident _____ in bed to avoid neck injury.

Making an Occupied Bed

Making an occupied bed is necessary when a resident is not able or permitted to be out of bed. The following steps are part of the procedure for making an occupied bed. For each set of steps, identify the proper order in which they should be completed by numbering them 1 through 5.

1. _____ Lock the bed wheels and then raise the bed to hip level. If there are side rails, raise and secure the rails on the opposite side of the bed from where you will be working. Lower the rail on the side you are working.

   _____ Arrange the clean linens in the order they will be used. Remove the call light from the bed. Make sure the bed is flat, unless otherwise indicated by the plan of care.

   _____ Provide privacy by closing the curtains, using a screen, or closing the door to the room.

   _____ Loosen the top linens from the foot of the bed. Place the bath blanket over the top linens and ask the resident to hold the top edge of the bath blanket. Remove the top linens from under the bath blanket, being careful not to expose the resident.

   _____ Bring the necessary equipment into the room. Place the following items in an accessible location: laundry hamper, 1 bath blanket, 1 bottom sheet, 1 top sheet, 1 cotton draw sheet, 1 disposable protective pad, 1 bedspread, 2 blankets, and pillowcases.

2. _____ Place the top linens in the laundry hamper. Make the bed one side at a time. If the mattress slips out of place, ask a coworker to help you move it to the head of the bed before continuing.

_____ Place a clean bottom sheet on top of the mattress. If using a fitted bottom sheet, pull the corners of the sheet tightly and smoothly over the corners of the mattress. Smooth the sheet and tuck it tightly under the top and side of the mattress.

_____ Ask the resident to turn toward the side of the bed farthest from you and grasp the side rail. Help the resident turn and keep the resident covered with the bath blanket. Move the pillow with the resident and adjust it under the head.

_____ Position the draw sheet with the center fold next to the resident. Tuck it under the mattress. Ask the resident to roll toward you and over all of the soiled linens. Move the pillow and bath blanket with the resident. If used, raise and secure the side rail on that side of the bed and lower the opposite side rail.

_____ Starting at the head of the bed, loosen the soiled bottom linens. Remove and dispose of the disposable protective pad. Roll the soiled bottom linens toward the resident and tuck them against his back.

3. _____ Pull the draw sheet tight and tuck it in. Place a disposable protective pad on top of the draw sheet and under the resident's buttocks.

_____ Remove the soiled bottom linens by rolling the edges inward and toward you. Put the soiled linens in the laundry hamper. Pull the clean bottom sheet into place as quickly as possible. If using a fitted bottom sheet, pull the corners of the sheet tightly and smoothly over the corners of the mattress. Smooth the sheet and tuck it tightly under the top and side of the mattress.

_____ Lower the bed. Follow the plan of care to determine if the side rails should be raised or lowered. Place the call light and personal items within reach, conduct a safety check, and perform hand hygiene.

_____ Place the clean top sheet over the resident. Remove the bath blanket and discard it in the laundry hamper. Place the blanket and bedspread on the resident. Tuck these in at the bottom of the bed and make mitered corners. Create room for the toes by making toe pleats in the top linens.

_____ Ask the resident to lie on his back in the center of the bed. Assist him if he cannot move himself. Change the pillowcases and place the pillows under the resident's head. Discard the used pillowcases in the laundry hamper.

Providing Comfort

Complete the following sentences.

1. The two aspects of _____ in healthcare are the resident's feeling of comfort and the actions a holistic nursing assistant takes to promote comfort.

2. For those who have _____ pain, a period of being pain free can bring comfort.

3. To promote and give comfort, holistic nursing assistants need to learn what is comfortable for _____.

4. Nursing theorist Katharine Kolcaba developed the _____ of Comfort, which describes comfort in three forms: relief, ease, and transcendence.

5. _____ occurs when comfort needs are met, and the resident experiences a sense of relief.

6. _____ is a feeling of contentment or peace (for example, after resolving a stressful issue).

7. _____ takes place when residents rise above challenges to achieve comfort (for example, by learning to walk after a paralyzing stroke).

8. Comfort is experienced in different _____, which can be physical, spiritual, sociocultural, or environmental.

9. Holistic nursing assistants help promote comfort by observing and _____ residents what is comfortable for them, being sensitive to culturally relevant issues, and identifying and performing actions that promote comfort.

10. _____-relief approaches for residents include being sensitive to and aware of residents experiencing pain, keeping the licensed nursing staff informed of resident pain levels, and making use of relaxation activities.

11. _____ is an important aspect of healing that reduces stress hormones and provides a healthy internal and external environment.

12. _____ presence is the practice of checking one's body for stress and consciously letting go of stressful feelings and thoughts.

13. Holistic nursing assistants can relax by showing residents they feel _____ for each day, laughing aloud, giving a reassuring smile, and simply providing a human touch.

14. Rest can occur at any time and can be the result of _____, or extreme tiredness.

15. _____ is necessary for survival and must occur daily to restore the body's energy, help repair muscle tissue, and release hormones that promote growth.

16. The body's natural sleep-wake cycle, called _____ rhythm, is controlled by structures in the brain that regulate sleepiness and wakefulness over 24 hours.

17. Circadian rhythm responds to _____, causing people to sleep when it is dark and be awake when it is light.

18. Ongoing sleep _____ can lead to impaired memory and unsafe physical performance.

19. Sleep deprivation can increase a person's risk for obesity, headaches, epileptic seizures, and _____ (visual, verbal, or physical perceptions that are not real, but are mistaken for reality).

20. Sleeping problems are common among people with heart disease, diabetes, Alzheimer's disease, stroke, cancer, and mental disorders such as _____ and schizophrenia.

Sleep Recommendations

Identify the recommended hours of sleep for each age group in the table.

Recommended Hours of Sleep by Age Group	
Age Group	**Recommended Hours of Sleep**
Infants	1. _____
Toddlers	2. _____
School-age children	3. _____
Adolescents	4. _____
Adults	5. _____

Sleep Stages

Identify whether each statement is true or false.

_____ 1. Sleep quality is associated with how much time a person spends in the nonREM (NREM) stage of sleep.

_____ 2. There are five stages of sleep: four stages of REM sleep and one stage of NREM sleep, which is the most restorative.

_____ 3. The number of sleep cycles a person has is affected by a person's age, the time of day or night, recent amounts of sleep, exercise, stress, and environmental conditions such as room temperature and lighting.

_____ 4. NREM stage 4 is the lightest stage of sleep, in which people feel they are drifting in and out of sleep.

_____ 5. NREM stage 2 is considered light sleep, in which the body continues to relax in preparation for deeper sleep in later stages.

_____ 6. If a person awakes during NREM stage 3, he or she will likely feel groggy, be confused, and have difficulty focusing.

_____ 7. The deepest stage of the sleep cycle is REM stage 4, which involves no eye movement or muscle activity.

_____ 8. During REM sleep, the muscles in the arms and legs become periodically paralyzed, possibly to prevent people from acting out their dreams.

Healthy Sleep Habits

Select the *best* answer.

_____ 1. Healthy sleep habits
   A. can help people get the sleep deprivation they need
   B. include a regular schedule for waking up, but not for going to sleep
   C. involve increasing the number and length of naps during the day
   D. include relaxation before bed and a comfortable, quiet, and dark environment

_____ 2. Which of the following is true of sleep disorders?
   A. They affect nearly one million people in the United States.
   B. Insomnia, sleep apnea, narcolepsy, and restless legs syndrome (RLS) are some examples.
   C. They do not have significant effects on older adults.
   D. They affect the mobility of a resident, but are unrelated to overall well-being.

_____ 3. Insomnia is
   A. a sleep disorder characterized by the inability to fall or stay asleep
   B. defined as one episode of sleeplessness each year
   C. prescribed by a doctor to treat sleeplessness
   D. best managed by keeping the lights on all night

_____ 4. Sleep apnea
   A. is interrupted breathing while awake that causes a heart attack
   B. often causes periodic gasping, snorting, or snoring during meals
   C. can be treated by losing weight, sleeping on the side, or using a CPAP machine
   D. causes blood oxygen to increase

_____ 5. Which of the following is true of narcolepsy?
   A. It causes slow loss of involuntary muscle control.
   B. It is a sleep attack that may last several seconds or days.
   C. It cannot be treated with prescription medications.
   D. It is severe daytime sleepiness with uncontrollable, sometimes sudden periods of sleep.

_____ 6. Restless legs syndrome (RLS)
   A. causes unpleasant creeping, crawling, and prickling sensations in the legs and feet
   B. makes people want to keep their legs still
   C. cannot be inherited
   D. cannot be treated with prescription medications

_____ 7. A restful environment
   A. helps promote hypertension in the resident
   B. can create a healing environment
   C. is most important for the nursing staff
   D. includes a noisy environment

_____ 8. How can holistic nursing assistants help promote sleep?
  A. avoiding giving a back rub prior to sleep
  B. providing fresh drinking water if the resident is NPO (nothing by mouth)
  C. providing evening, or p.m., care
  D. explaining surgical procedures prior to bedtime

_____ 9. Which of the following is true of back rubs?
  A. They should not be performed without permission from the resident.
  B. They should be performed on burns to increase circulation.
  C. They should be avoided during evening, or p.m., care.
  D. They do not require privacy with a curtain or bath blanket.

_____ 10. While giving care, a nursing assistant should
  A. talk with the resident about the experiences of the resident's roommate
  B. immediately document the resident's answers to questions
  C. be gentle and mumble in soft tones
  D. ask the resident about any health or treatment gains made during the day

Giving a Back Rub

Back rubs stimulate circulation to the skin and muscles, relieve muscle tension and stiffness, promote comfort and relaxation, help relieve pain, and allow nursing assistants to observe a resident's skin for any redness or decubitus ulcers. In this activity, you will practice giving a back rub. To prepare for this activity, review the procedural checklist for Giving a Back Rub. Also have your FIRST CHECK procedural checklist nearby.

Form a group of three and assign each person a role. One person will be the nursing assistant, another a resident, and the third person will serve as the evaluator. Then complete each of the following steps:

1. Complete the FIRST, or Preparation, steps of the procedure, omitting any steps that are not applicable to the Giving a Back Rub procedure.

2. Did you omit any steps that are not applicable to the Giving a Back Rub procedure? If yes, explain which step(s) were omitted and why.

_____

_____

_____

3. Give the resident partner a back rub following the correct procedure. The evaluator should assess how well the nursing assistant follows the procedure during the back rub.

4. Complete the CHECK, or Follow-Up and Reporting and Documentation, steps of the procedure, omitting any steps that are not applicable to the procedure.

5. Did you omit any steps that are not applicable to the procedure? If yes, explain which step(s) were omitted and why.

_____

_____

_____

6. Switch roles with your partners so each partner has the opportunity to be the nursing assistant.

Name: _____ Date: _____

Matching Chapter 21 Key Terms

Match each definition with the key term.

A. anticoagulants
B. compresses
C. cryotherapy
D. cyanotic
E. emesis basin
F. gangrene
G. hemorrhoids
H. hydration
I. hygiene
J. pallor
K. perineal care
L. perineum
M. podiatrist
N. sitz bath
O. skin integrity
P. tepid
Q. therapeutic
R. thermotherapy
S. whirlpool

_____ 1. medications that prevent the formation of blood clots

_____ 2. a type of therapeutic bath in which a person's perineum, buttocks, and sometimes hips are soaked in warm water

_____ 3. a small, kidney-shaped bowl used for oral care or if a resident needs to vomit

_____ 4. hygiene care that involves cleansing the area between the thighs (the coccyx, pubis, anus, urethra, and external genitals)

_____ 5. the condition of the skin; healthy skin is whole or intact without irritation, inflammation, or damage

_____ 6. slightly warm

_____ 7. the area between the thighs; includes the coccyx, pubis, anus, urethra, and external genitals

_____ 8. pads of material; can be warm, cold, dry, or moist

_____ 9. the death and decay of body tissue

_____ 10. swollen, inflamed veins found under the skin around the anus (external) or inside the rectum (internal); may be itchy or painful at times and can cause rectal bleeding

_____ 11. discolored and bluish due to insufficient oxygen in the blood

_____ 12. a sufficient amount of fluid in body tissues

_____ 13. the use of heat applications to increase circulation and ease pain

_____ 14. a doctor who specializes in diagnosing and treating diseases and conditions that affect the feet

_____ 15. a type of bathtub used for therapeutic purposes; has small spray jets that swirl water

_____ 16. routine actions such as bathing that promote and maintain cleanliness and health

_____ 17. the use of cold applications to reduce swelling and ease pain

_____ 18. having a healing effect on the body and mind

_____ 19. an unusually pale color of the skin

Understanding Hygiene

Complete the following sentences.

1. Personal _____ and grooming are essential to promoting healing and providing an environment of cleanliness, relaxation, and comfort.

2. Hygiene helps maintain a resident's physical and _____ well-being and enhances quality of life.

3. Nursing assistant hygiene responsibilities include morning care, bathing, shaving, oral care, fingernail and foot care, dressing or undressing, perineal care, and _____ care.

4. _____ care is care of the perineum, or the area between the thighs (the coccyx, pubis, anus, urethra, and external genitals).

5. _____ care, or a.m. care, is usually performed in the early morning hours, when residents first awake.

6. Morning care duties include taking _____ signs; assisting with transfers and elimination; measuring output; collecting specimens ordered by the doctor; helping residents wash their faces, comb their hair, and perform oral care; providing meal assistance; and changing linens.

7. Some residents require assistance with toileting and _____ their hands before lunch and dinner.

8. _____ is a part of hygiene that helps maintain cleanliness and keeps residents free from perspiration, irritation, and possible bacterial growth.

9. Baths can be pleasant, relaxing, and _____ (healing).

10. Bathing provides an opportunity for the nursing assistant to observe a resident's skin _____, or the condition of the skin.

11. During bathing, the nursing assistant observes a resident's level of _____ (amount of fluid in body tissues) and muscle and joint movement.

12. _____ and tub baths promote skin cleanliness and healing and control odors.

13. Some residents need a shower _____ so they can safely sit in the shower and not fall.

14. Water temperature for a shower or tub bath should be adjusted to _____ or as directed by the licensed nursing staff.

15. Grab bars in a shower or tub must be easily accessible, and a resident should never be left _____.

Bathing Residents with Limited Mobility
Identify whether each statement is true or false.

_____ 1. For residents who are not able to get out of bed or wash themselves, a doctor will typically order a tub bath.

_____ 2. During a total bed bath, a resident's entire body is washed by a nursing assistant, commonly using washcloths and warm, soapy water in a washbasin.

_____ 3. Sometimes, a liquid, no-rinse soap is used for a total bed bath.

_____ 4. A partial bed bath involves washing the face, hands, axilla, back, genitalia, and buttocks.

_____ 5. One responsibility of the nursing assistant is to ask and observe the extent to which residents can perform their own baths.

_____ 6. In a towel bath, a resident showers with a towel, which has been immersed in a warm, no-rinse soap solution. The resident is then dried with a bath blanket.

_____ 7. A bag bath is performed using a series of 30 washcloths that have been moistened with a no-rinse cleanser, placed in a bag, and warmed in a microwave.

_____ 8. The nursing assistant is responsible for purchasing a bag bath or assembling one using the facility's washcloths and no-rinse cleanser.

_____ 9. During a bag bath, each fresh washcloth is used for the same body area.

_____ 10. A sitz bath is a treatment in which a resident soaks in warm water up to his or her hips to promote healing for soreness and irritation from diseases and conditions.

_____ 11. A sitz bath generally lasts 10–20 minutes, and the temperature is determined by the nursing assistant's preference.

_____ 12. When giving a sitz bath, a nursing assistant should note the beginning time and check on the resident every 30 minutes or stay with the resident.

_____ 13. A whirlpool is a bathtub with small jets that move warm water to help decrease swelling and inflammation, ease muscle spasms and pain, and promote healing.

_____ 14. A resident may bathe or sit in a whirlpool as long as directed by the plan of care.

_____ 15. No matter what type of bath is ordered, nursing assistants should encourage residents to do as much of it themselves as they can.

Giving a Total Bed Bath
A nursing assistant gives a total bed bath when an entire bath must be performed for an immobile resident. The following steps are part of the procedure for giving a total bed bath. For each set of steps, identify the proper order in which they should be completed by numbering them 1 through 5.

1. _____ Keep the resident covered with the bath blanket as you remove the gown and put it in the laundry hamper.

_____ Arrange the towels, linens, and gowns in the order they will be used. Place a hand towel on the overbed table and place the following on the hand towel: a washbasin, liquid soap, personal hygiene products, and cotton-tipped applicators.

_____ Bring the necessary equipment into the room and place the following items in an accessible location: bath blankets, a disposable protective pad, disposable gloves, a laundry hamper, clean bed linens, several washcloths and hand towels, 2–3 bath towels, and 2 clean gowns.

_____ Put on disposable gloves. Loosen and pull the bed linens out from under the mattress and fanfold the bedspread and blanket to the foot of the bed. Place the bath blanket over the top sheet covering the resident. Have the resident hold the bath blanket while you pull the top sheet out from under the bath blanket. Fanfold the top sheet to the foot of the bed and place it in the laundry hamper.

_____ Provide privacy by closing the curtains, using a screen, or closing the door to the room. Lock the bed wheels and raise the bed to hip level. Wash your hands or use hand sanitizer to ensure infection control.

2. _____ Position the resident on the side of the bed closest to you. Make a bath mitt and wet the bath mitt using only water. Gently wash each eye from the inner corner to the outer corner. Use a different, clean part of the mitt for each swipe.

_____ Fill the washbasin about two-thirds full of warm water and check the water temperature. Place the washbasin on the overbed table, which should be covered with a hand towel.

_____ Place a dry bath towel across the resident's chest and fold the bath blanket down to the pubic area. Lift the dry bath towel slightly and wash, rinse, dry, and apply lotion to the chest and abdominal areas.

_____ Wash the entire face, ears, and neck and rinse. Gently pat-dry the face, ears, and neck with a dry towel. Before washing each arm, place a dry towel under it. Support the arm farthest from you and wash the shoulder, axilla, arm, hand, and fingers. Rinse and dry well, apply lotion, and place the dry arm under the bath blanket. Support the arm nearest to you. Wash, rinse, dry, and apply lotion to the shoulder, axilla, arm, hand, and fingers using the same procedure.

_____ Pull the bath blanket up and over the bath towel and remove the bath towel. Lower the bed, raise the side rails for safety, and give the resident the call light. Empty, rinse, and refill the washbasin about two-thirds full of warm water. Check the water temperature. Place the washbasin on the overbed table.

3. _____ Remove the washbasin and towel and cover the resident's legs and feet with the bath blanket. Lower the bed, raise the side rails for safety, and give the resident the call light. Place any soiled linens in the laundry hamper. Empty, rinse, and refill the washbasin about two-thirds full of warm water. Check the water temperature.

_____ Place a dry towel under the resident's leg farthest from you. Support and wash, rinse, dry, and apply lotion to the thigh and leg. Wash, rinse, dry, and apply lotion to the thigh and leg nearest you using the same procedure. Then cover both legs with the bath blanket.

_____ Help the resident onto his or her side and place a towel lengthwise next to the back. Wash, rinse, and dry the back of the neck, back, and buttocks. Give a back rub and help the resident onto his or her back with a towel under the buttocks and upper legs.

_____ Lower the bed, raise the side rails for safety, and give the resident the call light. Empty, rinse, and refill the washbasin about two-thirds full of warm water. Check the water temperature. Perform perineal care and then help the resident put on a clean gown or other clothing. Perform Follow-Up and Reporting and Documentation steps.

_____ Expose the foot and thigh nearest you and bend the knee. Place the washbasin on top of a towel near the foot, support the knee, and place the resident's foot in the water. Using a bath mitt, wash and clean between the toes and under the toenails, remove the foot from the water, and then rinse and dry it well. Apply lotion according to the plan of care (not between the toes). Wash, rinse, dry, and apply lotion to the other foot using the same procedure.

Practicing the Bed Bath

Many residents share rooms and bathrooms in long-term care facilities, making one of the most contaminated items the faucet handles of the sink. The bed bath procedure requires water changes at least four times. Nursing assistants use gloves for infection control, but must be aware that their gloved hands can contaminate items such as washbasins, side rails, and drawer handles. In this activity, you will practice giving a bed bath. To prepare for this activity, review the procedural checklist for Giving a Total or Partial Bed Bath. Also have your FIRST CHECK procedural checklist nearby.

Form a group of three and assign each person a role. One person will be the nursing assistant, another a resident, and the third person will serve as the evaluator. Then complete each of the following steps:

1. Prepare the faucet handles in the room with sticky jelly to illustrate the importance of not touching the handles at any time without a barrier.

2. Complete the FIRST, or Preparation, steps of the procedure, omitting any steps that are not applicable to the Giving a Total or Partial Bed Bath procedure.

3. Did you omit any steps that are not applicable to the Giving a Total or Partial Bed Bath procedure? If yes, explain which step(s) were omitted and why.

_____

_____

_____

4. The resident partner should remain clothed during this procedure, and the nursing assistant should only wash the areas specified. Wash the resident partner's eyes, face, ears, neck, and arms using the correct procedure. Change the water and wash the resident's feet. Change the water again and then wash the back of the resident's neck. Following procedure, change the water a final time. The evaluator should assess how well the nursing assistant follows the procedure and maintains infection control.

5. Complete the CHECK, or Follow-Up and Reporting and Documentation, steps of the procedure, omitting any steps that are not applicable to the procedure.

6. Did you omit any steps that are not applicable to the procedure? If yes, explain which step(s) were omitted and why.

_____

_____

_____

7. Switch roles with your partners so each partner has the opportunity to be the nursing assistant.

Providing Hair Care

Select the *best* answer.

_____ 1. Which of the following is true of hair?
A. Oily hair requires weekly shampooing.
B. Hair may be affected by age, genetics, medications, and skin conditions.
C. Dry hair needs extra moisture, so monthly shampooing is recommended.
D. Hair thickens as a person ages.

_____ 2. Alopecia is
A. not affected by genetics, hormones, or environmental factors
B. often caused by iron deficiency, poor diet, thyroid imbalance, or chemotherapy
C. more common in females over 50 years of age than in males
D. usually apparent after a person has grown 50 percent of their hair

_____ 3. What is canities?
A. the term for contaminated hair
B. a condition caused by age, but not by stress
C. a condition that affects most people 25 years of age or older
D. hair that turns gray or white due to changes in melanin production

_____ 4. The scalp
A. may have lesions that nursing assistants should scrub with their fingernails
B. normally has redness and irritation
C. needs extreme temperature variations to prevent skin breakdown
D. may have dandruff, which is the excessive flaking of dead skin cells

_____ 5. *Pediculus humanus capitis*
A. are parasites that crawl and can be spread by close human contact
B. are lice spread by contact with bodily fluids
C. are found inside the head
D. attach their eggs to the base of the hair shaft, but cannot be spread

_____ 6. Hair care
A. promotes cleanliness and comfort and stimulates circulation
B. includes frequent dry shampooing and coloring performed by the nursing assistant
C. includes shampooing, combing, or brushing the hair using the fingernails
D. promotes cleanliness, comfort, and hair loss

_____ 7. Which of the following is true of shaving?
A. Products and razors are selected by the nursing assistant.
B. Shaving over razor bumps may cause irritation.
C. Using shaving cream causes irritation, nicks, cuts, and razor bumps.
D. Very close shaving will prevent razor bumps.

_____ 8. Electric razors
A. should not be used with aftershave lotion
B. should be used if the resident is taking anticoagulant medications
C. should be plugged in and used for residents on oxygen therapy
D. tighten the skin and narrow the pores

_____ 9. Guidelines for shaving include
A. sterilizing the razor after use
B. shaving in the opposite direction of hair growth
C. starting under the sideburns and working downward over the cheeks
D. shaving all of the mustache and beard off for infection control

_____ 10. When shaving a resident, a nursing assistant should
A. shave over skin sores, moles, growths, acne, or bruises
B. use a disposable razor and throw it away in the resident's garbage
C. shave lightly and apply pressure if a nick or cut occurs
D. report any nicks or cuts to the licensed nursing staff after the work shift

Oral and Denture Care

Complete the following sentences.

1. Some residents do not have all of their natural _____ and have bridges, partial dentures, or full dentures.

2. A(n) _____ fills a gap between teeth and is anchored to the permanent teeth.

3. _____ dentures have a plastic base or metal structure that attaches to missing teeth.

4. _____, or complete, dentures replace all natural teeth on the upper and lower or both parts of the gums.

5. Dentures that have been properly cared for typically last about _____ year(s).

6. As the bones and gums age, dentures may become _____, resulting in an inability to chew well.

7. Residents with ill-fitting dentures may not receive adequate _____, which may cause lack of healing and weight loss.

8. Poorly fitting dentures can cause mouth and gum irritation, _____, and infections.

9. _____ care and teeth cleaning are a critical part of daily hygiene and reduce bacteria, provide moisture, freshen the mouth, and make food taste better.

10. Oral care can help prevent dental _____, or tooth decay that damages the hard surface of the teeth.

11. The term _____ refers to bad breath, which may indicate infection.

12. _____, also called *gum disease*, can be prevented with effective oral care.

13. _____ is an infection of the gums and bones that support the teeth.

14. Oral care may be needed as often as every _____ hour(s) if the resident is unable to take fluids by mouth.

15. Routine teeth cleaning consists of daily brushing and _____ in the morning and evening and after eating.

16. A(n) _____ should be replaced every three to four months and sooner if the bristles become frayed.

17. To perform the oral care procedure, the nursing assistant raises the _____ of the bed to at least 60–90°.

18. During oral care, the _____ should be brushed in addition to the teeth to remove bacteria and keep the breath fresh.

19. The licensed nursing staff should be notified of any complaints of pain or _____, sores on the lips or mouth, cracked or bleeding lips or gums, bad breath, and chipped or cracked teeth.

Cleaning and Storing Dentures

Cleaning dentures keeps them intact, freshens the mouth, removes remaining food particles, and reduces lingering bacteria. The following steps are part of the procedure for cleaning and storing dentures. For each set of steps, identify the proper order in which they should be completed by numbering them 1 through 5.

1. _____ Provide privacy by closing the curtains, using a screen, or closing the door to the room. If the resident can sit in a chair, assist to a chair and place the overbed table in a comfortable position so the resident may clean the dentures. If the resident is in bed, lock the bed wheels, use side rails according to the plan of care, and raise the bed to hip level. Raise the head of the bed.

    _____ Bring the necessary equipment into the room. Put a paper towel, towel, or disposable protective pad on the overbed table and place the following items: toothbrush or denture brush, denture cup and lid, toothpaste or denture cleaner, disposable cups, emesis basin, washcloths, mouthwash, denture solution, several towels, several packets of 2 × 2 gauze bandages, oral swabs, and disposable gloves.

    _____ Wash your hands or use hand sanitizer to ensure infection control. Put on disposable gloves and spread a towel across the resident's chest. Place a washcloth in the bottom of the emesis basin and ask the resident to remove the dentures and place them in the emesis basin. If the resident cannot remove the dentures, remove the dentures using a 2 x 2 gauze bandage.

    _____ Place a washcloth in the bottom of the sink and take one denture out of the emesis basin. Apply toothpaste or denture cleaner to the denture. Wet the toothbrush by immersing it in clean, running water. Hold the denture low in the sink in the palm of your hand. Brush all surfaces away from you until they are clean. Then rinse thoroughly using cool, running water. Repeat the same procedure for a second denture.

    _____ Place the dentures in the emesis basin on top of the washcloth. Place the emesis basin, toothbrush or denture brush, and toothpaste or denture cleaner next to the sink. If the resident wears full dentures, clean the resident's oral cavity after the dentures are removed with oral swabs and half-strength mouthwash.

2. _____ Remove and discard your gloves.

    _____ Wash your hands or use hand sanitizer to ensure infection control. Put on a new pair of gloves.

    _____ If the resident is in bed, check to be sure the bed wheels are locked. Then reposition the resident and lower the bed. If the resident is in a chair, help him or her back to bed, if desired.

    _____ To store dentures, fill the labeled denture cup with cool water, mouthwash, or denture solution. Place the dentures in the cup and close the lid. Leave the labeled denture cup with clean solution on the bedside stand or as indicated in the plan of care.

    _____ Check that the dentures are moist if reinserting them. Have the resident reinsert the dentures, if able, and assist, if needed. Check that the dentures fit correctly.

Identifying the Parts of a Nail

Apply the appropriate callouts to the image.

A. Nail groove
B. Cuticle
C. Nail bed
D. Root
E. Nail plate

1. _____
2. _____
3. _____
4. _____
5. _____

© Body Scientific International

Fingernail Care

Identify whether each statement is true or false.

_____ 1. Fingernails and toenails are composed of protein, keratin, and epithelial cells.

_____ 2. The hard surface of the nail is the nail slate.

_____ 3. The cubicle is the band of tissue at the sides and base of the nail plate.

_____ 4. The nail boot anchors the nail plate.

_____ 5. The pink color of the nail comes from blood vessels directly under the nail plate.

_____ 6. Nails need carbon dioxide because they are composed of living cells and tissue.

_____ 7. Routine fingernail care promotes cleanliness and prevents irritation or infection from torn or bleeding cuticles, cracked fingernails, or dirt under the fingernails.

_____ 8. Smooth fingernails prevent the skin from breaking if residents scratch themselves.

_____ 9. Nursing assistants shape and smooth residents' fingernails with a memory board.

_____ 10. The licensed nursing staff should be notified if a nursing assistant observes loose, dry, reddened, or irritated nails.

Foot Care

Select the *best* answer.

_____ 1. Which of the following happens with age?
A. The toenails become thin and yellow.
B. Feet become unattractive, but easy to keep clean.
C. Problems with feet may include calluses and corns.
D. Feet become less important for infection control.

_____ 2. Calluses are
A. rough areas on the skin caused by repeated friction or rubbing
B. caused by expensive shoes and walking barefoot
C. spots that normally appear on the top of the foot
D. vascular and more sensitive than surrounding skin

_____ 3. Which of the following is true of corns?
A. They cause increased circulation and sensation.
B. They often form on the bottoms and heels of the feet.
C. They are caused by lack of cushioning on the ankle.
D. They are small patches of thickened, dead skin with a central core.

_____ 4. A bunion
A. does not cause discomfort in enclosed shoes
B. creates a moist environment for bacterial growth
C. is an over-the-counter treatment for a foot problem
D. is a swelling on the joint of the big toe

_____ 5. What is a podiatrist?
A. a doctor who specializes in foot health
B. a doctor who specializes in diabetic nutrition
C. a resident with peripheral vascular disease (PVD)
D. a condition that can lead to serious nerve damage

_____ 6. Peripheral neuropathy
A. can result in unnoticed sores and swelling of the hands
B. promotes good blood circulation in residents
C. causes a loss of pain, heat, and cold sensitivity in the feet
D. cannot be prevented or improved

_____ 7. To care for the feet, a nursing assistant should
A. carefully check for signs of irritation, cuts, swelling, or blisters
B. wash feet weekly and apply lotion between the toes
C. provide daily toenail trims
D. order medicated powder to control odors

_____ 8. For good foot health, a resident should
A. wear tight shoes to prevent foot problems
B. wear shoes with a smooth lining and no irritating objects inside
C. wear socks without shoes
D. walk barefoot inside the facility

_____ 9. It is important to protect the feet
A. from hot and cold temperatures
B. by putting them in very hot water to prevent infection
C. with a hot water bottle, heating pad, or electric blanket
D. from routine foot care

_____ 10. Which of the following is true of foot care?
A. It is not essential for residents with diabetes.
B. The nursing assistant should inspect for redness and order treatment.
C. It is performed by a podiatrist and is outside a nursing assistant's scope of practice.
D. Observations should be documented and concerns reported to the licensed nursing staff.

Perineal Care

Complete the following sentences.

1. _____ care, sometimes called *peri care*, is the process of cleaning the genitals, the urethral opening, and the anus.

2. Perineal care is important for preventing infections, _____ breakdown, and possible odor.

3. Perineal care is typically performed after _____.

4. Perineal care is necessary each time a resident is _____, or unable to control elimination.

5. Residents who have a urinary _____ will require catheter care in addition to perineal care.

Female Perineal Care

The following steps are part of the procedure for providing female perineal care. Identify the proper order in which they should be completed by numbering them 1 through 5.

_____ Fill the washbasin with fresh, warm water and change your gloves, if needed. Using fresh water and a clean washcloth, rinse the area thoroughly. Gently pat the area dry with a towel. Turn the resident onto her side away from you.

_____ Apply soap to a wet washcloth. With one hand, lift the upper buttock to expose the anus. Wash the anal area using gentle, front-to-back strokes from the vagina to the anus. Rinse and gently pat the area dry. Remove and dispose of the protective pad. Remove and discard your gloves. Wash your hands or use hand sanitizer to ensure infection control.

_____ Wet a washcloth in the washbasin and apply a small amount of soap. Gently separate the labia with one hand. Wash the outer folds of the labia and the inner folds using single, downward strokes from top to bottom or front to back. With each downward stroke, turn the washcloth to a clean side or get a new washcloth. Clean from the clitoris to the anus.

_____ Put on a new pair of gloves and reposition the resident. Replace the top covers and remove the bath blanket. Check to be sure the bed wheels are locked and then lower the bed. Follow the plan of care for using side rails. Remove, clean, and store equipment in the proper location.

_____ After completing preparatory steps and filling a washbasin with warm water, ask the resident to bend her knees and separate her legs. The perineal area can also be accessed from a lateral position with the knees bent. Move the linens down to the foot of the bed to expose only the perineal area. Keep the legs covered.

Male Perineal Care

The following steps are part of the procedure for providing male perineal care. Identify the proper order in which they should be completed by numbering them 1 through 5.

_____ Put on a new pair of gloves and reposition the resident. Replace the top covers and remove the bath blanket. Check to be sure the bed wheels are locked and then lower the bed. Follow the plan of care for using side rails. Remove, clean, and store equipment in the proper location.

_____ Turn the resident onto his side away from you. Apply soap to a wet washcloth and wash the anal area using gentle, front-to-back strokes. Rinse and gently pat the area dry. Remove and dispose of the protective pad. Remove and discard your gloves. Wash your hands or use hand sanitizer to ensure infection control.

_____ Lift and wash the scrotum. Also wash the inner thighs. Fill the washbasin with fresh, warm water and change your gloves, if needed. Using fresh water and a clean washcloth, rinse the area thoroughly. Gently pat the area dry with a towel.

_____ After completing preparatory steps and filling a washbasin with warm water, ask the resident to bend his knees and separate his legs. The perineal area can also be accessed from a lateral position with the knees bent. Move the linens down to the foot of the bed to expose only the perineal area. Keep the legs covered.

_____ Wet a washcloth in the washbasin and apply a small amount of soap. Gently lift and hold the penis in one hand. Start at the tip and wash on each side in a circular motion down the shaft of the penis to the base. If the penis is not circumcised, pull back the foreskin while washing, rinsing, and drying. If it will not retract, report this to the licensed nursing staff.

Dressing and Undressing

Complete the following sentences.

1. A person's _____ is reflective of his or her personal preferences and image, so it is important for residents to choose what to wear.

2. Nursing assistants should encourage residents to be as _____ as possible during dressing and undressing.

3. Clothing with zippers, Velcro™ fasteners, _____ waistbands, and slip-on shoes can make it easier for residents to maintain some independence when dressing.

4. Shoes or slippers that fit well and have _____ soles or strips help maintain safety so residents do not slip or trip.

5. During dressing and undressing, disposable _____ are worn only if required for infection prevention and control.

6. To minimize stress, nursing assistants should put clothing on the weak or painful side of a resident's body _____.

7. Clothes should be _____ from the unaffected or strong side first.

8. It is important never to pull, push, or otherwise roughly handle the _____ when putting on or removing clothes.

9. When changing a hospital gown for a patient who has an IV catheter, a nursing assistant needs to ensure the IV catheter insertion and tubing are not _____.

10. If helping change a hospital gown for a patient who has an IV catheter, a nursing assistant should never lower the bag of IV fluid below the _____ site.

Understanding the Skin

Identify whether each statement is true or false.

_____ 1. The skin is the largest organ in the body and does not reflect health.

_____ 2. Moist skin is a sign of dehydration.

_____ 3. Skin types can be categorized as normal, dry, oily, or combination.

_____ 4. A person's skin type depends on the water content of the skin, which affects elasticity; oiliness, which affects texture; and sensitivity.

_____ 5. Skin type does not change over time due to personal care, cosmetics used, environment, medications taken, hormones, and aging.

Skin Types

Identify each skin type described in the table.

Characteristics of Skin Types	
Type	**Characteristics**
1. _____	Radiant complexion, balance between dryness and oiliness, few blemishes, little sensitivity, and barely visible pores
2. _____	Dry, rough complexion with lines; less elasticity; red, inflamed, peeling, and cracking skin; scaly, itchy patches, and invisible pores
3. _____	Shiny and dull complexion; blackheads, pimples, and blemishes; and enlarged pores
4. _____	Dryness and oiliness in different areas, blackheads, and larger-than-normal pores

Promoting Skin Integrity

Complete the following guidelines for promoting skin integrity.

1. Eat a healthy diet rich in fruits, whole grains, and _____ proteins.

2. If you are a man, drink _____ cup(s) of fluids each day.

3. If you are a woman, drink _____ cup(s) of fluids each day.

4. _____ the skin every morning and night and wash your hands before touching your face.

5. Apply _____ to keep skin hydrated.

6. Wear broad spectrum _____ that protects against UVA and UVB rays.

7. Make _____ a part of daily activities, sleep seven to eight hours every night, and manage stress using healthy strategies.

8. Avoid _____, which significantly advances aging of the skin and causes broken surface blood vessels.

Maintaining Residents' Skin Integrity

Complete the following sentences.

1. Holistic nursing assistants give excellent skin care and are vigilant about observing the skin, particularly when caring for older adults and residents with _____.

2. Residents require special skin care if they are taking _____, which prevent blood clot formation.

3. Nursing assistants should avoid giving residents long _____, as these can remove oils from the skin.

4. For skin care, mild cleansers should be used instead of strong soaps, which can remove _____ from the skin.

5. The skin should be patted _____ after a bath or shower to leave some moisture on the skin.

6. The skin requires routine moisturizing with lotion, especially if the skin is _____.

7. Lotion should not be applied between the _____, where fungus can grow.

8. If a resident is _____ of urine or feces, the skin should be cleaned immediately with mild soap and water and gently patted dry.

9. It is important to keep _____ neat, free of wrinkles, and free from food crumbs and any other items that could place pressure on the skin.

10. Nursing assistants should avoid dragging or pulling a resident during positioning, as _____ can cause the skin to become red or irritated.

Pressure Points and Decubitus Ulcers

Identify whether each statement is true or false.

_____ 1. Residents who are immobile, use wheelchairs, or need to use assistive devices are more vulnerable to changes in skin integrity.

_____ 2. Pressure points can be found where skin covers the soft areas of the body.

_____ 3. The severity of decubitus ulcers ranges from stage 1 to stage 10.

_____ 4. In stage 1 of a decubitus ulcer, the skin is somewhat red. Stage 4 is characterized by deep skin damage, exposed muscle and bone, necrotic tissue formation, and bleeding ulcers.

_____ 5. The best way to detect decubitus ulcers and ensure skin integrity is to observe the skin carefully while performing personal hygiene activities, grooming, and other procedures.

Observation of the Skin

Complete the following guidelines for observing the skin.

1. When observing the skin, notice whether the skin is cool, warm, hot, moist, or dry and the _____ of the skin, lips, and nail beds.

2. Report to the licensed nursing staff if you observe pallor or if the skin is flushed (red) or _____ (blue due to insufficient oxygen).

3. Report and document abrasions, tears, bruises, rashes, blisters, lumps, swollen or _____ areas, and drainage or bleeding.

4. Inform the licensed nursing staff of unusual _____ and resident complaints of itching, burning, or scratching.

5. Regularly check the skin for red areas, irritation, or skin breakdown at _____ points and immediately remove whatever is causing the pressure.

6. Do not _____ reddened areas. Instead, recheck the skin for redness after 15 minutes.

7. _____ a resident's position at least every two hours.

8. Help residents ambulate and perform _____ (ROM) exercises according to the plan of care.

9. Keep pressure _____ dry and clean.

10. Ensure any decubitus _____ are cleaned and dressed with bandages according to the plan of care.

Heat and Cold Applications

Identify whether each statement most relates to heat treatment (*H*) or cold treatment (*C*).

_____ 1. Thermotherapy increases circulation, eases pain, and promotes healing.

_____ 2. Cryotherapy is used to reduce swelling and ease pain for acute injuries.

_____ 3. Treatment applications include a tepid sponge bath and a hypothermia blanket.

_____ 4. Applications have the potential to cause severe frostbite, which can cause infection and gangrene.

_____ 5. Treatment opens or dilates blood vessels, which increases the circulation of oxygen and nutrients and reduces pain.

_____ 6. Treatment relaxes muscles, improves flexibility, and lessens spasms.

_____ 7. Applications are most effective if used early and often during the first 24–48 hours after an injury.

_____ 8. Applications must be immediately stopped if the resident complains of burning pain, which can indicate a lack of blood supply to the skin (called *ischemia*).

_____ 9. Applications on the surface of the skin are used to treat chronic injuries or later-stage acute injuries, such as dislocation of a joint or a contusion.

_____ 10. Treatment decreases blood flow to the injury, lessening inflammation and swelling.

_____ 11. Treatment helps residents with arthritis, tendonitis, and muscle tension and warms up the muscles before exercise.

_____ 12. Compresses are applied to injured areas for no more than 20 minutes at a time or as long as ordered by the doctor. They should be removed for 10 minutes and then reapplied for 10 minutes.

_____ 13. Treatment should be avoided after exercise and during the acute phase of an injury.

_____ 14. Cryotherapy is most effective for sprains, bumps, bruises, and soft-tissue injuries.

_____ 15. Applications should not be used if the resident cannot feel or is sensitive to the application or has infections, tumors, open wounds, or stitches.

_____ 16. Applications cause vasoconstriction (the shrinking of blood vessels), which slows the demand for oxygen.

_____ 17. Applications may include moist compresses (pads), soaks, and an aquathermia pad.

_____ 18. Treatment can slow or stop bleeding and ease pain.

_____ 19. Treatment can be provided with an aquathermia pad, or K-pad, which promotes skin circulation by applying a constant temperature to a body part.

_____ 20. Applications include moist compresses and different types of ice packs.

_____ 21. Applications must be immediately stopped if the resident complains of numbness or if the skin appears white or spotty.

_____ 22. Treatment must be monitored for signs of frostnip, which can lead to frostbite.

_____ 23. Treatments should be applied for 15–20 minutes, unless the doctor orders a shorter or longer time, and should be checked every five minutes to see how well the resident's skin tolerates the application.

_____ 24. Applications require maintenance of resident hydration, proper body position, comfort, and documentation of response to treatment.

_____ 25. Treatment may include an ice cap used specifically for the head.

_____ 26. Moist compresses may be wrapped with plastic wrap and then a bath towel to reduce inflammation, muscle contractions and spasms, and swelling.

_____ 27. Treatment may include an ice collar specialized to fit the neck.

Name: _____   Date: _____

Matching Chapter 22 Key Terms

Match each definition with the key term.

A. alternative feeding therapy
B. aspirate
C. botanicals
D. calories
E. carbohydrates
F. dietary fats
G. dysphagia
H. eating disorder
I. electrolytes
J. enteral
K. herbals
L. hydrated
M. legumes
N. malabsorption
O. metabolism
P. minerals
Q. nutrition
R. obesity
S. parenteral
T. patent
U. proteins
V. Recommended Dietary Allowances (RDAs)
W. sedentary
X. therapeutic diets
Y. triglycerides
Z. vitamins

_____ 1. a health condition characterized by a body weight greater than what is considered healthy for a certain height

_____ 2. having sufficient fluids in the body over a 24-hour period

_____ 3. plants with pods (long cases) that contain edible seeds

_____ 4. daily levels of nutritional intake needed to maintain good health

_____ 5. the reduced ability of the intestine to take in essential nutrients and fluids and transfer them to the bloodstream

_____ 6. plant-based substances

_____ 7. the chemical process by which nutrients are converted into energy in the body

_____ 8. eating plans that cause healing

_____ 9. units of energy

_____ 10. inorganic substances in the body that regulate and assist in metabolism

_____ 11. the ingestion of foods that maintain the health of the body

_____ 12. calories stored in a person's fat cells

_____ 13. the body's main source of energy; includes three types: starches, sugars, and fiber

_____ 14. organic compounds needed for cell development and growth; must be ingested from foods in a person's diet or from supplements

_____ 15. substances in the blood and bodily fluids that carry electrical charges when dissolved in water

_____ 16. by way of the gastrointestinal system

_____ 17. lipids; provide energy for the body and include saturated fat, *trans* fat, and unsaturated fat

_____ 18. by way of the veins or intravenous infusion

_____ 19. the practice of delivering food intravenously or through a gastrointestinal tube due to a resident's inability to ingest food through the mouth

_____ 20. substances containing herbs

_____ 21. open

_____ 22. an abnormal pattern of eating that leads to serious and often fatal medical consequences

_____ 23. strings of amino acids that are vital to cell structure, contribute to energy production, build body tissue, and promote growth and repair

_____ 24. to inhale a foreign object or substance, such as food or liquid, when eating

_____ 25. difficulty or discomfort when swallowing

_____ 26. inactive

Understanding Nutrition

Complete the following sentences.

1. Good nutrition makes a positive difference in growth and development and can significantly influence the _____ of people's lives as they age.

2. Eating healthfully is a key contributor to the _____ process and a vital ingredient for those who have chronic illnesses such as diabetes.

3. If they do not make appropriate food selections, residents with diabetes can experience _____ imbalances.

4. Good nutrition gives a nursing assistant the _____ needed to provide safe, quality care.

5. Food _____ are shaped by a family's access to food, dietary traditions, age, diseases, medications, and ethnic or religious origins.

6. Knowledge of _____, which encompasses ingesting foods that maintain the health of the body, influences food preferences.

7. Aside from food preferences, people often select foods based on food _____ or sensitivities, physical disabilities, amount of time, financial resources, or special diets.

8. Foods may be selected based on how they are _____ or arranged in a food market.

9. Eating _____, which describe how often and fast people eat, are affected by childhood experience and usually become more established during adulthood.

10. Eating patterns become habits, guide choice of foods, influence how foods are eaten, affect digestion, and can cause _____ disorders.

11. Eating a healthy diet means including the proper amounts of essential _____, or substances needed for normal body function.

12. The six _____ nutrients are carbohydrates, dietary fats, proteins, vitamins, minerals, and water.

13. Essential nutrients are required for _____, the chemical process by which nutrients are converted into energy.

14. During the process of metabolism, _____ in food and fluids combine with oxygen to release energy.

15. A person's metabolic _____ is the number of calories the body uses to carry out its basic function.

16. Factors such as biological sex, body size and composition, and age all affect how calories are _____.

17. Metabolic rate accounts for about _____ percent of the calories burned daily.

18. Thirty percent of calories are burned daily through the normal processes of digesting, absorbing, transporting, and storing food and through _____.

19. General guidelines for the number of calories needed daily are based on _____ and activity levels.

20. According to the NIH, a person's activity level can be described as _____ (inactive), moderately active, or active.

21. The role of a holistic nursing assistant is to be aware of and sensitive to residents' food preferences and follow the _____.

Calorie Needs

Identify the calorie needs for females and males at each age and activity level.

Calorie Guidelines by Sex, Age, and Activity Levels				
		Activity Level		
Sex	Age	Sedentary	Moderately Active	Active
Female	19–30	1. _____ calories	7. _____ calories	13. _____ calories
	31–50	2. _____ calories	8. _____ calories	14. _____ calories
	51+	3. _____ calories	9. _____ calories	15. _____ calories
Male	19–30	4. _____ calories	10. _____ calories	16. _____ calories
	31–50	5. _____ calories	11. _____ calories	17. _____ calories
	51+	6. _____ calories	12. _____ calories	18. _____ calories

Energy Balance and Nutrients

Identify whether each statement is true or false.

_____ 1. Understanding energy balance is important for determining how best to consume and burn calories.

_____ 2. Energy *in*, or calories from food and fluids, should balance energy *out*, or calories burned as a result of metabolic rate, body functions, and physical activity.

_____ 3. If energy (calories) *in* is greater than energy (calories) *out*, weight stays the same.

_____ 4. UIf energy (calories) *in* is less than energy (calories) *out*, weight is gained.

_____ 5. If energy (calories) *in* is greater than energy (calories) *out*, weight is lost.

_____ 6. Calories that are consumed, but not used, are stored in a person's fat cells as triglycerides and may be released later as needed between meals.

_____ 7. High levels of unused triglycerides lead to a condition known as *hypertriglyceridemia*.

8. People have different nutritional needs based on their ages, life events (such as pregnancy and breast-feeding), body types, and levels of physical activity.

9. Malabsorption occurs if the intestine fails to take in essential nutrients and fluids and transfer them to the bloodstream.

10. Malabsorption can result from intestinal diseases, infections, inflammation, trauma, surgery, or nutritional deficiencies and can lead to weight loss and dehydration.

Carbohydrates

Complete the following sentences.

1. _____ are the body's main source of energy and contain carbon, hydrogen, and oxygen.

2. Carbohydrates are a(n) _____ because large amounts need to be obtained from nutritious food for the body to function properly.

3. There are three types of carbohydrates found in food: starches, which are also known as *complex carbohydrates*; _____, which are also known as *simple carbohydrates*; and fiber.

4. Starch is found in _____ and grains.

5. There are two types of grains: whole grains, which contain the entire grain _____, and refined grains, which have had part of the kernel removed.

6. _____ naturally occurs in milk and fruit and can also be added to foods during canning or baking.

7. Lactose is sugar found in milk, fructose is _____ sugar, and sucrose is table sugar.

8. _____ is found only in fruits, vegetables, whole grains, nuts, and legumes.

9. Dietary fiber cannot be _____, so the majority of it passes through and out of the body as feces.

10. Fiber is important for digestive health, helps a person feel full after eating, and assists with _____.

Dietary Fats and Proteins

Select the *best* answer.

1. What are dietary fats?
   A. micronutrients that provide energy for the body
   B. nutrients composed of carbon monoxide, hydrogen, and oxygen
   C. lipids that are unrelated to essential body functions
   D. nutrients that assist in the absorption of vitamins A, D, E, and K

2. Saturated fats
   A. are packed with hydrogen molecules and are considered "liquid" fats
   B. are chemically processed using partially hydrogenated vegetable oil
   C. raise total blood cholesterol and low-density lipoprotein (LDL), or bad cholesterol, levels
   D. do not increase the risk of type 2 diabetes

3. *Trans* fats
   A. increase levels of low-density lipoprotein (LDL) and lower levels of high-density lipoprotein (HDL)
   B. are chemically processed to shorten shelf life
   C. are usually found in homemade cakes or cookies containing soybean oil
   D. decrease the risk of cardiovascular disease

4. Unsaturated fats
   A. include saturated fats and polyunsaturated fats
   B. are found in olive, canola, safflower, peanut, and corn oils; nuts; mayonnaise; and avocados
   C. are found in salmon, bacon, T-bone steak, sardines, and whole milk
   D. increase the risk of cardiovascular disease and type 2 diabetes

5. Proteins are
   A. a major contributor to waste production
   B. the main builders of body tissue
   C. not responsible for the growth and repair of body tissues
   D. vital to cell structure and destroy oxygen and enzymes

6. What are electrolytes?
   A. amino acids that pose risks to the environment
   B. substances the body can synthesize on its own
   C. substances that must be ingested through a person's airway
   D. substances that carry electrical charges when dissolved in water

Vitamins, Minerals, and Water

Identify whether each statement is true or false.

1. Vitamins are organic compounds important for the development and growth of cells.

2. Some vitamins are fat soluble, meaning they cannot be stored in the body.

3. Recommended Dietary Allowances (RDAs) for vitamins are the same for each life stage.

4. International units (IUs) are part of the metric system, the official system of measurement in the United States.

5. Minerals are inorganic substances essential for body function.

6. Vitamin and mineral supplements take the place of healthy food selections in a person's diet.

_____ 7. Probiotics are microbes that stimulate the growth of beneficial microorganisms.

_____ 8. Water makes up 25 percent of the body's total weight.

_____ 9. Hydration improves a person's energy, mood, and clarity in thinking.

Choosing Safe and Healthy Foods

Complete the following sentences.

1. Both MyPlate and the *Dietary* _____ *for Americans* help people choose healthy foods in appropriate amounts.

2. When selecting foods, people can use food _____ to determine what nutrients are in a food.

3. _____ is a government resource that helps people learn about food groups, the proper proportions of food groups in a healthy diet, and food selections.

4. For maximum health, people should vary fruit selections and pick fruits rich in _____ (bananas, oranges, prunes, peaches, and apricots).

5. The best canned fruits are those with 100 percent fruit _____ or water instead of syrup.

6. _____ are categorized into five groups: dark green, starchy, red and orange, beans and peas, and other.

7. In place of refined _____, one should select whole grains, such as whole-wheat flour, bulgur, oatmeal, whole cornmeal, and brown rice.

8. Some people are _____ sensitive or intolerant and have an abnormal immune response to gluten during digestion.

9. The healthiest protein selections are _____ meat, beans, peas, soy products, nuts, and seeds.

10. The _____ food group includes healthy choices such as low-fat milk, yogurt, cheese, soy milk, and lactose-free milk products.

Five Food Groups

List the five MyPlate food groups and give an example of a food in each group.

1. Food group: _____

   Example: _____

2. Food group: _____

   Example: _____

3. Food group: _____

   Example: _____

4. Food group: _____

   Example: _____

5. Food group: _____

   Example: _____

Dietary Guidelines for Americans

Complete the following pieces of guidance from the *Dietary Guidelines for Americans*.

1. _____ should account for 45 to 65 percent of a person's total daily intake.

2. Eat 25 to 30 grams of _____ each day.

3. _____ should be restricted to less than 30 percent of a person's daily caloric intake, and saturated fats should account for less than 10 percent.

4. Select a variety of _____, including at least 8 ounces of cooked seafood per week.

5. At least one-half of all grains consumed should be _____ grains.

6. During _____, select foods that have the vitamins and minerals needed for a healthy pregnancy.

Food Labels

Identify whether each statement is true or false.

_____ 1. The 1990 Nutrition Labeling and Education Act (NLEA) requires most foods to include labels showing nutritional information.

_____ 2. The Nutrition Facts label must be adhered to every canned, boxed, or packaged food and provide information about how food products meet RDAs and dietary guidelines.

_____ 3. One should start at the bottom of a food label to identify a single serving size and the total number of servings in the food item.

_____ 4. It is important to check the total number of calories per serving because the number of servings eaten affects the number of calories consumed.

_____ 5. A food label typically lists a food's fat, sugar, dietary fiber, protein, calcium, iron, vitamins, minerals, and total carbohydrates (which encompasses all three types of carbohydrates).

_____ 6. % Daily Values (DVs) identify what percentage of a nutrient's recommended weekly amount a single serving contains.

Food Safety

Complete the following sentences.

1. _____ safety is an important aspect of healthy eating and dietary awareness.

2. Foodborne illnesses are diseases caused by pathogens or _____ (such as pesticides) that contaminate food.

3. In a(n) _____ illness, a pathogen enters the body with food that is ingested, causing cramping, nausea, vomiting, and diarrhea.

4. In the United States, government laws regulate food ingredients, food _____, dietary supplements, agricultural chemicals, and water.

5. The Food Safety Modernization Act (FSMA) strengthened the food safety system by having the FDA focus more on _____ foodborne illnesses than on reacting to food safety issues.

6. Washing your _____ and the surfaces used for food often can help prevent foodborne illness.

7. One can prevent cross-_____ by washing a knife before using it to cut another food.

8. Using a food _____ is the best way to check a food's temperature.

9. _____ (raw) milk, cheese, and juices or raw or undercooked animal foods can carry foodborne illnesses.

Overweight, Obesity, and Underweight

Select the *best* answer.

_____ 1. Which of the following is true of obesity?
   A. It is an epidemic, or an insignificant health problem.
   B. It is a body weight much greater than what is healthy for a certain height.
   C. It affects adults, but not children.
   D. It improves diseases such as diabetes and cardiovascular health.

_____ 2. Body mass index, or BMI, is
   A. a way to measure if a person is underweight, at a healthy weight, overweight, or obese
   B. used to calculate a person's height
   C. based on an adult's height (in meters) and current age
   D. measured using kilograms to calculate weight

_____ 3. Being underweight
   A. is not as serious a condition as being overweight
   B. can be related to an overproduction of essential nutrients
   C. is due to a heightened sense of smell and taste
   D. can be related to a lack of appetite and reduced sense of taste

_____ 4. Which of the following is true of weight loss?
   A. It typically occurs as a person becomes less mobile.
   B. Extreme weight loss is normal and always happens as a person ages.
   C. Sudden, unintentional, and unexplained weight loss usually indicates an underlying disease.
   D. If intentional and related to a healthy diet and exercise, it needs to be treated by a doctor.

Calculating BMI

Calculate the BMI for the following residents and identify each resident's BMI category.

A. A BMI less than 18.5 falls within the underweight range.
B. A BMI between 18.5 and 24.9 indicates a healthy weight.
C. A BMI between 25.0 and 29.9 falls within the overweight range.
D. A BMI between 30.0 and 34.9 falls within the class 1 obesity range.
E. A BMI between 35.0 and 39.9 falls within the class 2 obesity range.
F. A BMI of 40.0 or higher falls within the class 3 obesity range.

_____ 1. A male resident is 183 cm tall and weighs 127 kilograms.

_____ 2. A female resident is 168 cm tall and weighs 82 kilograms.

_____ 3. A male resident is 6 feet, 5 inches tall and weighs 150 pounds.

_____ 4. A female resident is 5 feet, 3 inches tall and weighs 120 pounds.

Eating Disorders

Complete the following sentences.

1. Some people develop dysfunctional eating behaviors, or eating _____, as a way to deal with their perceptions of their bodies.

2. Eating disorders affect both males and females, but rates among _____ are twice that of males.

3. People with eating disorders often engage in secretive behaviors, such as hiding food to be eaten later or _____ (evacuating food from the body) after eating.

4. Risk factors for eating disorders include genetics, physical or sexual abuse, perfectionism, high achievement, low self-esteem, and sports or activities that emphasize _____.

5. _____ nervosa is an intense fear of gaining weight, resulting in extreme weight loss and life-threatening medical symptoms.

6. _____ disorder is a condition in which a person loses control, excessively overeats, and becomes overweight or obese.

7. _____ nervosa is a condition characterized by recurring episodes of binge eating and purging, resulting in decaying teeth, severe dehydration, and electrolyte imbalance.

8. Treatment approaches for eating disorders include counseling to ensure adequate nutrition, therapy (individual or family), medical supervision, and sometimes medications such as _____.

Name: _____ Date: _____

Eating and Nutritional Assistance

Identify whether each statement is true or false.

_____ 1. The only purpose of eating is to provide what is physically essential to the body.

_____ 2. Dietitians create special diets that residents require due to an illness or disease.

_____ 3. Some residents require therapeutic diets, or diets that promote healing.

_____ 4. Mindful eating involves eating as quickly as possible with many interruptions and distractions.

_____ 5. In long-term care facilities, many residents eat in dining rooms and sit with particular people during mealtimes.

_____ 6. Seniors are vulnerable to malnutrition due to the aging process, in which metabolic rate and lean body mass increase.

_____ 7. Significant weight loss constitutes losing 1–2 pounds in one week and 5 pounds in one month.

_____ 8. Weight loss becomes severe when a resident loses even more than 1–2 pounds in one week or 5 pounds in one month.

_____ 9. Licensed nursing staff members and dietitians usually conduct a nutritional status assessment to determine a resident's plan of care and assess how well a resident eats and drinks.

_____ 10. Holistic nursing assistants do not need to know about or follow residents' special diets.

_____ 11. Supplemental nutrition drinks are fortified with vitamins and are given to those who have specific diseases, such as cancer or COPD.

_____ 12. Formulas can be consumed orally, but are often delivered via feeding tubes following a doctor's order.

Therapeutic Diets

Match each description with the correct therapeutic diet. Some answers may be used more than once.

A. soft or mechanical soft diet
B. bland diet
C. full liquid diet
D. low-sodium diet
E. renal diet
F. liberalized diet
G. clear liquid diet
H. cardiac or heart-healthy diet
I. high-fiber diet
J. regular diet
K. diabetic or carbohydrate-controlled diet
L. low-fiber diet

_____ 1. diet used by doctors and dietitians to find more creative ways of managing diseases, improve resident compliance, and increase enjoyment

_____ 2. diet with no food restrictions

_____ 3. diet ordered when a resident has difficulty chewing or swallowing due to weakness or dental problems

_____ 4. diet that transitions residents from clear liquids to a soft diet; is ordered when residents have undergone special procedures (such as GI surgery) or have dental issues

_____ 5. diet ordered prior to tests, medical procedures, or surgeries that require the gastrointestinal system to be free from food; is also ordered for residents with digestive problems such as nausea, vomiting, or diarrhea

_____ 6. diet that does not provide sufficient calories and nutrients; is usually transitional after a procedure or illness

_____ 7. diet that helps treat ulcers, heartburn, nausea, vomiting, diarrhea, and gas; may also be ordered after stomach or intestinal surgery

_____ 8. diet for residents who have kidney or cardiac disease

_____ 9. diet for residents who have cardiovascular diseases; promotes overall health and weight loss

_____ 10. diet for residents who have diabetes; ensures steady blood sugar levels

_____ 11. diet for residents who have kidney disease; prevents or slows further kidney damage by restricting phosphorus, potassium, sodium, and fluids

_____ 12. diet for residents who have chronic constipation, irritable bowel syndrome, or an elevated risk for colon cancer

_____ 13. diet ordered when a resident is experiencing GI problems, such as abdominal pain, diarrhea, diverticulitis, and stricture

Alternative Feeding Therapies

Complete the following sentences.

1. Residents who cannot eat food through their mouths may require nutrition to be delivered using a(n) _____ feeding therapy.

2. _____ nutrition provides nutrients such as sugar, carbohydrates, proteins, and electrolytes to the body via an intravenous (IV) line.

3. _____ nutrition delivers a formula containing proteins, carbohydrates, fats, vitamins, and minerals by way of the gastrointestinal system.

4. _____ tubes are inserted or surgically placed depending on the doctor's order, the function of the GI system, and the length of time the tube will be used.

5. A(n) _____ tube is inserted through the nose and runs down the esophagus into the stomach.

6. A(n) _____ tube is inserted through the nose and ends in the first portion of the small intestine (duodenum), bypassing the stomach.

7. Residents who have stomachs that don't empty well, who are chronically vomiting, or who _____ (inhale) stomach contents into the lungs benefit from an ND tube.

8. A(n) _____ tube is inserted through the nose and ends in the second portion of the small intestine (jejunum).

9. _____ tubes are surgically inserted through the abdominal wall into the stomach and are commonly used for residents who receive long-term enteral nutrition.

10. A G tube often consists of a long tube, sometimes called a _____ *endoscopic gastronomy (PEG) tube*, and a skin-level button device.

11. A(n) _____ tube is surgically placed directly into the intestine.

12. In some states, nursing assistants can be delegated the responsibility of giving tube _____ and removing NG tubes.

13. Tube feedings may be scheduled or _____ (given slowly over a 24-hour period).

14. Formula should be given at _____ temperature and will only last eight hours after being opened.

15. During tube feeding, the _____ of the resident's bed should be elevated at least 30–45°, or as specified in the plan of care, and should remain elevated at least one hour after each feeding.

16. Licensed nursing staff members regularly check a feeding tube's placement to be sure the feeding tube is _____ (open).

17. If a feeding tube looks displaced, a nursing assistant should immediately notify the licensed _____ staff.

18. Nursing assistants should check the area around a feeding tube insertion site for _____, swelling, drainage, or odor and report concerns to the licensed nursing staff.

19. During tube feeding, it is important to notify the licensed nursing staff immediately if there is nausea, abdominal _____ (a swollen abdomen), complaints of pain, coughing, vomiting, respiratory distress, increased pulse rate, flatulence, diarrhea, or constipation.

20. To improve a resident's comfort and hygiene, a nursing assistant can provide frequent oral and nasal care and _____ the lips often.

Feeding Tubes

Apply the appropriate labels to the images.

A. Gastrostomy tube
B. Jejunostomy tube
C. Nasoduodenal tube

D. Nasogastric tube
E. Nasojejunal tube

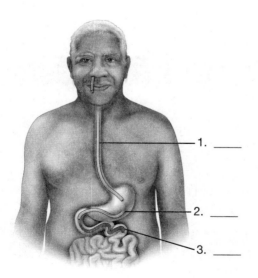

1. _____
2. _____
3. _____

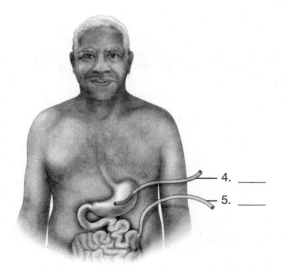

4. _____
5. _____

© Body Scientific International

Adaptive and Assistive Eating Equipment

Identify whether each statement is true or false.

_____ 1. Adaptive and assistive eating equipment helps residents be as independent as possible during meals.

_____ 2. Equipment to promote resident independence includes special plates and bowls, utensils, utensil holders, cups, and mugs.

_____ 3. Commercially available thickening products aid in safe swallowing and help prevent aspiration.

_____ 4. The thinner a liquid is, the less risk there is of choking.

_____ 5. Nursing assistants sometimes need to thicken fluids for residents who have dysphagia, or difficulty swallowing.

_____ 6. Signs of dysphagia include food spilling out of the mouth or coming up through the nose, coughing or choking during or after swallowing, complaints that food will not go down or feels stuck in the throat, and avoidance of foods that require chewing.

_____ 7. Adaptive equipment includes nonskid plates and bowls that prevent foods from slipping off.

_____ 8. Weightless knives, forks, and spoons help the hands of residents remain steady.

_____ 9. Utensil holders such as clips, straps, and foam handles help residents achieve better grip.

_____ 10. Cup holders, weighted mugs, nonslip bases, and no-spill lids should be avoided since they cause spills.

_____ 11. The role of the holistic nursing assistant is to prepare residents for meals, help residents to the dining room, and force residents to eat.

_____ 12. One of the most important aspects of caring for residents during mealtime is preventing independence.

_____ 13. Slightly extending the resident's head to achieve a chin-up position helps reduce aspiration and some types of dysphagia.

_____ 14. Nursing assistants should offer all liquid foods and then all solid foods.

_____ 15. Food should be placed in the weakest side of a resident's mouth.

Understanding Liquid Consistency

Identify the level of consistency for each description in the table.

Liquid Consistencies	
Level of Consistency	Description
1. _____	Puddinglike; holds shape and can be served with a spoon
2. _____	Honeylike; will not flow freely, but will run off a spoon
3. _____	Nectarlike; does not hold shape and will run off a spoon
4. _____	Free-flowing liquids, such as water, soda, coffee, or juice

Recording Food and Fluid Intake

Identify the equivalencies for recording food and fluid intake in the table.

Food Intake	
Percentage	Description
1. _____	Consumed none or only bites (but less than 25%)
2. _____	Consumed 1/4 of all item(s)
3. _____	Consumed 1/2 of all item(s)
4. _____	Consumed 3/4 of all item(s)
5. _____	Consumed all item(s)

Fluid Intake	
Cups and Bowls	Milliliters
1 oz. Cup	6. _____
4 oz. Cup	7. _____
5 oz. Cup	8. _____
6 oz. Cup/Bowl	9. _____
8 oz. Cup/Bowl	10. _____

Assisting with Meals

Due to diseases or conditions, some residents require help from nursing assistants to eat comfortably and consume sufficient amounts of their meals. In this activity, you will practice portions of the procedure for assisting with meals in the room. To prepare for this activity, review the procedural checklist for Assisting with Meals in the Room. Also have your FIRST CHECK procedural checklist nearby.

Form a group of three and assign each person a role. One person will be the nursing assistant, another a resident, and the third person will serve as the evaluator. Then complete each of the following steps:

1. To prepare for this activity, acquire a pair of eyeglasses, place tape over them, and have the resident partner wear them to simulate vision impairment. Have the resident partner bring in a food he or she would like to be fed and bring in assistive equipment for the feeding. Use a commercially prepared thickener to thicken liquids that will be offered and print two intake forms to record food and fluid intake.

2. Complete the FIRST, or Preparation, steps of the procedure, omitting any steps that are not applicable to the Assisting with Meals in the Room procedure.

3. Did you omit any steps that are not applicable to the Assisting with Meals in the Room procedure? If yes, explain which step(s) were omitted and why.

_____

_____

_____

4. Complete the procedure for assisting the resident with a meal in the room. Follow guidelines for offering food and placing foods in the resident's mouth. The resident should not assist with the procedure. The nursing assistant should complete all of the feeding, and the evaluator should observe and take notes about how well the procedure is followed.

5. On the intake form, record food and fluid intake. The evaluator should also complete the intake form and compare with the nursing assistant for accuracy.

6. Complete the CHECK, or Follow-Up and Reporting and Documentation, steps of the procedure, omitting any steps that are not applicable to the procedure.

7. Did you omit any steps that are not applicable to the Assisting with Meals in the Room procedure? If yes, explain which step(s) were omitted and why.

_____

_____

_____

8. Switch roles so each partner has the opportunity to be the nursing assistant.

Name: _____ Date: _____

Matching Chapter 23 Key Terms

Match each definition with the key term.

A. constipation
B. defecate
C. dehydration
D. diarrhea
E. enema
F. flatus
G. graduate
H. hernia
I. impaction
J. motility
K. ostomy
L. stoma
M. suppositories
N. void

_____ 1. gas or air in the gastrointestinal tract; is expelled via the anus

_____ 2. small, meltable, solid cones or cylinders that may be medicated and are inserted into a body passage such as the rectum or vagina

_____ 3. a protrusion or bulge of an organ through the wall of the body cavity or structure that contains it

_____ 4. to expel urine from the body

_____ 5. a condition in which bowel movements occur fewer than three times a week and contain hard, dry stools that are difficult to evacuate; can be an acute or chronic condition

_____ 6. a procedure in which liquid is inserted into the rectum to clean the lower intestine

_____ 7. container used to measure intake and output

_____ 8. a surgical procedure that creates an opening in the abdominal wall so that stool can be eliminated from the intestines to the outside of the body

_____ 9. blockage of hard stool in the rectum

_____ 10. to have a bowel movement

_____ 11. movement of substances through the GI system

_____ 12. lack of adequate body fluids

_____ 13. a surgically created abdominal opening, through which stool are eliminated

_____ 14. a condition in which bowel movements have stool with excess water and occur frequently; can be an acute or chronic condition

Hydration

Complete the following sentences.

1. Fluids in the body moisten tissues in the eyes, nose, and mouth; protect organs; regulate body _____; lubricate joints; and flush toxins.

2. Excess fluid can lead to _____, or swelling in the body tissues.

3. If a person does not take in enough fluids, _____, or lack of adequate fluids in the body tissue, can occur.

4. Infants, children, and older adults have _____ risk for dehydration.

5. Dehydration occurs when the body lacks adequate body _____ due to decreased consumption, excessive perspiration, or a disease or injury.

6. The _____ in the body's systems caused by dehydration can become so severe it leads to death.

7. Dehydration may occur if a person consumes insufficient fluids due to lack of access, inability to consume fluids, _____ (difficulty swallowing), or unconsciousness.

8. Exposure to excessive or long-lasting heat, exercise, or a high _____ may cause dehydration.

9. Constant vomiting, _____ (frequent, watery stools), and extreme skin injuries such as burns can cause significant loss of fluids.

10. The first signs of dehydration are increased _____ and dry mouth, leading to dizziness or weakness.

11. As dehydration becomes more severe, symptoms include tongue swelling, _____ palpitations, headaches, confusion, and fainting.

12. Advanced dehydration can cause chest pain, difficulty breathing, inability to sweat, _____ (infrequent, hard, dry stools), and a noticeable decrease in urinary output.

13. When fluids are lacking, urine becomes more _____ and becomes dark yellow or orange in color.

14. Increasing the amount and variety of fluids and water-concentrated _____ and vegetables (such as oranges, tomatoes, and pineapple) can increase fluid intake to prevent dehydration.

15. To ensure hydration, holistic nursing assistants should discourage caffeinated beverages, which have a(n) _____ effect.

Parenteral IV Infusion

Identify whether each statement is true or false.

_____ 1. Parenteral IV infusion restores fluids and electrolytes and ensures adequate intake of fluids.

_____ 2. In parenteral IV infusion, fluid is administered through an open system consisting of a bag of fluid, tubing, and a needle or catheter.

_____ 3. In the IV system, the bag of fluid hangs on a pole below the patient's head. The pole may be attached to the head of the bed or stand next to the bed.

_____ 4. When the bag of IV fluid is hanging, gravity aids the flow of the fluid through the system.

_____ 5. Tubing attaches the bag of IV fluid to a catheter, which is inserted into the body with a needle by the licensed nursing staff.

_____ 6. An IV catheter is usually inserted into a peripheral vein in the patient's arm, but can also be inserted into the leg, foot, or scalp.

_____ 7. An IV pump is a programmable medical device that delivers fluids into a patient's body in a controlled manner to improve the accuracy and continuity of IV infusions.

_____ 8. The type and amount of IV fluid is ordered by the nurse and is infused at an appropriate rate based on the resident's condition.

_____ 9. Patients with NPO restrictions can drink fluids while undergoing parenteral IV infusion.

_____ 10. Licensed nursing staff members ensure that the tubes and catheters of the closed IV system remain patent and that the flow rate is accurate.

_____ 11. Nursing assistants should observe the IV insertion site for swelling and puffiness, which indicate dehydration.

_____ 12. Nursing assistants need to regularly monitor the IV system to make sure the IV fluid bag remains below the patient's heart and that there is no fluid leaking.

_____ 13. Complaints of discomfort, such as pain or burning at or near the IV site, should be reported to the licensed nursing staff.

_____ 14. Fever, itching, shortness of breath, chest pain, irregular pulse, and a drop in blood pressure are examples of systemic symptoms.

_____ 15. Nursing assistants should monitor patients' vital signs, know abnormal ranges, and alert the licensed nursing staff immediately of VS outside normal range.

_____ 16. Nursing assistants ensure the security of the IV dressing and maintain the position of the tubing and the extremity in which the IV needle or catheter is inserted.

Understanding the IV System

Apply the appropriate labels to the image.

A. IV catheter
B. Drip chamber
C. Closed clamp
D. IV bag
E. IV tube

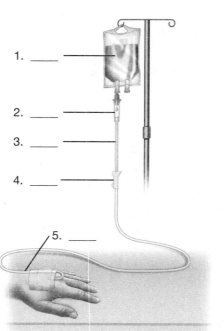

1. _____
2. _____
3. _____
4. _____
5. _____

© Body Scientific International

Common IV Insertion Sites

Apply the appropriate labels to the image.

A. Basilic vein
B. Cephalic vein
C. Dorsal metacarpal veins
D. Median cubital vein

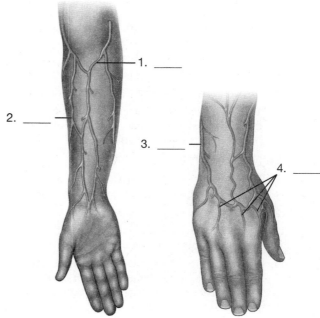

1. _____
2. _____
3. _____
4. _____

© Body Scientific International

Measuring Fluid Intake and Output

Select the *best* answer.

_____ 1. Fluid intake and output (I&O) is
   A. not as important as the meal intake of solids
   B. measured as an important monitor of hydration
   C. measured for patients in hospitals, but not for residents in long-term care facilities
   D. a rough estimation of fluids consumed

_____ 2. What is included in fluid intake?
   A. all oral fluids, IV fluids, and tube feedings
   B. all oral fluids, but not IV fluids or tube feedings
   C. all solids consumed between meals
   D. all solids consumed during meals and between meals

_____ 3. What is included in fluid output?
   A. urine from a urinary drainage bag, but not emesis
   B. diarrhea, colostomy bag drainage, and all liquids consumed
   C. formed feces as part of regular elimination
   D. any urine that is voided from the body

_____ 4. I&O is measured
   A. by pouring all leftover liquids into a graduate while residents are in the dining room
   B. on a 24-hour schedule using a graduate
   C. for fluids, but not for wound drainage
   D. using a urinary hat for leftover IV fluids

_____ 5. The I&O form
   A. can be obtained from the housekeeping or maintenance department
   B. can be a paper, but not an electronic, checklist
   C. is used to record intake and output throughout each shift
   D. is subtotaled at the end of each shift and doesn't continue to the next shift

Standard Measurements

Identify the standard measurements for each container.

Standard Volumes for Intake and Output		
Item	Volume in Ounces (oz)	Volume in Milliliters (mL)
Drinking glass	1. _____	6. _____
Cup	2. _____	7. _____
Teacup	3. _____	8. _____
Styrofoam cup	4. _____	9. _____
Popsicle	5. _____	10. _____
Ice cube	Melts to 1/2 the original volume	

Recording Fluid Intake and Output

For this activity, print the intake and output (I&O) form shown in the text. Then, read the following scenario and fill out the I&O form based on the scenario. Compare forms with a partner and print out another copy of the I&O form to record your own fluid intake and output.

Scenario

At 0200, a resident in a long-term care facility turned on her call light. The nursing assistant promptly answered the call and found the resident vomiting into her bath basin. The nursing assistant observed the color, odor, and consistency and measured the emesis as 350 mL. The resident requested assistance to the bathroom at 0300 and voided 650 mL into a urinary hat. She drank 150 mL of water. The resident went back to bed until 0500, when she requested assistance to the bathroom due to cramping, but did not have diarrhea. She returned to bed and vomited 400 mL. The resident drank a 6-oz can of clear soda at 0730. At 0830, she requested a light breakfast and consumed one-half an 8-oz carton of apple juice and 8 oz of water. At 1100, she voided 100 mL, returned to her bed, and had another episode of vomiting measured at 300 mL. She slept quietly until 1600 and then requested coffee. While waiting for the coffee, she vomited 100 mL. Over the course of the next hour, she sipped two 8-oz cups of coffee. She voided 375 mL at 1900, and upon feeling much better, ordered a turkey sandwich during the evening news and drank another 8-oz cup of coffee.

Measuring and Recording Fluid Intake

Careful and accurate measurement of intake and output (I&O) is essential to maintaining the body's fluid balance. The following steps are part of the procedure for measuring and recording fluid intake. Identify the proper order in which they should be completed by numbering them 1 through 5.

_____ Provide privacy by closing the curtains, using a screen, or closing the door to the room. Wash your hands or use hand sanitizer. Put on disposable gloves, if needed for infection prevention and control.

_____ Immediately record the amount consumed on the intake side of the I&O form. All other intake, such as from IV fluids or liquids given by tube, will be measured and recorded by the licensed nursing staff.

_____ For each container, note the amount of liquid that the resident was served and the amount the resident consumed by measuring the amount left in each container at eye level.

_____ Bring the necessary equipment into the room. Place the following items in an accessible location: disposable gloves (if needed), pen and form or digital device for recording I&O, appropriate measuring containers, and a graduate.

_____ Subtract each amount measured from the full amount the resident was served. Add all of these amounts together for the total amount the resident drank.

Measuring and Recording Urinary Output

The following steps are part of the procedure for measuring and recording urinary output. For each set of steps, identify the proper order in which they should be completed by numbering them 1 through 5.

1. _____ If the resident is ambulatory, place a urinary hat in the commode or toilet and instruct the resident to urinate into the hat, not into the commode or toilet. A bedpan, urinal, or urinary catheter with a drainage bag may also be used to collect urine. To empty a urinary drainage bag, begin by placing a disposable protective pad on the floor underneath the drainage bag. Place a graduate on top of the protective pad.

   _____ Close the drain on the urinary drainage bag. Wipe the drain with an antiseptic swab or according to facility policy. Replace the drain in the holder on the urinary drainage bag.

   _____ Provide privacy by closing the curtains, using a screen, or closing the door to the room. Wash your hands or use hand sanitizer. Put on disposable gloves.

   _____ Place a paper towel on a level surface and put the graduate used to measure output on top. If a bedpan or urinal was used, carefully pour the urine into the graduate. Note the color, odor, clarity, and amount. Measure the amount of urine at eye level and make note of this amount.

   _____ Clean the tubing of the urinary drainage bag with an antiseptic swab and open the drain at the bottom of the bag. Empty the urine into a graduate. Make sure the urine does not splash and the drainage tube does not touch the sides of the graduate.

2. _____ Dispose of urine in the toilet and avoid splashes. Carefully rinse the graduate and pour the rinse water into the toilet as well. All other output, such as the contents of a colostomy drainage bag, will be observed and measured by the licensed nursing staff.

   _____ Remove, clean, and store equipment in the proper location. Remove soiled linens and discard disposable equipment. Remove and discard your gloves. Wash your hands to ensure infection control.

   _____ Check to be sure the bed wheels are locked. Then reposition the resident and lower the bed.

   _____ Follow the plan of care to determine if the side rails should be raised or lowered. Ensure the call light is in place and conduct a safety check before leaving the room.

   _____ Record the urine output amount and characteristics on the paper or electronic I&O form. At the end of the shift, or as ordered, record the total urine output on the output side of the I&O form.

Assisting with Urinary Elimination

Complete the following sentences.

1. When a resident has limited _____, holistic nursing assistants need to frequently assist with elimination needs.

2. Urine is primarily _____ and a waste product produced by the kidneys. It passes through the bladder to the urethra, where it is expelled from the body.

3. Changes in the normal composition of urine are usually due to medications, urinary disorders, infection, or _____.

4. Some residents need to void during the night, which is called _____.

5. A resident with mobility challenges may use a bedside _____ for urinary and bowel elimination needs.

6. There are two types of bedpans: a regular bedpan and a(n) _____ bedpan.

7. A(n) _____ bedpan fits the contour of the buttocks and has a shallow bowl that collects urine and stool.

8. A(n) _____ bedpan is used when a resident has limited mobility, casts, traction, missing limbs, or spinal cord injuries or surgeries.

9. Men who have limited mobility may use a handheld _____ for urinary elimination while in bed.

10. Nursing assistants must be observant of changes in urine color, urgency, burning, and _____ (painful or difficult urination).

11. An abnormally small amount of urine is called _____.

12. _____ is an excessive amount of urine.

Name: _____   Date: _____

13. Infection control and prevention procedures should always be followed, as urine and stool may contain _____.

14. When assisting residents to the toilet, nursing assistants should make sure the area contains _____ paper and a clean hand towel or paper towels.

15. When helping a resident stand and walk to the bathroom, a nursing assistant should be safe and apply a(n) _____ belt for ambulation, if appropriate.

Assisting with a Bedpan

Proper bedpan use provides a safe means of urinary and bowel elimination for residents who cannot ambulate to the bathroom. The following steps are part of the procedure for assisting with a bedpan. For each set of steps, identify the proper order in which they should be completed by numbering them 1 through 5.

1. _____ Put a disposable protective pad under the resident's hips and position the bedpan under the buttocks. Position a standard bedpan like a regular toilet seat. Position a fracture bedpan with the thin edge facing the head of the bed. If necessary, roll the resident onto the side facing away from you and place the bedpan against the resident's buttocks. Then have the resident roll back with the bedpan underneath the buttocks.

   _____ Wash your hands or use hand sanitizer and put on disposable gloves. Fold the top linens back and raise the resident's gown. Ask the resident to bend his or her knees, put the feet flat on the mattress, and raise the hips.

   _____ Place the toilet paper and call light within reach. Instruct the resident to use the call light when finished. Remove and discard your gloves and wash your hands before leaving the room. Follow the plan of care for using side rails. If the resident cannot be left alone, stay in the room to ensure safety.

   _____ Bring the necessary equipment into the room and place in an accessible location. Provide privacy by closing the curtains, using a screen, or closing the door to the room. Lock the bed wheels and raise the bed to hip level. If there are side rails, raise and secure the rail on the opposite side of the bed from where you will be working. Lower the rail on the side you are working.

   _____ Put a bath blanket over the resident and raise the head of the bed. Ask the resident not to put toilet paper in the bedpan. Provide a waste container for the toilet paper.

2. _____ Check to be sure the bed wheels are locked, then reposition the resident and lower the bed. Follow the plan of care for using side rails. Take the bedpan to the bathroom. Check the stool and urine for unusual appearance or odor.

   _____ Help the resident put on clean briefs or undergarments. Change the resident's gown, if needed. Cover the resident with the top linens and place the bath blanket in the laundry hamper. Straighten or change bed linens, as needed.

_____ Return to the room when the resident uses the call light or within five minutes. Wash your hands or use hand sanitizer and put on disposable gloves. Assist with wiping and perineal care, as needed. Remove and discard your gloves. Wash your hands or use hand sanitizer.

_____ Put on a new pair of disposable gloves. Help the resident raise the hips or roll to the side so you can remove the bedpan. Remove and discard the protective pad and cover the bedpan immediately. Place the bedpan on top of a paper towel or barrier in a secure place.

_____ Remove and discard your gloves, wash your hands or use hand sanitizer, and put on a new pair of disposable gloves. Fill a washbasin with warm water and help the resident wash his or her hands. Remove the washbasin and place the used towels in the laundry hamper.

3. _____ Remove and discard your gloves and wash your hands. If I&O is being monitored, record the amount of output on the paper or electronic I&O form. If there was a bowel movement, record it in the form provided or in the electronic record.

   _____ Empty the contents of the bedpan into the toilet. Avoid splashes. Carefully rinse the bedpan and pour the rinse water into the toilet. Using disinfectant spray or wipes, clean and then dry the bedpan and cover. Store the clean bedpan and cover in the appropriate storage location.

   _____ Communicate any specific observations, complications, or unusual responses to the licensed nursing staff. Record this information, along with the care provided, in the chart or EMR.

   _____ Make sure the resident is comfortable and place the call light and personal items within reach. Conduct a safety check before leaving the room. The room should be clean and free from clutter or spills.

   _____ Wash your hands or use hand sanitizer before leaving the room.

Assisting with Urinary Catheters

Identify whether each statement is true or false.

_____ 1. An inability to eliminate urine can cause bladder distention.

_____ 2. Urinary elimination problems can be caused by surgery, childbirth, blockage, and certain diseases and conditions.

_____ 3. A urinary catheter works by evaporating urine from the body.

_____ 4. An indwelling urinary catheter is a catheter inserted into the urethra and left inside the bladder.

_____ 5. A catheter is held in place by a balloon inflated with sterile water in the kidney.

_____ 6. A suprapubic catheter is surgically inserted into the bladder through the abdominal wall below the pubic area.

Name: _____   Date: _____

_____ 7. Gravity helps urine in the urinary bladder flow into the catheter tubing and empty into a drainage bag inside the body.

_____ 8. To prevent backwash of urine, the urinary drainage bag should always be positioned above the bladder, even when a resident is ambulating.

_____ 9. A urinary drainage bag should be attached to a movable part of the bed, be clear of any wheels, and never touch or rest on the floor.

_____ 10. Nursing assistants are typically responsible for providing proper catheter care every eight days, or as required by facility policy.

_____ 11. Proper catheter care is key to preventing catheter-associated urinary tract infections (CAUTIs).

_____ 12. Catheter care involves cleansing the catheter at the insertion site and perineum, checking the catheter and drainage bag for leaks or kinks, making sure the resident is not lying on the catheter, and observing any other problems.

_____ 13. If residents are experiencing pain, this should be reported to the licensed nursing staff.

_____ 14. A catheter care kit includes disposable gloves, a disposable protective pad, and applicators with antiseptic solution.

_____ 15. For catheter care, nursing assistants can use clean washcloths and mild soap in place of applicators and antiseptic.

Providing Catheter Care

Proper catheter care ensures consistent hygiene, maintains skin integrity, and helps prevent CAUTIs. The following steps are part of the procedure for providing catheter care. For each set of steps, identify the proper order in which they should be completed by numbering them 1 through 5.

1. _____ Check the catheter insertion area for crusting, lesions, discharge, or anything abnormal. Notify the licensed nursing staff if you observe any of these conditions.

   _____ Provide privacy by closing the curtains, using a screen, or closing the door to the room. Lock the bed wheels and then raise the bed to hip level. If using side rails, raise and secure the side rail on the side opposite where you will be working. Lower the side rail on the side you are working. Wash your hands or use hand sanitizer and put on disposable gloves.

   _____ Bring the necessary equipment into the room and place the following items in an accessible location: a catheter care kit, disposable gloves, bath blanket, washcloths, soap, towels, washbasin, disposable protective pad, plastic bag, and laundry hamper.

   _____ Position the resident on his or her back and cover the resident with a bath blanket. Without exposing the resident, fanfold the top linens to the foot of the bed.

   _____ Open the catheter kit and remove the disposable protective pad. If there is no kit, use the protective pad you brought into the room. Place the protective pad under the resident's buttocks.

2. _____ Clean the catheter. Start near the meatus and move down the catheter about 4 inches. Rinse using a new washcloth and dry with a fresh towel.

   _____ Remove the applicators from the kit. If there is no kit, fill a washbasin with warm water (between 100–105°F) and use a washcloth and soap. Using a circular motion, apply the antiseptic solution to the entire catheter insertion area. If there is no kit, use a clean part of the washcloth for each stroke.

   _____ Secure the catheter and tubing to the resident's upper thigh. Leave some slack in the catheter tubing.

   _____ Remove the disposable protective pad and cover the resident with the top linens. Remove the bath blanket, check to be sure the bed wheels are locked, then reposition the resident and lower the bed. Remove, clean, and store equipment in the proper location. Perform hand hygiene and document.

   _____ Coil the remaining tubing and be sure it is not under the resident, twisted, or bent. Secure the drainage bag to the bottom of the bedframe using the bag ties.

Urinary Drainage Bags

Complete the following sentences.

1. When changing a urinary drainage bag, a nursing assistant should clamp the catheter to prevent _____ from draining into the drainage tubing.

2. The _____ cap and catheter plug must not be touched while they are being opened.

3. When disconnecting the old drainage bag tubing, a nursing assistant should be careful not to let anything _____ the end of the catheter.

4. A nursing assistant should hold the sterile catheter _____, but should not touch the end that goes inside the catheter.

5. A sterile _____ should be placed on the end of the old drainage bag tubing without the nursing assistant touching the end of the tubing.

6. To change a urinary drainage bag, a nursing assistant should remove the cap from the end of the new _____ bag tubing and remove the sterile plug from the catheter.

7. The end of the new drainage bag tubing should be _____ into the flexible catheter.

8. The _____ should be removed from the catheter to ensure the free flow of urine into the new bag.

9. A(n) _____ bag may be used as an alternative to a urinary drainage bag when a resident is ambulatory.

10. A leg bag must be checked regularly for proper drainage and _____ more frequently.

Understanding Incontinence

Select the *best* answer.

_____ 1. Urinary incontinence
   A. prevents the loss of bladder control
   B. is more common in men than in women
   C. often relates to disease and the age-related weakening of bladder muscles
   D. develops when residents drink too much alcohol

_____ 2. Stress incontinence
   A. often occurs during coughing, sneezing, or laughing
   B. lessens stress on the bladder sphincter
   C. strengthens the muscle that holds urine
   D. is always permanent

_____ 3. Which of the following is true of urge incontinence?
   A. It is not the same as an overactive bladder (OAB).
   B. It occurs when the bladder contracts with enough force to override urethral sphincter muscles.
   C. It cannot cause the involuntary loss of urine.
   D. It has no known treatment.

_____ 4. Overflow incontinence
   A. occurs when the bladder is not completely emptied
   B. causes urine to remain in the bladder and not leak
   C. is unaffected by urinary obstructions and weak sphincter muscles
   D. is sometimes called *scribbling*

_____ 5. What is the goal of treating urinary incontinence?
   A. to help residents increase bladder control
   B. to force residents to perform pelvic-floor muscle training
   C. to cure incontinence with biofeedback
   D. to limit fluid intake throughout the entire day and evening

_____ 6. Caring for residents who are incontinent involves
   A. showing empathy and support and rushing residents to the bathroom
   B. using diapers to reduce feelings of embarrassment and guilt
   C. lecturing residents about smoking, alcohol, and spicy foods
   D. showing respect and compassion

_____ 7. To prevent resident embarrassment, a nursing assistant should
   A. tell residents not to feel angry
   B. force residents to wear incontinence briefs
   C. not use the term *diaper* when referring to an incontinence brief
   D. apply double briefs and remove briefs correctly

_____ 8. If a resident is incontinent, a nursing assistant should
   A. pack the resident's brief with foam padding to prevent skin irritation
   B. perform careful perineal care after every episode
   C. clean perineal skin with disinfecting wipes
   D. avoid using soap-free cleansers if the skin is dry

_____ 9. Incontinence care includes
   A. ordering a skin sealant or moisture barrier
   B. applying cream or ointment before perineal care
   C. liberally applying baby powder to dry skin
   D. checking clothing and bed linens for dampness

_____ 10. Which of the following is true of fluid intake for incontinent residents?
   A. It is restricted to 100 mL if residents are NPO.
   B. It is stopped after lunch.
   C. It may be reduced in the evening to decrease incontinence overnight.
   D. It is forced in the evening to prevent UTIs.

Bowel Elimination

Identify whether each statement is true or false.

_____ 1. Stool is a waste product composed primarily of undigested food and is produced from digestion.

_____ 2. Stool is expelled from the large intestine via the urethra and contains bacteria, dead cells, and mucus.

_____ 3. Typical stool is brown in color because of the presence of ketones found in bile.

_____ 4. Bilirubin is produced through the synthesis of hemoglobin and is unrelated to digestion.

_____ 5. The Bristol Stool Chart indicates standard sizes, shapes, and consistencies for stool.

_____ 6. Observation of stool consistency is helpful in identifying gastrointestinal diseases or disorders.

_____ 7. Helpful bacteria found in the intestines give stool its normal odor.

_____ 8. Changes in diet, vitamins, medications, food allergies, infections, and diseases that cause malabsorption do not affect stool odor.

_____ 9. A healthy individual typically has a bowel movement from 10 times a day to once every four weeks.

_____ 10. Changes in stool or bowel habits are important and should be reported to the licensed nursing staff.

Stool Color

Match each factor with the stool color it produces.

A. black stool
B. red stool
C. orange stool
D. gray, clay-colored, or pale stool
E. green stool
F. black, sticky (tarry), and foul-smelling stool

_____ 1. naturally or artificially colored foods or blood

_____ 2. red or orange foods and some medications

_____ 3. green foods or iron supplements

_____ 4. vitamins that contain iron or other medications

_____ 5. the presence of blood in the stool, which is a serious condition

_____ 6. some diagnostic tests, a blockage in the flow of bile, or liver disease

Bowel Observations and Treatments

Complete the following sentences.

1. It is important that nursing assistants measuring I&O wash their hands to ensure infection control and wear disposable _____.

2. Nursing assistants may need to use a disposable stick or wooden _____ blade to examine stool closely.

3. If nursing assistants observe excessive _____ (gas), diarrhea or constipation, undigested food, blood or mucus in the stool, or unusual color (particularly black or dark green foul-smelling stool), they should report it to the licensed nursing staff immediately.

4. Nursing assistants help maintain residents' _____ integrity, provide proper hygiene, and achieve an odor-free environment.

5. Nursing assistants assist with procedures that alleviate pain due to excessive flatus or evacuate the bowels of a resident who has a(n) _____ (a blockage of hard stool in the rectum).

6. A(n) _____ tube and its connected bag can be used once every 24 hours to help relieve flatus, which can build up in the lower intestine.

7. Fecal or bowel _____ is the accidental leaking or passing of solid or liquid stool or mucus, usually due to diarrhea, constipation, or sometimes muscle or nerve damage.

8. Risk factors for fecal incontinence include age and diseases or conditions such as _____.

Diarrhea

Complete the following sentences.

1. _____ occurs when food and waste move so rapidly through the gastrointestinal system that the large intestine does not absorb fluids before expulsion.

2. Diarrhea is often _____, but can become chronic with serious complications that may lead to death.

3. Some causes of diarrhea are infection, parasites, tainted food, some diseases and medications, and bowel and gastrointestinal _____ or movement disorders.

4. Celiac disease and _____ bowel disease (IBS) can cause chronic diarrhea.

5. Symptoms associated with diarrhea may include a fever of _____°F or higher, nausea, vomiting, and abdominal pain.

6. Complications of diarrhea may include mild to severe _____ (lack of body fluids), lack of adequate nutrition, and extreme weight loss.

7. One treatment goal for diarrhea is to manage dehydration and nutrition through sufficient oral intake to provide more bulk to the _____.

Constipation

Identify whether each statement is true or false.

_____ 1. Constipation is characterized by difficult and infrequent bowel movements that can be acute or chronic.

_____ 2. Infrequent bowel movements can result in major or minor blockages in the intestines, causing waste to move very quickly through the gastrointestinal system.

_____ 3. Risk factors for constipation include a very young age, pregnancy, a high-fiber diet, and excellent hydration.

_____ 4. Symptoms of constipation often include a bloated feeling, swollen abdomen, feeling that there is a blockage in the rectum, or inability to empty the bowel.

_____ 5. Complications of constipation include internal or external hemorrhoids and a hernia, which is the protrusion of an organ through the wall of the body cavity or structure that contains it.

_____ 6. An anal fissure is a break or tear in the lining of the anal canal.

_____ 7. Colitis is an inflammation of the small intestine.

_____ 8. Laxative dependency, bowel impaction, obstruction, and rectal prolapse (in which a small amount of the rectum protrudes from the anus) are possible complications of constipation.

_____ 9. In a barium enema, a liquid containing a metallic substance is injected into the lower colon to coat its lining.

_____ 10. Treating chronic constipation usually begins with encouraging residents to decrease fluid and fiber intake and ignore the urge to have a bowel movement.

_____ 11. Laxatives, fiber supplements, stimulants, lubricants, stool softeners, and suppositories are often used to treat constipation.

_____ 12. A rectal suppository is used primarily to block bowel elimination, but may also be used to administer medications that relieve pain and promote healing.

_____ 13. Prior to the insertion of a suppository, a small amount of lubricating gel is applied to the anus and suppository.

_____ 14. A suppository is typically inserted about 2 inches beyond the anal sphincter.

_____ 15. After suppository insertion, residents should be encouraged to relax by taking slow, deep breaths until they feel the need to have a bowel movement.

Enemas

Complete the following sentences.

1. Enemas are used to help initiate _____ movements.

2. A(n) _____ enema introduces tap water, water with soapsuds, or saline into the rectum and colon via the anus.

3. A(n) _____ enema uses oil to soften and lubricate stool for easy elimination.

4. A disposable enema kit typically contains an enema bag with tubing, _____, and disposable protective pad.

5. Residents often experience _____ when the enema solution flows into the rectum and colon.

6. To prepare an enema, a nursing assistant should _____ the clamp on the enema bag tubing, fill the enema bag with the amount of water ordered, and seal the bag.

7. Before an enema is used, the tubing should be unclamped to run a small amount of enema solution through the tubing to eliminate _____ and warm the tube.

8. Before an enema is administered, the _____ of the enema solution should be checked to be sure it is not too warm.

9. The enema bag should be hung on the IV pole not higher than _____ inch(es) above the mattress to avoid discomfort.

10. The best resident position for an enema is _____ position.

11. The enema tubing should be lubricated _____ inch(es) from the tip for comfortable insertion.

12. The tip of the enema tubing should be gently inserted 2–4 inches into the _____.

13. After enema tubing is inserted, it can be _____ to let the enema solution flow slowly.

14. A resident should take slow, deep _____ to relax and help relieve any cramps caused by the enema.

15. When most of the enema solution has flowed into the rectum, the clamp should be _____ to prevent air from entering the bowel.

16. A nursing assistant should hold toilet paper around the enema tubing against the _____ as the tubing is slowly withdrawn.

17. Residents should _____ their buttocks to hold the solution in the rectum for as long as possible.

18. When the resident is no longer able to hold the solution, a nursing assistant should assist the resident to a bedpan, bedside _____, or bathroom.

19. If a commercially prepared small-volume enema is ordered, the container should be gently _____ at the bottom and rolled until almost all of the solution goes into the rectum.

Ostomies and Stoma Care

Identify whether each statement is true or false.

_____ 1. Diseases such as diverticulitis, Crohn's disease, and colon cancer may require a surgical procedure called an ostomy.

_____ 2. An ostomy procedure creates a *stoma*, or an artificial opening between the surface of the abdomen and the intestine to eliminate waste.

_____ 3. An ostomy bag is applied to a stoma to collect blood.

_____ 4. If a stoma extends from the surface of the abdomen to the large intestine, the procedure to create it is called a colostomy.

_____ 5. If a stoma extends between the surface of the abdomen and the ileum, the procedure to create it is called an ileostomy.

_____ 6. Stomas are always permanent and give the intestines rest.

_____ 7. Some residents find colostomies or ileostomies traumatic and embarrassing.

_____ 8. Residents with stomas never worry about soiling themselves or about odor.

_____ 9. Holistic nursing assistants need to be patient and supportive with ostomy care.

_____ 10. Caring for a stoma and emptying and changing an ostomy bag are outside a nursing assistant's scope of practice.

Name: _____ Date: _____

Providing Ostomy Care

Regular ostomy care keeps the skin around a stoma clean and prevents irritation and breakdown from contact with stool. The following steps are part of the procedure for providing ostomy care. For each set of steps, identify the proper order in which they should be completed by numbering them 1 through 5.

1. _____ Wash your hands or use hand sanitizer and put on disposable gloves. Position the resident on his or her back and place a disposable protective pad under the resident's buttocks. Cover the resident with a bath blanket. Without exposing the resident, fanfold the top linens and move clothing to expose the stoma. Place another protective pad alongside the resident and cover the resident with the bath blanket from the waist down.

_____ Disconnect the ostomy bag from the ostomy belt and remove and inspect the belt. If the belt is soiled, dispose of it. Remove the ostomy bag and skin barrier by gently stretching the skin and pulling the ostomy bag away. Use warm water or adhesive remover, if necessary. Place the ostomy bag in a bedpan and cover the bedpan. Neutralize any odor, following facility policy.

_____ Bring the necessary equipment into the room and place on a paper towel, towel, or disposable protective pad on the overbed table. Provide privacy by closing the curtains, using a screen, or closing the door to the room. Lock the bed wheels and raise the bed to hip level. If using side rails, raise and secure the rail on the side opposite where you will be working. Lower the rail on the side you are working.

_____ Remove the clamp at the bottom of the ostomy bag and let stool drain into a graduate. Wipe the open end of the ostomy bag with an antiseptic wipe, following facility policy. Fold the end of the ostomy bag and close it with the clamp.

_____ Note the color, odor, consistency, and amount of stool, measuring stool and drainage if recording I&O. Empty the stool and drainage into a toilet or bedpan. Remove and discard your gloves. Wash your hands or use hand sanitizer and put on a new pair of gloves.

2. _____ Remove any stool or drainage by gently wiping the stoma with a 4 × 4 gauze pad or toilet paper. Discard the dirty gauze pads and your gloves in a disposable trash bag. Wash your hands or use hand sanitizer and put on a new pair of gloves.

_____ Gently press around the edges of the ostomy bag to seal it to the skin. Add deodorant to the bag and make sure the skin around and under the bag is smooth and wrinkle free. Close the ostomy bag at the bottom using the clamp or clip. Attach the ostomy belt to the ostomy bag.

_____ Wash the stoma and the skin around it using a 4 × 4 gauze pad or washcloth mitt, soap, and water or a cleansing agent. Rinse and thoroughly dry the skin around the stoma. Observe the stoma and the skin. Immediately report any skin irritation, breakdown, or bleeding to the licensed nursing staff.

_____ Remove the protective pads and change any soiled linen. Remove the bath blanket and replace the top linens. Check to be sure the bed wheels are locked, then reposition the resident and lower the bed. Follow the plan of care for using side rails. Remove, clean, and store equipment in the proper location. Perform hand hygiene and report and document care given.

_____ Apply the correctly sized skin barrier, according to the manufacturer's instructions. Position the clean ostomy belt and remove the adhesive backing from the ostomy bag. Make sure the drain or end of the bag is pointing downward and then center the bag over the stoma.

Bladder and Bowel Retraining

Complete the following sentences.

1. Bladder and bowel _____ are ordered by a doctor to help residents gain greater independence and self-reliance with elimination.

2. Retraining includes changing diet, tracking elimination to determine individual patterns, scheduling toileting to increase _____ between visits, determining any obstacles to toileting, modifying medications contributing to the issue, learning pelvic-floor exercises, and rehabilitating muscles.

3. Bladder and bowel retraining require persistence and concentration by residents, and retraining may continue up to _____ month(s) or more before any progress is made.

4. Retraining orders are written by the _____, and guidance is given by the licensed nursing staff.

5. Nursing assistants document resident urination and episodes of incontinence to contribute to a(n) _____ diary.

6. Residents should toilet before _____ and empty the bladder as soon as they get up in the morning to start the retraining schedule.

7. Toileting visits are typically increased by intervals of _____ minute(s) until the resident reaches three to four hours between each bathroom visit.

8. Every time residents feel an urge to urinate, they should wait _____ minute(s) before going and increase that time gradually by 10 minutes.

9. _____ exercises strengthen the pelvic muscles for starting and stopping the flow of urine.

10. _____ drinks such as sodas, coffee, and tea should be avoided before bedtime.

11. A regular time should be set to encourage daily bowel movements, usually _____ minute(s) after a meal.

12. High-fiber foods such as _____ grains, fresh vegetables, and beans promote a healthy bowel.

13. Residents should drink _____ liters of fluid daily, unless contraindicated by the doctor.

Name: _____ Date: _____

Matching Chapter 24 Key Terms

Match each definition with the key term.

A. acuity
B. asylums
C. bipolar disorder
D. cerebral palsy (CP)
E. cues
F. cystic fibrosis (CF)
G. delusions
H. hydrocephalus
I. intoxication
J. legal blindness
K. neural tube
L. paralysis
M. paranoia
N. post-traumatic stress disorder (PTSD)
O. retinal detachment
P. schizophrenia spectrum disorder
Q. scoliosis
R. self-harm
S. spina bifida (SB)
T. stigma
U. suicide
V. ventilator

_____ 1. places offering safety and shelter

_____ 2. a condition of reduced control caused by the overuse of a chemical substance

_____ 3. a serious mental health condition characterized by changes in mood, energy, and activity levels; a person with this condition may swing from mania to depression

_____ 4. a refractive error of 20/200, even after vision correction

_____ 5. a condition that affects movement, muscle tone, and posture; is typically caused by damage to the developing fetal brain

_____ 6. a stress-related mental health condition that occurs after a person experiences or witnesses a traumatic or stressful event

_____ 7. actions that can cause a response

_____ 8. a severe and chronic mental health condition in which a person experiences a loss of reality; has delusions, hallucinations, and thought disorders; and displays agitated body movements

_____ 9. intentional death caused by fatal, self-inflicted injuries

_____ 10. clearness

_____ 11. a device used to mechanically aid breathing

_____ 12. a genetic disorder that changes how the body makes mucus and sweat

_____ 13. a congenital disorder resulting in incomplete development of the spinal cord

_____ 14. irrational beliefs that something is true, even when there is overwhelming proof that it is not

_____ 15. the structure from which the nervous system develops; consists of the brain and spinal cord

_____ 16. a condition of fluid in the brain

_____ 17. the loss of function and feeling in one or more muscle groups

_____ 18. condition of a spine curved sideways

_____ 19. a negative perception that causes others to think less of an idea or person

_____ 20. unsupported or exaggerated distrust of others

_____ 21. the act of hurting one's self on purpose

_____ 22. the separation of the retina from the back of the eye

Disabilities and Cognitive Disorders

Complete the following sentences.

1. A(n) _____ is a limitation of a person's function that occurs due to aging, a disease process, congenital or genetic disorders, developmental disorders, injury, or trauma.

2. A(n) _____ disorder is a limitation of a person's ability to remember, learn, process, and understand information and display appropriate behavior in social settings.

3. Cognitive disorders are the result of organic changes in the _____.

4. Reversible cognitive disorders are treatable and are usually called _____.

5. Delirium may be caused by electrolyte imbalance or _____ (a condition resulting from the overuse of a prescription medication or drug).

6. Progressive, permanent cognitive disorders are called _____.

7. Types of dementia include _____ disease, Lewy body dementia, and dementia caused by HIV/AIDS.

Refractive Errors

Match each definition with the refractive error.

A. presbyopia
B. astigmatism
C. myopia (nearsightedness)
D. hyperopia (farsightedness)

_____ 1. clear near vision and blurry far vision

_____ 2. blurry near vision and clear far vision

_____ 3. age-related inability to focus on a single, close object or page of text

_____ 4. problems with focus

Assisting with Vision Impairment

Complete the following sentences.

1. People who have refractive errors often use _____-correction devices.

2. Eyeglass lenses are often prescribed to correct refractive errors and make a person's vision as close to _____ as possible.

3. People who have both near- and farsightedness may have _____ lenses that accommodate both errors.

4. _____ lenses sit on the surface of the eye and are prescribed to correct refractive errors and help people achieve 20/20 vision.

5. _____ surgery permanently reshapes the cornea and restores the eye's ability to focus.

6. People with _____ vision typically have partial blindness, blurry vision, poor night vision, or tunnel vision; see only shadows; or are not able to distinguish shapes or objects.

7. Unlike refractive errors, low vision cannot be _____ and interferes with a person's ability to perform ADLs.

8. _____ blindness is a refractive error of 20/200 even after vision correction.

9. People who have _____ blindness cannot see even light.

10. In the absence of vision, _____ is the most important sense.

11. Low vision or vision loss can occur at birth, be caused by injury to the brain or eyes, or result from emergencies such as _____ detachment (separation of the retina from the back of the eye).

12. Low vision and vision loss can be caused by diabetic _____, stroke, tumors or inflammation in the optic nerve, surgery, and aging.

13. Three vision-related diseases and conditions that can lead to low vision or vision loss are cataracts, glaucoma, and _____ degeneration.

14. A primary responsibility of a nursing assistant caring for a resident with vision impairment or loss is to maintain a(n) _____ environment.

15. It is important for residents with vision impairment to have lives filled with enjoyable _____.

16. Eyeglasses should be washed with a soft, clean _____ at least once a day or whenever they are dirty.

17. Eyeglasses should be stored in a sturdy _____ to protect against scratching, bending, or breaking.

18. _____ hygiene is important before handling contact lenses to remove dirt, oils, and lotions.

19. An ocular prosthesis, or _____ eye, is fitted to the inner eye socket and is held in place by the upper and lower eyelids.

20. A nursing assistant should follow the resident's _____ and facility policy for care of an ocular prosthesis.

Supporting and Promoting Self-Reliance and Independence

Select the *best* answer.

_____ 1. Self-reliance and independence
   A. are not achievable for an aging person with a vision impairment
   B. may take longer and require written instructions if a resident has a vision impairment
   C. are important and must be supported for residents with vision impairments
   D. can be encouraged by using a loud tone of voice and speaking slowly to residents with vision impairments

_____ 2. Which of the following ensures safety for a resident with a vision impairment?
   A. checking on the resident every two hours in a new setting
   B. having the resident touch areas surrounding him or her, especially handrails
   C. telling the resident not to hit or fall over objects
   D. offering an arm or hand and walking behind the resident

_____ 3. Nursing assistants can help residents with vision impairments eat by
   A. performing hand hygiene and touching residents' food instead of utensils
   B. identifying each utensil and where it is in the kitchen
   C. explaining the position of food on a plate using the hands of a clock
   D. cutting up large pieces of food and filling cups to the top

Name: _____   Date: _____

_____ 4. Which of the following should nursing assistants do to help residents with vision impairments?
  A. help with daily activities, as needed
  B. use assistive devices to restore blindness
  C. do all ADLs for residents to prevent falls
  D. buy residents large-print books and magazines

_____ 5. Which of the following is true of Braille?
  A. It is the name of the first guide dog.
  B. It is required for residents with legal blindness.
  C. It may not be allowed by facility policy.
  D. It is a reading system of raised dots.

Hearing Impairment
Identify whether each statement is true or false.

_____ 1. Hearing impairments are characterized by increased hearing.

_____ 2. The structures of the ear receive and convert vibrations into sound waves, which are interpreted by the heart.

_____ 3. The intensity of sound is measured in milliliters (dB).

_____ 4. Sounds between 80 and 90 dB increase risk for hearing impairment, and injury to the ear occurs at 120 dB.

_____ 5. A rapid loss of 30 dB or more of hearing ability is chronic hearing loss and requires immediate attention from a doctor.

_____ 6. Lengthy exposure to loud noises is a key factor that causes hearing impairment.

_____ 7. Factors that lead to hearing impairment include certain medications, illnesses, head trauma, heredity, and aging.

_____ 8. Permanent hearing impairment occurs when there is damage to the inner ear or nerves.

_____ 9. Reversible hearing impairment (for example, a punctured eardrum) occurs when sound waves cannot reach the inner ear.

_____ 10. Hearing impairments often continue over time and have a significant impact on a person's quality of life.

_____ 11. Symptoms of hearing impairment include not understanding words, asking others to speak more loudly and slowly, turning up the volume of a television or radio, hearing muffled words, and experiencing tinnitus.

_____ 12. Tests used to diagnose hearing impairment include a physical examination, screening, the use of a kitchen fork, and audiometer testing.

_____ 13. Levels of hearing impairment are mild, moderate, severe, and profound.

_____ 14. A person who has moderate hearing impairment needs words to be repeated during conversations and has a hard time keeping up without a hearing aid.

_____ 15. Severe hearing loss makes it hard to hear a conversation without a powerful hearing aid and the use of lip reading.

_____ 16. In profound hearing impairment, a person is very hard of hearing and relies on lip reading and American Sign Language (ASL).

_____ 17. ASL uses hand signs combined with facial expressions and body postures to communicate.

_____ 18. Treatments for hearing impairment include the removal of earwax blockage, hearing aids, surgery, or cochlear implants.

_____ 19. Cochlear implants amplify sounds directly into the ear canal and bypass any damaged or dysfunctional parts of the inner ear.

_____ 20. A hearing aid is a small, electronic device worn in or behind the ear that helps the hearing of those whose inner ears are damaged.

_____ 21. A hearing aid can restore lost hearing ability.

_____ 22. A hearing aid converts sound waves into signals that are transmitted to an amplifier, which increases the power of signals and sends them to the ear.

_____ 23. An analog hearing aid converts sound waves into numerical signals and then amplifies sound.

_____ 24. A digital hearing aid converts sound waves into electrical codes and then amplifies sound.

Assisting with Hearing Impairment
Complete the following guidelines for assisting residents with hearing impairments.

1. Turn off background _____ when conversing.
2. Speak _____ and do not shout.
3. Position yourself so you are _____ the resident.
4. Provide proper maintenance and care of hearing aids by keeping hearing aids away from _____, moisture, or hair-care products and cleaning hearing aids per the manufacturer's instructions.
5. Never stand over a resident. Instead, position yourself at the same _____.
6. Turn hearing aids _____ when they are not in use and immediately replace dead batteries.
7. Gain a resident's _____ before talking.
8. Use _____ listening devices, such as TV-listening systems, telephone-amplifying devices, and Internet telephone services.

Speech Impairment

Match each description with the speech impairment.

A. receptive aphasia (fluent)
B. aphasia
C. global aphasia
D. anomic aphasia
E. expressive aphasia (nonfluent)

_____ 1. an inability to understand and use words

_____ 2. knowing what to say, but having difficulty communicating with others

_____ 3. hearing a voice or reading, but not understanding the meanings of words

_____ 4. struggling to find the right words to speak or write

_____ 5. having difficulty speaking and understanding words and being unable to read or write

Assisting with Speech Impairment

Select the *best* answer.

_____ 1. Which of the following is true of speech impairment?
   A. It affects a resident's ability to urinate.
   B. It results from damage or injury to the part of the brain that controls breathing.
   C. Causes include a stroke, brain tumor, brain injury, infection, or dementia.
   D. Severity depends on the extent of damage and the area of the heart affected.

_____ 2. Treatment for aphasia
   A. may include speech and language therapy
   B. cannot help residents improve their communication abilities
   C. cures the reason for the loss of language and identifies other methods of communication
   D. is often a quick process and starts long after the impairment or loss

_____ 3. How can a nursing assistant assist a resident with a speech impairment?
   A. by not providing care
   B. by speaking slowly and softly
   C. by using complex sentences to enhance recovery
   D. by using simple sentences

_____ 4. When communicating with a person who has a speech impairment, a nursing assistant should
   A. use gestures, point to objects, and avoid talking
   B. give the resident time to communicate and avoid finishing the resident's sentences
   C. shout instructions clearly and simply
   D. use a notepad to write instructions and wait for the resident to respond verbally

Down Syndrome

Complete the following sentences.

1. _____ disorders are caused by problems during fetal development prior to birth.

2. Some congenital disorders can be observed at _____, but others are detected later in a person's life.

3. _____ disorders develop due to changes or mutations in the normal sequence of a person's DNA.

4. _____ syndrome is a genetic disorder in which a baby is born with an extra full or partial copy of chromosome 21.

5. The presence of extra genetic material in Down syndrome results in _____ changes related to brain and body development.

6. Two risk factors for Down syndrome are a mother over age _____ and a history of Down syndrome in the family.

7. A person with Down syndrome will often live to _____ year(s) of age, have a full life, establish relationships, marry, and develop skills to work with some assistance.

8. Children who have Down syndrome have distinctive facial and body features, including a flat _____; small ears; slanted eyes; a small mouth; and a short neck, arms, and legs.

9. Children with Down syndrome experience physical _____ related to poor muscle tone and loose joints.

10. In addition to physical disabilities, Down syndrome causes _____ disabilities and respiratory, cardiac, GI, and hearing problems.

11. _____ is a resource that can help the child with Down syndrome and his or her family deal with socioemotional issues.

12. Adults who have Down syndrome experience premature aging and may show symptoms of early-onset _____ disease.

13. Symptoms of early-onset Alzheimer's disease include a decline in the ability to pay attention, less interest in social activities and interaction, changes in coordination, fearfulness, irritability, and _____ loss.

Spina Bifida (SB)

Identify whether each statement is true or false.

_____ 1. Spina bifida (SB) is a congenital disorder that results in incomplete development of the spinal cord.

_____ 2. A history of developmental changes in the neural tube and folic acid (vitamin B$_9$) deficiency are risk factors for SB.

_____ 3. The severity of SB depends on the size and location of incomplete spinal cord development, the presence of skin covering the affected area, and any protrusion of the spinal nerves.

_____ 4. Visible signs of SB at birth include an abnormal clump of hair or fat, a small dimple, or a birthmark on the baby's forehead.

_____ 5. The least severe form of SB results in a myelomeningocele, in which vertebrae do not cover the spinal cord, and the spinal cord may protrude through the vertebrae.

_____ 6. Common impairments associated with SB are leg muscle weakness and paralysis, bowel and bladder problems, and hydrocephalus.

_____ 7. SB can cause seizures, developmental changes in the feet, and scoliosis (a condition of a straight spine).

_____ 8. Most people with SB can walk for long distances and do not need braces, canes, crutches, or wheelchairs.

_____ 9. People with SB often experience challenges related to learning and emotional health due to physical disabilities and may benefit from therapy.

_____ 10. With recent treatment methods, some adults with SB can live 60 or more years.

_____ 11. Treatments for SB include surgery to close the sac of a myelomeningocele, a surgically placed ventricular shunt to drain fluid from the brain into the abdomen, and the management of paralysis and bladder and bowel problems.

Cystic Fibrosis

Select the *best* answer.

_____ 1. Cystic fibrosis (CF) is a genetic disorder that
A. changes how the body makes mucus and sweat
B. leads to the deterioration of leg muscles
C. damages nerves in the peripheral nervous system
D. causes a myelomeningocele

_____ 2. Which of the following is a symptom of CF?
A. very thin mucus that affects the respiratory system
B. a flat face
C. intellectual disabilities
D. congestion in the lungs

_____ 3. How does CF affect the GI system?
A. The mucus produced eases digestion.
B. Salty sweat increases perspiration.
C. Salty sweat interferes with electrolytes.
D. A stoma is necessary.

_____ 4. The average life expectancy for people with CF is
A. 10 years
B. 37 years
C. 72 years
D. 90 years

_____ 5. Treatments to ease CF include
A. monthly postural drainage
B. anaerobic exercise
C. percussion to help mucus drain from the airways in the lungs
D. inhaled medications to increase inflammation

Developmental Disabilities

Complete the following sentences.

1. _____ disabilities are a group of conditions that occur during a child's development and result in physical, learning, language, or behavioral impairment.

2. Cerebral _____ is a nonprogressive disability that affects movement, muscle tone, and posture.

3. Cerebral palsy (CP) is typically caused by damage to the developing fetal _____.

4. Risk factors for CP include infections during pregnancy; birth injuries; poor _____ supply to the baby's brain before, during, and immediately after birth; and prematurity.

5. Rh blood _____, in which the mother has a negative Rh factor and the baby has a positive Rh factor, is a risk factor for CP.

6. CP can develop during early childhood as a result of _____ injury due to severe illnesses such as meningitis, extensive physical trauma, or serious dehydration.

7. If CP develops during early childhood, it will usually appear by age two or _____.

8. Symptoms of CP include abnormal posture, impaired mobility, muscle _____ and stiffness, abnormal reflexes and involuntary movements, and imbalance of the eye muscles.

9. The goal of CP treatment is to maximize abilities and physical strength, prevent _____, and improve quality of life.

10. The use of _____ equipment, such as special shoes, crutches, orthotics, casts, special seats, walkers, and wheelchairs, is a treatment for CP.

11. _____ spectrum disorder is a developmental disability that can cause considerable social, communication, and behavioral challenges.

12. A person with autism spectrum disorder (ASD) does not exhibit any distinguishing physical characteristics, but ASD does affect how a person _____, behaves, and learns.

13. Symptoms of ASD include having trouble _____ to others, avoiding eye contact, wanting to be alone, repeating or echoing communicated words, and engaging in repetitive actions.

14. People with ASD often have trouble understanding other people's _____, prefer not to be held, and struggle to express needs using typical words or emotions.

15. Treatments for ASD include auditory training; music, occupational, and physical _____; dietary changes; and medications to manage symptoms.

16. _____ syndrome is a genetic disorder with no cure and is caused by a change in the FMR1 gene.

17. Symptoms of fragile X syndrome (FXS) include _____ delays, trouble learning new skills, lack of eye contact, and difficulty paying attention.

18. Treatment for FXS includes therapies that help with walking, talking, and communication and _____ to help control behavioral issues.

Traumatic Brain Injury (TBI)

Identify whether each statement is true or false.

_____ 1. Trauma and injury can have a significant impact on a person's physical and cognitive abilities.

_____ 2. In the event of trauma, soft tissues and organs can be injured, and neurological and skeletal damage can lead to amputation.

_____ 3. The goal of treatment for trauma is the restoration and rehabilitation of function.

_____ 4. Traumatic brain injury (TBI) can result in loss of consciousness, partial or total paralysis, and the need to use a mechanical ventilator to breathe.

_____ 5. Traumatic brain injury (TBI) is a chronic and acquired injury to the brain.

_____ 6. Causes of TBI include a vehicular accident, a bullet from a firearm, a fall, carbon monoxide or lead poisoning, tumors, infections, stroke, deceleration injuries, and hypoxia.

_____ 7. The extent of a brain injury is immediately apparent and always improves after several days, weeks, or months.

_____ 8. Brain injury causes mental and cognitive disabilities, but not physical disabilities.

_____ 9. TBI can lead to limited function or paralysis of the arms and legs, abnormal speech or language patterns, and coma.

_____ 10. TBI can lead to secondary brain injuries caused by bleeding in the skull, increased pressure and fluid in the skull, and infection.

_____ 11. Loss of consciousness and level of confusion have no impact on the level of a TBI.

_____ 12. Recovery after TBI is consistent, short, and usually challenging.

_____ 13. The goal of treatment for TBI is to provide support and minimize function and independence.

Levels of Consciousness

Identify the level of consciousness for each status in the table.

Levels of Consciousness	
Level	**Status**
1. _____	A person experiences loss of consciousness and confusion lasting fewer than 30 minutes.
2. _____	A person experiences loss of consciousness lasting longer than 30 minutes and physical and cognitive disabilities, but can still live independently.
3. _____	A person is conscious, but is dependent on others for care.
4. _____	A person has minimal consciousness, but follows a sleep/wake cycle and opens and closes the eyes.
5. _____	A person is in a true coma or altered state of consciousness, has no voluntary responses to pain stimuli and does not move the limbs voluntarily.
6. _____	A person's eyes may be open, but the person displays no interaction with the environment.
7. _____	A person exhibits no brain function.

Spinal Cord Injury (SCI)

Select the *best* answer.

_____ 1. Spinal cord injury (SCI)
- A. occurs if there is damage to any part of the spine, vertebrae, or discs
- B. is not as traumatic as TBI
- C. may cause permanent changes such as paralysis
- D. is always accompanied by loss of bladder or bowel control

_____ 2. Which of the following can cause SCI?
- A. a fall or a blow to the back from a vehicular accident
- B. increased bone density and regeneration of the vertebral discs
- C. inflammation or swelling in the lower extremities
- D. excess fluid in the frontal lobe of the brain

_____ 3. Signs and symptoms of SCI include
- A. effortless breathing and coughing
- B. increased bladder or bowel control and changes in sexual function
- C. mild pain or pressure in the feet and hands and ringing in the ears
- D. weakness, numbness, loss of movement and sensation, and spasms

_____ 4. The location of an SCI
- A. affects respiratory function if the injury is in the lumbar spine
- B. determines what functions below the site of the injury may be lost
- C. cannot affect arm movement and respiratory ability
- D. will not determine how much arm or leg control is lost

_____ 5. Which of the following refers to paralysis of the arms, trunk, legs, and pelvic organs?
- A. quadriplegia
- B. hemiplegia
- C. paraplegia
- D. omniplegia

_____ 6. When a patient is intubated,
- A. an endotracheal (ET) tube is inserted into the trachea through the mouth
- B. a tube is inserted directly into the lungs
- C. the spine is immobilized to prevent injury
- D. first responders breathe into the patient's mouth

_____ 7. The creation of a surgical opening in the trachea is a(n)
- A. ostomy
- B. colostomy
- C. tracheostomy
- D. SCI

_____ 8. When caring for a patient with a mechanical ventilator, a nursing assistant should
- A. document, but not report, if the patient is in pain
- B. assist with introducing mucus into the ET tube
- C. respond to the ventilator alarm immediately
- D. order enteral feedings

Care Considerations for TBI and SCI

Complete the following sentences.

1. Nursing assistants should establish a calm, supportive, respectful environment when caring for someone in a coma and always respect patient _____.

2. The nursing assistant should observe for small _____ over time, which can be very subtle (such as a small movement of a finger or toe, a quick noise, or the opening or closing of eyes).

3. Comatose patients may still be able to _____, so nursing assistants should respectfully communicate with them as they would with any patient.

4. Therapeutic touch, such as holding _____ and massage, may be helpful for a person in a coma.

5. As nursing assistants care for patients in comas, they should ask whether patients are in _____ and observe for subtle responses.

6. Computer adaptations and voice-controlled devices can make _____ easier after a TBI or SCI.

7. It is important to understand that a period of _____ and mourning usually follows a TBI or SCI.

8. When caring for patients who are paralyzed, nursing assistants should always focus on the patient, not on the _____.

9. Nursing assistants should maintain _____ eye contact with a patient who is paralyzed during longer conversations.

10. When caring for a patient with paralysis, nursing assistants should always ask if assistance is needed _____ attempting to help to preserve the patient's independence.

11. Nursing assistants should never hang or _____ on a patient's wheelchair, as the wheelchair is an important part of the patient's personal life space.

Delirium

Identify whether each statement is true or false.

_____ 1. A cognitive disorder is characterized by difficulty thinking, remembering, learning, processing, and understanding information and displaying appropriate behavior in public settings.

_____ 2. Cognitive disorders are the result of organic changes in the brain and may be reversible or permanent.

_____ 3. Irreversible cognitive disorders are called delirium.

_____ 4. Delirium is usually caused by acute medical conditions, such as meningitis, UTIs, electrolyte imbalances, metabolic and endocrine disorders, heatstroke, medications, and intoxication.

_____ 5. Delirium improves the brain's ability to create and use energy and alter chemical messengers in the brain and nervous system.

_____ 6. Delirium not otherwise specified (NOS) is often the result of sensory deprivation or can follow the use of general anesthesia.

_____ 7. A person with delirium is confused; has a distorted sense of time; and experiences severe attention, memory, language, and perception problems.

_____ 8. Delirium, when treated effectively, will last no longer than one year after the onset of symptoms.

_____ 9. If left untreated, delirium can cause more serious and permanent brain damage.

_____ 10. Care considerations for delirium are similar to those for residents with dementia.

Dementia

Select the *best* answer.

_____ 1. What is dementia?
   A. a progressive, semi-permanent cognitive disorder
   B. a range of symptoms that begin slowly and gradually get worse
   C. the most common form of Alzheimer's disease
   D. a genetic disorder with no modifiable risk factors

_____ 2. Alzheimer's disease (AD)
   A. is the most common form of dementia
   B. is always followed by vascular dementia
   C. is caused by a sudden lack of blood flow to the brain
   D. has no relationship to genetics, lifestyle, or environmental factors

_____ 3. Which of the following is true of vascular dementia?
   A. It develops gradually over time due to stress.
   B. An acute event such as a stroke can cause it.
   C. It is not affected by blockages or the slowing of blood flow.
   D. Symptoms will appear more slowly than symptoms of AD.

Stages of Dementia

Match each characteristic with the stage of dementia in which it begins.

A. early-stage or mild
B. middle-stage or moderate
C. late-stage or severe

_____ 1. memory lapses

_____ 2. need for full-time care for all ADLs

_____ 3. wandering and becoming lost

_____ 4. repetitive and compulsive behaviors

_____ 5. problems planning and organizing information

_____ 6. inability to effectively interact with the environment

_____ 7. aggressive behavior

_____ 8. difficulty doing daily activities

_____ 9. inability to control movements

_____ 10. ability to function independently

Psychological Changes of Dementia

Complete the following sentences.

1. Psychological changes associated with dementia include alterations that lead to resistance, anxiety, agitation, depression, and _____ (irrational beliefs).

2. Dementia may cause _____, which are false or distorted sensory experiences.

3. _____ is an unsupported or exaggerated distrust that residents with dementia may experience.

4. Psychological changes may lead to _____, hoarding items, and sundowning.

5. _____ is characterized by increased confusion, inability to follow directions, and anxiety (demonstrated by pacing and wandering) at the end of the day.

6. Residents with dementia may become physically _____ and express themselves by hitting, pinching, scratching, biting, and hair pulling.

7. Dementia can cause _____ aggressive behaviors such as screaming, swearing, shouting, and making threats.

8. Aggression can be the result of insufficient _____; pain; side effects from medications; a distracting, disorganized environment; loud noises; and confusion.

9. _____ is characterized by an uncontrollable need to repeat a word, phrase, or gesture for no apparent reason.

10. Psychological changes during dementia can cause inappropriate _____ behavior such as disrobing, exposure, masturbation, and fondling.

11. If a resident displays an inappropriate sexual behavior, a nursing assistant should be respectful, guide the resident to a private area, use _____ to redirect the resident to more positive activities, and report to the licensed nursing staff.

12. _____ occurs when a resident follows a caregiver's every move due to growing feelings of dependency and the need for comfort and safety.

Treatment and Care for Dementia

Identify whether each statement is true or false.

_____ 1. Maintaining a safe environment is a primary focus of care for residents with dementia.

_____ 2. Treatment for dementia focuses on the management of symptoms, the restoration of as many daily functions as possible, and palliative care.

_____ 3. The goal of care for dementia is to align with and support the disabilities of the resident.

_____ 4. Many residents with dementia stay in either long-term care facilities or special memory care units.

_____ 5. Prescribed medications can cure symptoms related to dementia.

_____ 6. Physical activity and massage, light, toy, music, art, pet, and aroma therapy can help manage the symptoms of dementia.

_____ 7. Holistic nursing assistants respect the individuality of residents with dementia, use the plan of care to guide activities, provide as much independence as possible, and keep residents safe.

_____ 8. When caring for residents with dementia, nursing assistants should maintain a calm, professional manner; smile; and avoid eye contact.

_____ 9. Simple verbal, visual, and manual cues can be used to demonstrate the steps to complete actions.

_____ 10. Nursing assistants should make the personal items belonging to residents with dementia difficult to find using labels and memory cues.

_____ 11. Monitoring systems allow residents freedom to move, but alert caregivers when a resident is wandering out of bounds.

_____ 12. Involving residents in cognitive and sensory stimulation can improve memory, communication skills, and social interaction and decrease boredom, inactivity, and sensory deprivation.

_____ 13. When caring for a resident with dementia, nursing assistants can use *reminiscence*, or a recollection of memories to increase pleasurable experiences and improve mood.

_____ 14. In validation therapy, a nursing assistant tries to convince the resident of present reality.

_____ 15. Maintaining an erratic schedule for ADLs reduces the confusion of residents with dementia.

Caring for a Resident with Dementia

People with dementia experience incessant, noisy thoughts they cannot turn off, which interferes with ADLs. To prepare for this activity, review the guidelines for caring for a resident with dementia. Also have your FIRST CHECK procedural checklist nearby.

Form a group of three and assign each person a role. One person will be the nursing assistant, another a resident, and the third person will serve as the evaluator. Then complete each of the following steps:

1. Separate the nursing assistant and the resident partner. The nursing assistant should choose a procedure he or she would like to practice and should tell the evaluator, but not the resident. The resident should put on headphones poorly tuned to an AM radio station with the volume just loud enough to disrupt understanding what the nursing assistant says.

2. Complete the FIRST, or Preparation, steps of the procedure, omitting any steps that are not applicable to the chosen procedure.

3. How difficult was it for the nursing assistant to communicate with the resident? How difficult was it for the resident to understand what was happening?

_____

_____

_____

4. Perform the chosen procedure, being extra careful to follow the guidelines for caring for a resident with dementia. The evaluator should assess how well the nursing assistant is following the guidelines and keeping the resident's attention.

5. Complete the CHECK, or Follow-Up and Reporting and Documentation, steps of the procedure, omitting any steps that are not applicable.

6. How difficult was it for the nursing assistant to perform the procedure? How difficult was it for the resident to follow along with the procedure?

_____

_____

_____

7. Switch roles with your partners and then discuss any difficulties encountered while performing the chosen procedure for a resident with dementia. Discuss what it was like to be the resident with dementia.

Mental and Emotional Health

Complete the following sentences.

1. Mental and emotional health are built on needs; growth and development; links between the body, mind, and _____; and levels of wellness and illness.

2. _____ health encompasses a person's ability to function productively by processing and storing information, shaping the environment to meet needs, making voluntary choices, taking action, initiating and maintaining satisfying and meaningful relationships, engaging in creative work, adapting to change, being flexible, having resilience, and coping with challenges.

3. _____ health involves feeling good about and having respect for one's self and others, enjoying life, giving and receiving love, and positively expressing and managing emotions.

4. Mental and emotional health require _____ interactions among physical, social, family, psychological, and environmental factors throughout life.

5. Sometimes mental and emotional health can be at _____ due to life changes, aging, and limited coping mechanisms.

6. _____ symptoms of stress include moodiness, short temper, agitation, loneliness, or depression.

7. _____ symptoms of stress include aches and pains, dizziness, nausea, rapid heartbeat, or frequent colds.

8. _____ symptoms of stress include procrastination, isolation, nervous habits, or the use of alcohol or drugs to relax.

9. Good stress, called _____, helps motivate people to learn or change.

10. When stress becomes harmful, it is called _____.

11. Sources of stress, or _____, that a person experiences need to be identified before they can be handled.

Mental Health Conditions

Identify whether each statement is true or false.

_____ 1. Mental health conditions are the most common cause of disability in the United States.

_____ 2. Risk factors for mental health conditions include stressful living conditions, overcrowding, abuse, adverse childhood experiences, learning disorders, congenital disorders, low birthweight, and chronic illnesses.

_____ 3. People who have experienced physical and mental trauma and older adults who have dementia are at decreased risk for mental health conditions.

_____ 4. During the mid-1800s, US activist Dorothea Dix vigorously worked to improve living conditions for people with mental health conditions.

_____ 5. In 1900, government-funded psychiatric hospitals were adequately staffed and well-funded.

_____ 6. In asylums, mental health treatment teams typically included a psychiatrist, orthopedist, counselor, licensed social worker, and psychiatric mental health nurse practitioner.

_____ 7. People with mental health conditions who experience stigma feel they are negatively labeled because of their conditions.

_____ 8. The categories of mental health conditions most often used by psychiatrists, psychologists, and researchers come from the American Psychiatric Association's Diagnostic and Statistical Manual of Mental Disorders (DSM-5).

Anxiety Disorders

Select the *best* answer.

_____ 1. Anxiety disorders are characterized by
　　A. persistent, excessive worry or fear of nonthreatening situations
　　B. intense worry about a threatening situation
　　C. normal anxiety
　　D. hallucinations

_____ 2. Which of the following are symptoms of anxiety disorders?
　　A. intense energy, excitement, and nervousness over important events
　　B. shortness of breath, fatigue, an upset stomach, and diarrhea
　　C. a deep sense of calm
　　D. a slow heart rate and apprehensiveness

_____ 3. What are panic attacks?
　　A. episodes of normal anxiety
　　B. sudden feelings of terror that happen without warning
　　C. bouts of indigestion
　　D. fighting or fleeing in a dangerous situation

_____ 4. Which of the following is true of phobias?
　　A. Phobias are rational fears.
　　B. People cannot have phobias of animals.
　　C. Examples include claustrophobia and acrophobia.
　　D. Phobias do not make functioning difficult.

_____ 5. Uncontrollable, recurrent, interfering thoughts and urges that result in repetitive behaviors are characteristic of
　　A. phobias
　　B. generalized anxiety disorder
　　C. depression
　　D. obsessive-compulsive disorder (OCD)

Trauma- and Stress-Related Disorders

Complete the following sentences.

1. Trauma- and stress-related disorders can develop after a person experiences or witnesses a traumatic or stressful _____.

2. _____ stress disorder is caused by childhood neglect or physical abuse, sexual assault, physical attacks, or combat exposure.

3. People with post-traumatic stress disorder (PTSD) have a variety of disruptive symptoms, which may begin within _____ month(s) after the event or not emerge until years later.

4. A person with _____ stress disorder develops severe anxiety and dissociation within one month after an extreme traumatic event.

5. _____ disorder or stress-response syndrome lasts no longer than six months and is characterized by extreme difficulty coping with or adjusting to a particular source of stress.

Depressive Disorders

Identify whether each statement is true or false.

_____ 1. Persistent depressive disorder, major or clinical depression, perinatal depression, and seasonal affective disorder (SAD) are all examples of depressive disorders.

_____ 2. Depression only develops during childhood and adolescence and is caused by a combination of biological, genetic, environmental, and psychological factors.

_____ 3. Depressive disorders are characterized by feelings of sadness, anxiety, hopelessness, helplessness, and guilt.

_____ 4. Bipolar disorder is a serious mental health condition characterized by swings from extreme happiness to sadness, fatigue, and depression.

_____ 5. Risk factors for bipolar disorder include family history, genetics, and being male.

_____ 6. There is only one type of bipolar disorder.

Personality and Substance Use Disorders

Complete the following sentences.

1. _____ disorders are characterized by trouble sensing and relating to everyday situations and other people.

2. A person with borderline personality disorder (BPD) experiences extreme swings in _____, is uncertain about his or her identity, and has an intense fear of abandonment.

3. _____ use disorders are characterized by the excessive use of caffeine, alcohol, tobacco, cannabis, hallucinogens, inhalants, opioids, sedatives, hypnotics, and stimulants such as cocaine.

4. _____ drinking involves consuming five or more alcoholic drinks for males or four or more alcoholic drinks for females in a short period of time.

5. Excessive _____ use involves consuming five or more drinks at the same event on five or more days in the past 30 days.

6. Alcohol use disorder, or _____, is characterized by problems controlling alcohol intake, alcohol tolerance that leads to dangerous risks, withdrawal symptoms, and the continuation of drinking even with serious physical consequences.

7. People with a(n) _____ use disorder consume amphetamines, methamphetamines, and cocaine to increase energy, alertness, and attention.

8. _____ use disorder involves using the illegal drug heroin, synthetic opioids such as fentanyl, and pain relievers.

9. Opioids relieve pain and can lead to a sense of _____ (joy and excitement), but can also depress respirations and cause death.

Schizophrenia Spectrum Disorder, Self-Harm, and Suicide

Select the *best* answer.

_____ 1. Schizophrenia spectrum disorder is
A. an acute mental health condition
B. a minor mental health condition that affects thoughts, but not feelings
C. a severe and chronic mental health condition that affects a person's entire life
D. a developmental disability

_____ 2. Which of the following is a risk factor for schizophrenia spectrum disorder?
A. chemical imbalances in the brain
B. a healthy pregnancy
C. excellent nutrition
D. a lack of family history

_____ 3. Symptoms of schizophrenia
A. begin between the ages of 7 and 30
B. lead to a firm grasp of reality
C. include hallucinations and thought disorders
D. include an expressive affect

_____ 4. Which of the following is true of self-harm?
A. People who self-harm never inflict fatal injuries.
B. Self-harm is characteristic of good mental and emotional health.
C. People self-harm to gain attention.
D. Self-harm is a coping mechanism for dealing with emotional pain.

_____ 5. If a resident practices self-harm or expresses suicidal thoughts, a nursing assistant should
A. leave the resident to inform the licensed nursing staff
B. tell the resident to stop and leave the room
C. ignore the behavior
D. inform the licensed nursing staff without leaving the resident alone

Treatment for Mental Health Conditions

Complete the following sentences.

1. _____ behavioral therapy helps a person develop mastery over thoughts and feelings.

2. Phobias are often treated with _____ therapy, which involves gradual, repeated exposure to the source of fear.

3. Medications for mental health conditions often have _____ that need to be monitored.

4. Brain stimulation therapies such as _____ therapy are sometimes used to treat depression.

5. Holistic nursing assistants can help residents with mental health conditions by recognizing the resident's _____ are very real to him or her.

6. A nursing assistant should never take a resident's behavior _____, but should step back if a resident is physically aggressive.

7. Nursing assistants need to understand that mental health conditions do not affect a resident's _____.

CHAPTER 25 Caring for Special Populations and Needs

Name: _____ Date: _____

Matching Section 25.1 Key Terms

Match each definition with the key term.

A. amniocentesis
B. antepartum
C. colostrum
D. ectopic pregnancy
E. embryo
F. fetus
G. hemophilia
H. infertility
I. intrapartum
J. lochia
K. miscarriage
L. natal
M. ovulation
N. placenta
O. placental abruption
P. placenta previa
Q. postpartum
R. preeclampsia
S. stillbirth

_____ 1. a disk-shaped organ that develops temporarily and attaches to the uterus during pregnancy; transfers oxygen and nutrients from the woman to the fetus via the umbilical cord

_____ 2. a diagnostic procedure in which a small amount of fluid is withdrawn from the amniotic sac to identify genetic abnormalities or determine the sex of a fetus

_____ 3. spontaneous loss of a fetus before the twentieth week of pregnancy

_____ 4. relating to birth

_____ 5. a blood disorder caused by changes in a gene on the X chromosome; characterized by an inability of the blood to clot

_____ 6. during labor and delivery

_____ 7. vaginal discharge composed of blood, mucus, and uterine tissue

_____ 8. before labor or childbirth

_____ 9. fetal death after 20 weeks of pregnancy

_____ 10. a thin, milky fluid discharged from the breasts; contains antibodies that provide passive immunity for the newborn; develops by the end of the third month of pregnancy

_____ 11. a condition in which the placenta separates from the uterine wall before delivery, resulting in a lack of oxygen and nutrients for the fetus and severe bleeding for the mother

_____ 12. a continued inability to reproduce after trying to conceive for one year or repeated miscarriages

_____ 13. after childbirth

_____ 14. a condition in which a fertilized ovum implants outside the uterus in the fallopian tube, abdominal cavity, ovary, or neck of the uterus (cervix)

_____ 15. the process by which a mature ovum is released from an ovary

_____ 16. the fertilized ovum from implantation until the end of the eighth week of pregnancy

_____ 17. a condition in which the placenta covers part of, or the entire, opening of the cervix; can cause the mother to have severe vaginal bleeding or hemorrhage

_____ 18. the fertilized ovum from the ninth week of pregnancy until birth

_____ 19. a condition characterized by high blood pressure and signs of organ damage during pregnancy; usually occurs after 20 weeks

Fertilization, Implantation, and Pregnancy

Complete the following sentences.

1. When a woman has a baby, the first _____ phase happens prior to labor and delivery.

2. The second phase, called the _____ phase, includes labor and delivery.

3. The final _____ phase takes place after childbirth and includes postnatal care.

4. Pregnancy most commonly occurs when a man ejaculates _____ into a woman's vagina and the sperm travel into the uterus and fallopian tubes.

5. In artificial _____, sperm are inserted into a woman's vagina or uterus using a syringe or similar device.

6. During in vitro fertilization (IVF), ova are combined with sperm in a petri dish, allowing _____ (the union of an ovum and sperm).

7. _____ is the release of an ovum from a woman's ovary.

8. _____ occurs when the fertilized ovum attaches to the lining of the uterus.

9. After implantation, an organ called the _____ forms from uterine and fetal tissue.

10. A fertilized ovum from the ninth week of pregnancy until birth is called a(n) _____.

11. One side of the placenta is connected to the fetus via the _____ cord, and the other side is connected to the wall of the uterus.

12. The placenta produces hormones that provide passive _____ for the fetus and help regulate the woman's responses to pregnancy.

13. The _____ sac is filled with a clear, slightly yellowish fluid that surrounds the growing fetus.

14. The fetus swallows and inhales amniotic fluid, and fluid is then replaced through fetal exhalation and _____.

15. The cervix is sealed by a plug of _____ until the fetus is ready to be born.

16. _____ age is calculated using the first day of the woman's last menstrual period (LMP).

17. The sex of a fetus is determined by whether a sperm carries the _____ chromosome, which causes a fetus to be male.

18. If two ova are fertilized and implanted during the same cycle, _____ twins develop.

The Developing Fetus

Apply the appropriate callouts to the image.

A. Amniotic cavity
B. Placenta
C. Cervix
D. Uterus
E. Umbilical cord

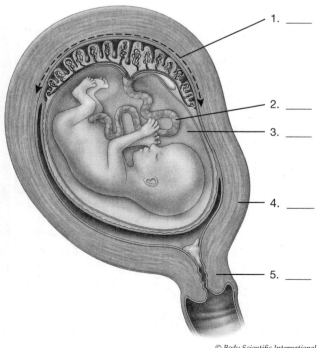

1. _____

2. _____

3. _____

4. _____

5. _____

© Body Scientific International

Preconception Care

Select the *best* answer.

_____ 1. What is preconception care?
A. healthcare designed to help women and men have healthy babies
B. care that is not wise for women who plan their pregnancies
C. standard care for each woman or man
D. discussions with a healthcare provider about starting birth control

_____ 2. Birth control methods
A. can be discontinued immediately without consulting a healthcare provider
B. include natural family planning, barrier, and hormonal methods
C. should not include an intrauterine device (IUD)
D. must be discontinued immediately to prevent pregnancy

_____ 3. During preconception care, healthcare providers and partners discuss
A. family history, but not medical conditions
B. any history of sexually transmitted infections (STIs)
C. the importance of not having genetic counseling
D. medications that will not affect the pregnancy

Prenatal Care

Identify whether each statement is true or false.

_____ 1. Prenatal care occurs after a baby is born, or after pregnancy.

_____ 2. The goal of prenatal care is to monitor progress and ensure early treatment for any problems.

_____ 3. At the first prenatal visit, a healthcare provider reviews any medications, performs a physical exam, tests blood to determine Rh factor, and tests urine to detect glucose or protein.

_____ 4. During subsequent prenatal visits, blood pressure and weight are checked, the abdomen is measured for growth, and fetal heart rate is monitored.

_____ 5. Genetic testing can include blood tests, ultrasounds, or amniocentesis (in which a small amount of amniotic fluid is withdrawn and tested to identify genetic abnormalities).

_____ 6. Most women gain 2 to 4 pounds during the first trimester and 8 pounds per week thereafter.

_____ 7. An obstetrician-gynecologist (OB/GYN) provides pregnancy care, but does not deliver babies.

_____ 8. A perinatologist helps women who have high-risk pregnancies or problems during pregnancy.

_____ 9. A family practitioner (FP) provides care for the whole family and may offer OB/GYN services.

_____ 10. A certified nurse midwife (CNM) is a specially trained licensed nurse experienced in providing obstetric and newborn care.

Name: _____   Date: _____

_____ 11. A certified midwife (CM) is not certified, but has received informal training through self-study or apprenticeship.

_____ 12. A women's health nurse practitioner or family nurse practitioner has advanced education and training and can provide pre- and postnatal care.

_____ 13. A doula specializes in providing emotional, physical, and educational support before, during, and after childbirth.

_____ 14. A pediatrician specializes in gynecological exams and contraceptive counseling.

_____ 15. A pediatric nurse practitioner (PNP) has advanced education and training in the care of newborns, infants, children, and adolescents.

_____ 16. Labor, delivery, and postnatal care usually all occur in a neonatal intensive care unit (NICU).

_____ 17. Birthing centers are specially prepared to handle complicated pregnancies.

_____ 18. Home birth is an option if a pregnancy has been progressing well and there are no risk factors.

Stages of Pregnancy

Match each characteristic with the appropriate stage of pregnancy.

A. First trimester
B. Second trimester
C. Third trimester

_____ 1. Hemorrhoids may develop.
_____ 2. Menstrual period stops.
_____ 3. The stage includes weeks 13–28.
_____ 4. Nausea and fatigue lessen.
_____ 5. The mother may experience morning sickness.
_____ 6. The hands may feel numb and tingle.
_____ 7. Colostrum may leak out of the breasts.
_____ 8. The stage includes weeks 1–12.
_____ 9. The linea negra may become visible.
_____ 10. The stage includes weeks 29–40.

Labor and Delivery

Complete the following sentences.

1. The physical signs of impending _____ include lightening, diarrhea, bloody show, ruptured membranes, effacement, and labor contractions.

2. _____ occurs when the fetus starts to drop into the pelvis in preparation for delivery.

3. Bloody show is caused by the release of the mucus _____, which seals off the cervix to prevent infection.

4. The tearing of the _____ sac, which causes fluid to leak from the vagina, is commonly referred to as the water breaking.

5. _____, also known as the thinning of the cervix, begins the birthing process.

6. False labor pains called _____ Hicks contractions can start as early as the second trimester.

7. True labor contractions come in a wavelike motion, starting at the top of the _____ and moving to the bottom.

8. Regular intervals of _____ minute(s) between contractions mean labor has begun.

9. Stage one of labor contains _____ phase(s).

10. The _____ phase of stage one is often the longest and least intense.

11. During the _____ phase of stage one, dilation progresses quickly, contractions are more intense, and the woman feels an urge to push, even though the cervix is not yet fully dilated.

12. In the _____ phase of stage one, the cervix is fully dilated, and contractions become strong and painful.

13. During labor, _____ relieve pain without total loss of feeling or movement.

14. _____ used during labor block all feeling and muscle movement.

15. The second stage of labor begins when the cervix is completely _____ and ends with the expulsion of the fetus.

16. During the second stage of labor, women are urged to _____ or bear down during contractions.

17. The soft spots, or _____, on a fetus's head allow it to fit through the birth canal.

18. When a newborn is fully delivered, the umbilical _____ is clamped and cut, usually 30 to 60 seconds after birth.

19. During stage three contractions, the _____ is delivered.

Recovery After Delivery

Identify whether each statement is true or false.

_____ 1. Bonding gives the newborn a sense of security and self-esteem and also creates a strong attachment between the parents and newborn.

_____ 2. Bonding is not helped when the mother touches, feeds and cares for, rocks, and interacts with the newborn.

_____ 3. Right after delivery, the mother's vital signs are checked, and she receives assistance with ambulation and toileting.

_____ 4. New mothers may experience contractions and pains for a few months until the uterus returns to its normal size.

_____ 5. Cochlea is vaginal discharge composed of blood, mucus, and uterine tissue.

_____ 6. Lochia typically disappears after four to six years.

_____ 7. Vaginal birth sometimes requires an episiotomy to prevent tearing during delivery.

_____ 8. After delivery, a new mother's breasts may feel painful and swollen until the milk comes in.

_____ 9. Once a baby is born, a mother may experience short-term hair loss due to hormonal changes, and stretch marks will fade from reddish purple to silver or white.

_____ 10. After giving birth, new mothers may experience urinary or fecal incontinence when laughing or sneezing.

_____ 11. Irritability, sadness, and crying, known as the *baby blues*, may occur within a few weeks after delivery.

Problems and Complications of Pregnancy and Childbirth

Complete the following sentences.

1. Placenta _____ is a condition in which the placenta covers the opening of the cervix, causing severe bleeding for the mother.

2. In placental _____, the placenta separates from the uterine wall before delivery, resulting in a lack of oxygen and nutrients for the fetus and severe bleeding for the mother.

3. _____ is a condition characterized by high blood pressure and signs of organ damage during pregnancy.

4. The spontaneous loss of a fetus before the twentieth week of pregnancy is a(n) _____.

5. _____ pregnancy is a condition in which a fertilized ovum implants outside the uterus in the fallopian tube, abdominal cavity, ovary, or cervix.

6. _____ labor begins before the fetus can survive outside the mother's body.

7. Fetal death after 20 weeks of pregnancy is called a(n) _____.

8. A(n) _____ delivery is the delivery of the fetus by means of a surgical incision in the woman's abdomen and uterus.

9. After a baby is delivered via a C-section, the _____ is removed from the uterus, and surgical incisions are closed with sutures or staples.

10. Sometimes a C-section is performed if _____ is prolonged, has stopped, or has complications.

11. Recovery from a C-section takes longer than recovery from a(n) _____ delivery.

12. Postpartum _____ can cause severe mood swings, intense irritability, anger, excessive crying, loss of appetite, overwhelming fatigue, insomnia, withdrawal, difficulty bonding with the newborn, and thoughts of harming one's self or the newborn.

13. Postpartum depression (PPD) is associated with _____ changes that occur after childbirth.

14. Risk factors for PPD include depression or anxiety during _____, a traumatic childbirth experience, an ill newborn, and lack of support.

Postnatal Care

Select the *best* answer.

_____ 1. After delivery, mothers and their caregivers should
   A. neglect personal hygiene
   B. attend to postnatal care
   C. eat without concern for nutrition
   D. treat the newborn like a small adult

_____ 2. Six weeks after delivery, a healthcare provider
   A. does not ask questions about sexual activity
   B. assumes the mother already knows everything about breast-feeding
   C. examines the mother's vagina, cervix, uterus, and breasts
   D. does not take vital signs

_____ 3. Well-baby exams
   A. monitor an infant's physical, developmental, and emotional growth
   B. determine whether a woman is pregnant
   C. track physical, but not emotional, growth
   D. are performed by nursing assistants

Breast-Feeding

Complete the following sentences.

1. The first milk released from the breasts is colostrum, which contains _____ that provide passive immunity for the newborn.

2. Approximately two to four days after childbirth, _____ milk replaces colostrum.

3. Ten to 15 days after childbirth, the production of _____ milk begins.

4. Some infants have trouble _____, or connecting with the breast.

5. A certified _____ consultant may help the mother and infant experience successful breast-feeding.

6. Breast-feeding provides protection against infections and helps the mother's _____ contract and return to normal size.

7. Exclusive breast-feeding is recommended for the first _____ month(s) of an infant's life.

8. Ideally, a mother will continue breast-feeding until the infant reaches _____ year(s) of age.

9. Breast-feeding frequently prevents the breasts from becoming _____, or filled with milk.

10. To ensure successful breast-feeding, a mother should perform hand hygiene and then bring her infant to her breast to feel the bare skin and trigger the _____ that causes the infant to latch on to the breast.

11. While breast-feeding, the mother should be in a comfortable position with a(n) _____ support.

12. To remove the infant from the breast, the mother can push _____ on the breast near the infant's mouth and break the suction by gently inserting her finger at the corner of the infant's mouth.

13. The infant should be _____ by gently rubbing or patting the infant's back in a circular motion for two to three minutes.

Bottle-Feeding
Identify whether each statement is true or false.

_____ 1. Commercial formulas have ingredients similar to breast milk.

_____ 2. Infants should be bottle-fed every six hours or whenever they appear hungry.

_____ 3. An infant will usually consume 2–3 ounces per feeding and should be encouraged to finish the entire bottle.

_____ 4. If an infant makes a noisy sucking sound, he or she may be taking in too much air.

_____ 5. A bottle should not be propped up, as this can cause choking.

_____ 6. Formula should be prepared at refrigerator temperature.

_____ 7. Formula that has not been consumed by the infant during a feeding can be saved.

_____ 8. New bottles, nipples, and rings should be sterilized by immersion in a pot of boiling water for a minimum of five minutes.

_____ 9. It is best to look for BPA-free bottles or use bottles made of opaque plastic.

_____ 10. When washing bottles, one should squeeze hot, soapy water through the nipples to remove the formula or breast milk.

Mother and Infant Hygiene
Select the *best* answer.

_____ 1. To maintain proper hygiene, mothers should
   A. shower weekly
   B. get rest, but not exercise
   C. invite unwell visitors
   D. wash hands or use hand sanitizer regularly

_____ 2. Which of the following is part of breast hygiene?
   A. changing the bra monthly
   B. not replacing breast pads
   C. washing the nipples gently each day
   D. using warm water on the breasts when bathing

_____ 3. Which of the following is part of toileting hygiene?
   A. wiping from back to front
   B. using used toilet paper to pat the area dry
   C. cleansing the area with warm water
   D. only wiping the genital area after urination

_____ 4. Care of the perineum includes
   A. taking a sitz bath
   B. performing perineal care twice weekly
   C. changing sanitary pads once a day
   D. taking out stitches

_____ 5. Providing hygiene for an infant
   A. promotes feelings of insecurity
   B. provides an opportunity to observe the skin
   C. is a poor time to hold the infant
   D. should not be part of a routine

Bathing Infants
Holistic nursing assistants may provide a full bath for an infant or assist the mother with this procedure. The following steps are part of the procedure for bathing infants. For each set of steps, identify the proper order in which they should be completed by numbering them 1 through 5.

1. _____ Wash your hands or use hand sanitizer before entering the room.

   _____ Introduce yourself using your full name and title. Explain that you work with the licensed nursing staff and will be providing care.

   _____ Identify the infant by name and check the infant's identification bracelet. In some facilities, the baby's identification bracelet is compared with the mother's.

   _____ Ask the licensed nursing staff or the mother if there are any special instructions or precautions regarding the procedure.

   _____ Knock before entering the room.

2. _____ Fill the bathtub with 1–2 inches of warm water. Check that the water temperature is 100–105°F.

   _____ Provide privacy by closing the curtains, using a screen, or closing the door to the room.

   _____ Explain the procedure to the mother in simple terms. Ask permission to perform the procedure.

   _____ Bring the necessary equipment into the room. Place the following items in an accessible location: infant-size bathtub, tub liner, 2 bath towels, paper towels, 2–3 washcloths, cotton balls, baby soap and shampoo, baby lotion or cream, baby nail scissors or clippers, and a clean diaper and clothes.

   _____ Wash your hands or use hand sanitizer to ensure infection control.

3. _____ Wet a washcloth and squeeze out the excess water. Wash and rinse the infant's face.

   _____ Moisten a cotton ball with warm water and squeeze out the excess water. Wipe the infant's eyes and eyelids, moving from the nose toward the ears. Use a clean cotton ball for each eye and eyelid.

_____ Place a towel or paper towel on a safe, flat surface. Place the bathtub on the towel or paper towel. Line the bottom of the bathtub with a foam liner or towel.

_____ Lay a bath towel on the counter next to the tub.

_____ Undress the infant and lay him or her on the clean towel. Keep one hand on the infant for safety.

4. _____ Wet a washcloth and put a small amount of baby shampoo on the infant's head. Squeeze a small amount of water from the washcloth onto the infant's head. Carefully wash the infant's hair and scalp using a circular motion. Rinse the infant's head and scalp by squeezing water from the washcloth. Make sure soapsuds do not get into the infant's eyes.

_____ Gently lower the infant, feet first, into the tub.

_____ Support the infant in an upright position with the infant's head and chest out of the water. Support the infant's head at all times in the tub.

_____ Wash the infant's neck and behind the ears with a small amount of baby soap and a washcloth. Rinse.

_____ Using a clean washcloth, clean the infant's gums and tongue.

5. _____ Cleanse the anal area with soap and water.

_____ Wash the infant's back and buttocks with a clean washcloth.

_____ Using a clean washcloth, gently wash the perineal area. For female infants, gently spread the labia and wash from front to back. For male infants, gently wash from the urethra to the scrotum with warm water. If the infant is uncircumcised, do not pull back the foreskin, as it will gradually loosen on its own.

_____ Wash the infant's chest, arms, hands, and between the fingers. Wash the legs and between the toes. After washing with the soapy washcloth, rinse the washcloth. Thoroughly rinse the infant.

_____ Clean the umbilical cord with a disposable wipe or cotton ball wet with soap and water. Make sure the umbilical cord is dry after cleaning.

6. _____ Lift the infant out of the tub and wrap with a bath towel.

_____ Carefully trim the infant's fingernails and toenails using baby scissors or clippers. Trim the fingernails following the natural shape of the nail. Trim the toenails straight across.

_____ Lightly apply lotion or cream to the skin, if appropriate.

_____ Diaper and dress the infant. Make sure the infant is safe and comfortable.

_____ Using the bath towel, gently pat the infant dry. Keep the infant covered and warm when wet.

7. _____ Wash your hands or use hand sanitizer before leaving the room.

_____ Communicate any specific observations, complications, or unusual responses to the licensed nursing staff. Record this information, along with the care provided, in the chart or EMR.

_____ Remove, clean, and store equipment in the proper location. Remove soiled linens and discard disposable equipment.

_____ Wash your hands to ensure infection control.

_____ Conduct a safety check before leaving the room. The room should be clean and free from clutter or spills.

Changing an Infant's Diaper

An infant's diaper must be changed whenever it becomes wet or soiled to reduce skin irritation. The following steps are part of the procedure for diapering. For each set of steps, identify the proper order in which they should be completed by numbering them 1 through 5.

1. _____ Bring the necessary equipment into the room. Place the following items in an accessible location: disposable gloves; clean, prefolded cloth or disposable diaper; diaper cover; disposable protective pad; washcloth; disposable wipes or cotton balls; basin of warm water; baby soap; and baby lotion or cream.

_____ Provide privacy by closing the curtains, using a screen, or closing the door to the room. Wash your hands or use hand sanitizer to ensure infection control. Put on disposable gloves.

_____ Wipe the perineal area with the clean front of the diaper from front to back. Remove as much stool as possible using the front of the diaper.

_____ Place a disposable protective pad under the infant. Unfasten the tabs or pins on the dirty diaper. If diaper pins are used, place them out of reach.

_____ Roll the soiled diaper so the urine and stool are inside. Set the diaper aside. Use disposable wipes or cotton balls wet with soap and water to clean the infant. If there is a large amount of stool, use a washcloth instead. Check for skin irritation, rashes, or lesions.

2. _____ Clean the umbilical cord with a disposable wipe or cotton ball wet with soap and water. If the infant is circumcised, gently clean the circumcision with a disposable wipe or cotton ball wet with soap and water. Apply a small amount of cream or lotion to the perineal area and buttocks, if needed.

_____ Raise the infant's legs. Slide a clean diaper under the infant's buttocks. For a boy, fold a cloth diaper for extra thickness at the front. For a girl, fold a cloth diaper for extra thickness at the back.

_____ Rinse thoroughly and pat the area dry. Remove and discard your gloves and put on a new pair of disposable gloves.

_____ Secure the diaper in place. Use the tape strips on a disposable diaper to secure at the hips. If pins are used, insert the pins sideways, with points away from the infant's abdomen. If using a cloth diaper, cover the diaper with a diaper cover.

_____ Bring the diaper up between the legs to cover the lower abdomen. Make sure the diaper is snug around the hips and abdomen. If an infant's circumcision is not healed, make sure the diaper is loose near the penis. If the cord stump has not healed, the diaper should be below the umbilicus.

3. _____ Wash your hands or use hand sanitizer before leaving the room.

_____ Make sure the infant is safe and comfortable. Rinse the stool from a cloth diaper into the toilet. Store the used cloth diaper in a covered pail or wet bag. Throw a disposable diaper in a covered waste container.

_____ Remove and discard your gloves. Wash your hands. Conduct a safety check before leaving the room. The room should be clean and free from clutter or spills.

_____ Remove and discard your gloves. Wash your hands or use hand sanitizer. Put on a new pair of gloves. Remove, clean, and store equipment in the proper location. Remove soiled linens and discard disposable equipment.

_____ Communicate any specific observations, complications, or unusual responses to the licensed nursing staff. Record this information, along with the care provided, in the chart or EMR.

Infant Safety

Complete the following guidelines for ensuring infant safety.

1. Use smooth, not jerky, movements to avoid _____ infants.

2. When lifting an infant, use both hands, one hand to support the _____ and upper back and the other hand to support the legs.

3. When laying an infant down for sleep, lay the infant on his or her _____ on a firm surface.

4. Respond quickly if an infant _____, as this can mean an infant is in discomfort or hungry.

5. Keep infants _____ and away from drafts.

6. Never leave an infant _____.

Clearing an Infant's Obstructed Airway

An obstructed airway blocks the flow of air to the lungs. The following steps are part of the procedure for clearing an infant's obstructed airway. For each set of steps, identify the proper order in which they should be completed by numbering them 1 through 5.

1. _____ Expose the infant's upper body.

_____ Observe the infant. Note if the infant has difficulty breathing, a weak or absent cry, choking, or wheezing. Call for help.

_____ Support the infant on your arm and turn the infant faceup. Rest your forearm on your thigh for support. The infant's head should be lower than the trunk. Using your index finger and middle finger, give five chest thrusts in the midsternal region. Give one thrust per second. Check for the object obstructing the airway. Stop if the object has been dislodged.

_____ Keep giving back blows and chest thrusts until the foreign object is expelled or until the infant loses consciousness.

_____ Position the infant over your forearm facedown with the head lower than the trunk. Support the infant's head and neck with one hand. Rest your forearm on your thigh for support. Using the heel of your hand, deliver five back blows between the infant's shoulder blades. Check for the object obstructing the airway. Stop if the object has been dislodged.

2. _____ Breathe in, but not deeply.

_____ Place the infant on his or her back.

_____ Open the infant's airway by tilting the head and lifting the chin. Do not hyperextend the infant's neck.

_____ Place your mouth over the infant's mouth and nose, making an airtight seal.

_____ If the infant becomes unconscious, observe the infant. Note if the infant has difficulty breathing, a weak or absent cry, choking, or wheezing. Call for help.

3. _____ Blow one small puff of air into the infant's mouth and nose. Observe if the chest rises.

_____ Observe for coughing or movement. Check the infant's brachial pulse. If pulse is absent, begin CPR.

_____ Remove your mouth to hear or feel an exhaled breath.

_____ If the infant's chest does not rise with each breath, reposition the infant's head by tilting it back slightly and lifting the infant's chin to open the airway.

_____ Replace your mouth over the infant's mouth and nose and blow another small puff of air.

4. _____ Open the infant's airway by tilting the head and lifting the chin. Do not hyperextend the infant's neck.

_____ Place two fingers on the sternum just below an imaginary line between the two nipples. Give 30 compressions to one-third the depth of the chest (about 1½ inches).

_____ Continue the cycle of 30 compressions and two breaths until the object is expelled or until medical professionals arrive and take over.

_____ Wash your hands to ensure infection control. Make sure the infant is safe and comfortable and report to the licensed nursing staff.

_____ Give two breaths (1 second per breath) so the chest rises.

Matching Section 25.2 Key Terms

Match each definition with the key term.

A. ablation
B. gurney
C. hypovolemic shock
D. intraoperative
E. laparoscopic surgery
F. meniscus
G. perioperative
H. polyp
I. postoperative
J. preoperative
K. prolapse
L. reservoir

_____ 1. a place in which fluid can collect

_____ 2. surgical removal of body tissue

_____ 3. after surgery, until recovery from the surgery

_____ 4. a flat, padded table with wheels; also called a *stretcher*

_____ 5. a minimally invasive surgical technique in which an operation is performed through a small incision in the body

_____ 6. a cartilage pad that creates a smooth surface for a joint such as the knee to move

_____ 7. during surgery, up until the patient's arrival in the recovery room

_____ 8. relating to the three phases of surgery

_____ 9. a condition in which an organ or body part sinks or falls out of place

_____ 10. growth or mass bulging from a mucous membrane

_____ 11. a life-threatening condition characterized by severe blood loss

_____ 12. before surgery, from the decision to have surgery until the surgery begins

Types of Surgery

Complete the following sentences.

1. _____ surgery is surgery that is planned.

2. Surgery performed as an emergency is called _____ surgery.

3. Surgery performed because a patient is critically injured is called _____ surgery.

4. _____ surgery is performed to obtain further information about a disease or condition.

5. Surgeries may be performed in a(n) _____ room in a hospital, in a hospital's outpatient surgical center, or in a freestanding surgery center.

6. _____ surgeries can respond to a broad range of conditions and disorders (for example, the repair of a hernia).

7. _____ surgeries typically focus on one organ or body system.

8. An example of a simple surgery is one that removes a(n) _____, or growth or mass.

9. Surgery may be performed to repair a(n) _____, or falling organ.

10. One example of a complex surgery is the repair of the _____, a cartilage pad in the knee.

11. _____ is the surgical removal of tissue, such as in the heart.

12. Laparoscopic surgery is a type of surgery that is minimally _____, leading to less blood loss and scarring, quicker recovery, and a reduced amount of pain.

13. Laparoscopic surgeries are performed using a(n) _____, which is a telescopic rod lens system connected to a video camera or digital camera.

14. _____ surgical procedures use light or electromagnetic radiation to cut, burn, or destroy tissue, lesions, and tumors.

The Phases of Surgery

Select the *best* answer.

_____ 1. The three phases of surgery are known collectively as
  A. natal
  B. perioperative
  C. intraoperative
  D. trauma

_____ 2. Which phase of surgery starts with the decision to have surgery and ends when surgery begins?
  A. preoperative
  B. perioperative
  C. postoperative
  D. intraoperative

_____ 3. The intraoperative phase of surgery ends when
  A. the surgeon inserts stitches
  B. the patient completely recovers
  C. the patient is moved to the recovery room
  D. family members can see the patient again

_____ 4. In a hospital, a recovery room is usually called a(n)
  A. intensive care unit (ICU)
  B. stepdown unit
  C. operating room (OR)
  D. post-anesthesia care unit (PACU)

_____ 5. Which phase of surgery begins after surgery and lasts until the patient returns to his or her optimal level of health?
  A. postoperative
  B. perioperative
  C. preoperative
  D. intraoperative

The Surgical Staff

Complete the following sentences.

1. _____ surgeons are licensed medical doctors who have advanced training in surgery.

2. Specialty surgeons pursue _____ training and credentials to specialize in surgeries on specific areas of the body.

3. An example of a specialty surgeon is a(n) _____ surgeon who operates on blood vessels.

4. In an OR, the _____ team is responsible for performing surgery within a limited area that must always be sterile.

5. A surgeon may have one or two _____ surgeons depending on the surgery.

6. Assistant surgeons arrange instruments for use, help maintain _____ of the surgical site, control bleeding, close wounds, and apply dressings.

7. Members of the _____ team in an OR are not allowed to enter the sterile field, but must still wear PPE.

8. An OR's unsterile team helps maintain the _____ field, provides the sterile team with wrapped sterile supplies, touches unsterile surfaces and equipment, and provides patient care outside the sterile field.

9. A(n) _____ is a licensed medical doctor with specialized training in the administration of anesthesia.

10. A nurse _____ is an RN who works under the supervision of an anesthesiologist or surgeon and has advanced credentials and training to administer anesthetics.

11. The _____ nurse on the unsterile team monitors all activities in the OR, manages the care and comfort of the patient, and ensures the sterile field is strictly observed.

12. In the PACU, _____ nurses help patients recover from anesthesia, monitor patients' vital signs, and provide postsurgical care.

Organization of the OR

Select the *best* answer.

_____ 1. The OR environment should be
   A. dimly lit
   B. very warm
   C. well-vented to prevent infection
   D. open to the public

_____ 2. Which of the following is true of the sterile field?
   A. The area around the patient is unsterile.
   B. Sterile drapes help establish the sterile field.
   C. There should be a 2-inch barrier between the sterile and unsterile fields.
   D. The unsterile team works in the sterile field.

_____ 3. The crash cart in an OR
   A. contains a defibrillator, airway intubation devices, a resuscitation bag or mask, and medications
   B. does not need to be accessible
   C. takes the place of monitoring a patient's vital signs
   D. is not used if the patient codes

Safety in the OR

Identify whether each statement is true or false.

_____ 1. Fires due to electrical units, high temperatures, smoke generated from lasers, and the oxygen-enriched atmosphere are OR safety hazards.

_____ 2. Electrical shocks are never the result of faulty equipment.

_____ 3. Slipping, falling, and tripping are safety concerns on the OR floor.

_____ 4. In the OR, lights should be kept out of the way unless they are in use.

_____ 5. Exposure to blood and body fluids from sharps is a risk when inserting IV lines, cutting, suturing, withdrawing needles, cleaning up, and disposing of equipment.

_____ 6. Using lasers involves the risk of exposure to pathogenic particulates in the water.

_____ 7. Exposure to waste anesthetic gases from leaks is a hazard in the OR.

_____ 8. Chemical cleaning agents do not pose a risk in the OR.

Preoperative Care

Complete the following sentences.

1. Before surgery, a(n) _____ will explain the surgery, review medications, and identify any risks associated with the procedure.

2. A patient signs an informed _____ form confirming he or she understands the risks associated with a procedure.

3. The day before surgery, patients should be _____, or not eat or drink anything, usually starting around 5:00 p.m.

4. NPO orders include mints and chewing _____.

5. On the day of surgery, patients take only those _____ advised by the surgeon with a sip of water.

6. When arriving at the surgery, the patient should bring his or her _____ card, personal identification, and medication list.

7. Prior to surgery, a patient will need to remove _____ polish so it does not interfere with oxygen delivery.

8. The role of a(n) _____ assistant is to help the patient with bathing; securing valuables; removing makeup, nail polish, hair-related items, contact lenses, hearing aids, prostheses, and dentures; maintaining NPO status; and completing the surgical preoperative checklist.

9. Transport staff members take the patient, usually via a(n) _____, to the preoperative section of the OR.

10. Before surgery, a(n) _____ catheter or needle is typically inserted, and medications may be given for specific health conditions and to relax the patient prior to surgery.

11. The _____ or anesthetist visits the patient to discuss the anesthesia being used, expectations for recovery, and any questions the patient might have.

12. In the OR, the patient is carefully transferred from the gurney or bed to the _____ table and positioned for surgery.

Intraoperative Care

Identify whether each statement is true or false.

_____ 1. The anesthesiologist or nurse anesthetist stands at the foot of the operating table and talks with the patient while attaching a blood pressure cuff.

_____ 2. Monitoring equipment, infusion pumps that deliver anesthesia, and any necessary medications or blood are placed nearby the patient.

_____ 3. If a patient is receiving general anesthesia, the patient will become conscious, and pain receptors to the brain will be enhanced.

_____ 4. A mask is often placed over the patient's nose and mouth, and the patient is asked to breathe deeply.

_____ 5. Anesthetic can only be delivered through the respiratory system.

_____ 6. An endotracheal tube is typically placed in the throat while the patient is still awake.

_____ 7. Just before surgery, the area where the surgery will take place is cleaned with an antiseptic solution and covered with a sterile drape, leaving only the site to be operated on uncovered.

_____ 8. During a pause or time-out right before surgery, the OR team double-checks the patient's identity, the procedure and site, the side and position, and necessary equipment.

_____ 9. If the surgery is long, compression boots or antiembolism stockings may be placed on the patient's lower legs to prevent blood clots.

_____ 10. The amount of time in the operating room depends on the type of surgery and any complications encountered.

Postoperative Care

Complete the following sentences.

1. On average, it takes one to three _____ to recover from anesthesia.

2. In the PACU, monitors are attached to the patient, and _____ signs are taken every 5 to 15 minutes.

3. A(n) _____ mask or nasal cannula helps patients with breathing after surgery.

4. After surgery, some patients may feel _____ and vomit, but medications can ease these feelings and provide pain relief for comfort and healing.

5. The timing of discharge from the PACU depends on the surgery and the patient's recovery from _____.

6. Patients who are going home or will be transferred to another facility must have _____ vital signs, manageable pain, and no nausea or vomiting.

7. If patients have had _____ anesthesia, which wears off slowly, they will usually move their toes and feet before they first feel them.

8. After spinal anesthesia, a patient is usually asked to remain in a(n) _____ position for six to eight hours.

9. After surgery, a patient is transferred to a hospital bed, which must be made as a(n) _____ bed.

10. Once the postoperative patient arrives in the hospital room, a licensed nursing staff member confirms his or her _____ by checking the identification bracelet.

11. After surgery, vital signs are measured frequently per the doctor's order, as often as every _____ minute(s) upon arrival, with decreasing frequency as the patient becomes stable.

12. If the postoperative patient does not have a catheter, the first _____ after surgery is critical to monitor.

Complications After Surgery

Identify whether each statement is true or false.

_____ 1. Possible complications after surgery include reactions to anesthesia, reactions related to the endotracheal tube, changes in vital signs, hemorrhage, shock, cardiac arrest, and urinary retention.

_____ 2. Hypovolemic shock is severe blood loss characterized by hypertension, a slow pulse, restlessness, and warm skin.

_____ 3. Deep vein thrombosis (DVT) poses the risk of blood clots traveling through the bloodstream to cause a pulmonary embolus.

_____ 4. To give compassionate, supportive care, holistic nursing assistants can recognize the patient's anxiety and stress before and after surgery.

5. When paying attention to a patient's pain, nursing assistants should observe verbal, but not nonverbal, communication and report pain levels to the licensed nursing staff.

6. After surgery, nursing assistants should reposition patients often according to the plan of care, pay special attention to tubing and dressings, and check for any signs of skin breakdown or infection.

7. It is important to check a postoperative patient's vital signs on schedule; check circulation; and observe the skin, lips, and fingernails for signs of cyanosis.

8. If a patient has had surgery, it is not important to observe, report, and document his or her level of pain.

9. Monitoring a postoperative patient's I&O accurately ensures proper hydration, and the time of the third, but not the first, urination should be noted.

10. If a patient vomits, a nursing assistant should turn the patient's head to the side to prevent aspiration.

11. If a patient has an abdominal incision, the incision site should be supported with a small pillow or folded towel.

12. Some patients use an inventive spirometer to breathe more deeply and prevent pneumonia.

13. Compression devices or antiembolism stockings, leg exercises, and early and frequent ambulation can help prevent DVT.

14. The application of heat compresses decreases swelling and speeds the healing process.

Drains and Evacuators

Complete the following sentences.

1. Postoperative patients often have drains and evacuators to help remove _____, or discharge such as blood or pus.

2. There are two types of drainage _____: open drainage and closed drainage.

3. In _____ drainage, a drain is placed within an incision, and a dressing may be applied to capture exudate.

4. A drain is a small, collapsible, plastic tube and is usually anchored with a(n) _____ pin so it does not slip into the incision.

5. _____ drainage involves evacuators that use compression and suction to collect drainage in a reservoir or drainage device.

6. Nursing assistants maintain strict standard precautions when handling drains, prevent kinking, report any possible clogging, ensure the drain is properly secured and is located _____ the insertion site, and observe and document the amount and type of fluid removed.

7. The licensed nursing staff should be notified immediately if the patient has a(n) _____, if there is extreme tenderness at the drainage site, or if there is increased drainage.

Abdominal Binders and Antiembolic Measures

Select the *best* answer.

1. An abdominal binder is
   A. fastened from the top down
   B. one-size-fits-all
   C. applied firmly enough to constrict circulation
   D. a wide, flat piece of fabric or elastic material applied to hold a dressing in place

2. Antiembolic measures
   A. do not reduce risks for DVT and PE
   B. include sequential compression devices (SCDs) and antiembolism stockings
   C. are not listed in the plan of care
   D. are never continued after the postoperative phase

Applying Antiembolism Stockings

When a patient has had surgery and is not active, antiembolism stockings are applied to promote circulation in the legs and feet and prevent life-threatening blood clots. In this activity, you will practice applying antiembolism stockings. To prepare for this activity, review the procedural checklist for Applying Antiembolism Stockings. Also have your FIRST CHECK procedural checklist nearby.

Form a group of three and assign each person a role. One person will be the nursing assistant, another a resident, and the third person will serve as the evaluator. Then complete each of the following steps:

1. Complete the FIRST, or Preparation, steps of the procedure, omitting any steps that are not applicable to the Applying Antiembolism Stockings procedure.

2. Did you omit any steps that are not applicable to the Applying Antiembolism Stockings procedure? If yes, explain which step(s) were omitted and why.

_____

_____

_____

3. Complete the steps of the Providing Foot Care procedure from Chapter 21. The nursing assistant should follow the steps of the procedure closely, and the evaluator should assess how well the nursing assistant is performing the procedure.

4. Complete the steps of the procedure for Applying Antiembolism Stockings.

5. Complete the CHECK, or Follow-Up and Reporting and Documentation, steps of the procedure, omitting any steps that are not applicable to the procedure.

6. Did you omit any steps that are not applicable to the procedure? If yes, explain which step(s) were omitted and why.

_____

_____

_____

7. Switch roles with your partners so each partner has the opportunity to be the nursing assistant.

Discharge After Surgery

Complete the following sentences.

1. After surgery, some patients are _____ to another facility for rehabilitation such as physical therapy or further care.

2. A discharge _____ provides instructions concerning medications, activity levels, treatments that need to be continued, and follow-up appointments with the doctor.

3. Depending on the complexity of the surgery, patients often need _____ at home and will likely become tired quickly.

4. After discharge, patients may need regular visits from a(n) _____ healthcare provider or nurse.

5. The goal of recovery is always to help the patient return to his or her _____ level of health.

Name: _____ Date: _____

Matching Chapter 26 Key Terms
Match each definition with the key term.

A. allergen
B. anaphylaxis
C. angina
D. antihistamine
E. asphyxia
F. automated external defibrillator (AED)
G. basic life support (BLS)
H. bioterrorism
I. cardiopulmonary resuscitation (CPR)
J. cyberattacks
K. evacuation
L. fibrillation
M. grand mal seizure
N. Hands-Only™ CPR
O. Heimlich maneuver
P. hemorrhage
Q. petit mal seizure
R. rule of nines
S. seizures
T. shock

_____ 1. excessive loss of blood over a short period of time due to internal or external injury

_____ 2. the intentional removal of people or objects from a dangerous area

_____ 3. a generalized seizure in which a person has impaired awareness and responsiveness, may stare, and may have facial or body twitches

_____ 4. any substance that the body perceives as a threat and that causes an allergic reaction

_____ 5. a method of calculating the surface area of the body affected by burns

_____ 6. care given to a person experiencing respiratory arrest, cardiac arrest, or airway obstruction; includes giving cardiopulmonary resuscitation (CPR), using an automated external defibrillator (AED), and relieving an obstructed airway

_____ 7. chest pain or discomfort; characterized by a sensation of squeezing, pressure, heaviness, or tightness in the center of the chest

_____ 8. an emergency procedure in which air is exhaled into a person's mouth or nose to provide ventilation and external chest compressions help oxygenated blood flow to the brain and heart

_____ 9. illegal attempts to gain access to a digital device or network to cause harm

_____ 10. a severe allergic reaction that can affect the whole body; characterized by skin reactions, swelling, trouble breathing, rapid pulse, nausea, and dizziness

_____ 11. the use of harmful agents and products with biological origins (including pathogens or toxins) as weapons

_____ 12. irregular heart rhythm

_____ 13. a medication that slows or stops the actions of histamine, a substance that causes inflammation

_____ 14. sudden changes in the brain's normal electrical activity that cause an altered or loss of consciousness

_____ 15. a medical device that delivers an electric shock to the heart to stop irregular heart rhythm and allow normal heart rhythm to resume

_____ 16. a generalized seizure in which a person may experience a loss of consciousness and violent muscle contractions

_____ 17. a lack of oxygen in the body; may be caused when breathing stops due to an obstruction or swelling in the trachea

_____ 18. a condition in which the organs and tissues of the body do not have sufficient oxygen

_____ 19. uninterrupted chest compressions given to restore heartbeat and promote blood circulation; a procedure for those not trained in conventional CPR

_____ 20. the procedure of placing one's fist just above the navel of a choking person, covering the fist with the other hand, and performing abdominal thrusts inward and upward

Understanding First Aid
Complete the following sentences.

1. A medical _____ is a sudden, acute, and serious illness or injury.

2. Medical emergencies can result from _____ (such as severe cuts, burns, and broken bones) or medical conditions such as strokes and heart attacks.

3. The United States has emergency _____ services accessible by calling 9-1-1.

4. First _____ are people who first arrive at an emergency.

Name: _____   Date: _____

5. If an emergency occurs, nursing assistants should immediately turn on the emergency call _____ to alert staff, always follow facility policy, and consider safety and comfort.

6. Outside a healthcare facility, the first actions for responding to an emergency should be calling for help and providing basic _____.

7. A person calling 9-1-1 should always give his or her name, _____, and all known factual information about the victim to the operator.

8. Good _____ laws protect people who voluntarily help during a medical emergency outside a healthcare facility.

9. _____ is the process of observing and responding to a medical emergency, such as an injury, poisoning, burn, or medical issue.

10. First aid begins with determining the _____ of the emergency and quickly taking the correct and best course of action based on standards of care.

11. When responding to an emergency, nursing assistants should pay attention to their own _____, notice their surroundings, evaluate the situation, and consider infection control.

12. It is best not to _____ a person except for safety reasons to prevent paralysis or death due to spinal cord damage.

13. During an emergency response, it is important to do no _____.

14. The area around an emergency situation should be kept free from distractions such as _____, noise, or other disturbances.

15. Basic life _____ includes giving cardiopulmonary resuscitation (CPR), using an automated external defibrillator (AED), and relieving an obstructed airway.

The Chain of Survival

List the links in the chain of survival.

Dzm1try/Shutterstock.com

1. _____

2. _____

3. _____

4. _____

Cardiopulmonary Resuscitation (CPR)

Identify whether each statement is true or false.

_____ 1. Cardiopulmonary resuscitation (CPR) is an emergency, lifesaving procedure for a person whose breathing or heartbeat has stopped.

_____ 2. The term *cardiopulmonary* means "pertaining to the heart and intestines," while *resuscitation* means "to revive."

_____ 3. CPR supports blood circulation and breathing with manual external chest compressions and rescue breaths.

_____ 4. CPR is often necessary after a person suffers an electric shock, drowning, or cardiac arrest.

_____ 5. A person's chance for survival increases 7 to 10 percent for every minute a normal heartbeat is not restored.

_____ 6. The best approach for CPR depends on the amount of training a person has.

_____ 7. People not trained in CPR should provide conventional CPR with mouth-to-mouth breathing.

_____ 8. People trained in CPR and confident in their ability should conduct Hands-Only™ CPR.

_____ 9. The acronym *CAB* represents the CPR steps of compressions, airway, and breathing.

_____ 10. Hands-Only™ CPR can be used for teens or adults, but is not recommended for infants and children.

Hands-Only™ CPR

The following steps are part of the procedure for performing Hands-Only™ CPR. Identify the proper order in which they should be completed by numbering them 1 through 7.

_____ Place the heel of one hand on the lower half of the person's sternum. Place your other hand on top and interlock your fingers. Keep your fingers off the chest and do not lean on the person.

_____ Expose the chest. Move clothing out of the way so you can see the skin.

_____ With your arms straight and your shoulders directly over your hands, use your body weight to push hard and fast in the center of the person's chest on the sternum.

_____ Call 9-1-1 (or send someone to do so) and follow first aid guidelines.

_____ Give 100–120 chest compressions per minute with no interruptions. The chest should be compressed to a depth of 2 inches and then released back. Do not remove your hands from the sternum. Continue chest compressions until the person starts to breathe, until an AED becomes available, or until trained healthcare providers arrive.

_____ Be sure the person is lying on his or her back (in the supine position), and if possible, on a hard surface. Get on your knees and bend over one side of the person.

_____ Check to see if the person is conscious. Look at the person's chest to see if he or she is breathing and check the person's carotid pulse. If the person has a weak or absent pulse, is unconscious, and is not breathing or is gasping, proceed.

Name: _____   Date: _____

Conventional CPR

Conventional CPR includes chest compressions, airway clearing, and rescue breathing (CAB). The following steps are part of the procedure for performing conventional CPR. Identify the proper order in which they should be completed by numbering them 1 through 7.

_____ Perform five cycles of CPR (lasting two minutes) before using an automated external defibrillator (AED). An AED can be used twice between a set of five CPR cycles. If an AED is not available, continue CPR until the person starts to move, until an AED becomes available, or until trained healthcare providers arrive.

_____ Check the carotid pulse located on the side of the person's neck. Place your index finger and middle finger on the neck to the side of the windpipe to feel the pulse. Check pulse for no more than 10 seconds.

_____ After clearing the airway, check for normal breathing for no more than 10 seconds. Assess breathing by looking for chest motion, listening for normal breath sounds, and feeling the person's breath. If the person is not breathing or is gasping, then begin rescue breathing.

_____ Using the heels of your hands, place one hand on top of the other. Interlock your fingers. Your dominant hand should touch the person's chest. With your arms straight and your shoulders directly over your hands, use your body weight to push hard and fast in the center of the person's chest on the sternum. Perform 30 chest compressions with no interruptions. For teens and adults, compress the chest 2 inches. For children, compress the chest 1½ inches.

_____ If there is no pulse, prepare to start chest compressions. Be sure the person is lying on his or her back (in the supine position), and if possible, on a hard surface. Get on your knees and bend over one side of the person.

_____ After 30 chest compressions, clear the airway by tilting the head and lifting the chin. Put your palm on the person's forehead and gently tilt the head back. With your other hand, gently lift the person's chin forward to open the airway.

_____ After clearing the airway and covering the mouth to form a seal, give two rescue breaths, each lasting one second. After the first breath, watch to see if the chest rises. Then give the second breath and resume chest compressions.

Automated External Defibrillator (AED)

Complete the following sentences.

1. Heart rate and rhythm are controlled by an internal _____ system in the heart.

2. An automated external _____ is a medical device that delivers an electrical shock through the chest to the heart.

3. An AED shock to the heart can stop _____, or irregular heart rhythm, and allow a normal heart rhythm to resume.

4. AEDs are lightweight, battery operated, and easy to use with _____ prompts and visual prompts that inform the user if and when a shock should be delivered to the heart.

5. One should provide _____ minute(s) of CPR at the appropriate level of training before using an AED.

6. Because an AED emits an electrical shock, it is important to check for any _____ nearby and carefully move the person, if needed.

7. Before applying the AED's pads, one should expose the person's _____ and quickly remove any metal and excess chest hair as needed.

8. AEDs have sticky pads with sensors called _____.

9. One pad should be placed on the _____ center of the person's chest above the nipple, and the other pad should be placed slightly below the other nipple and to the left of the rib cage.

10. Defibrillator pads should be moved at least 1 inch away from implanted devices such as a(n) _____.

11. Once the wires of the electrodes are connected to the AED and no one is touching the person, one can press the AED's _____ button.

12. If a shock is needed, the AED may prompt the user to press the _____ button.

13. After the AED delivers a shock, one can resume _____.

14. After delivering a shock, the AED will automatically reanalyze the person's heart _____ to determine if another shock is needed.

Chest Pain and Heart Attacks

Identify whether each statement is true or false.

_____ 1. Angina, or chest pain, is any major discomfort around the chest.

_____ 2. Chest pain is located in the chest area and does not radiate to the back, neck, lungs, esophagus, or abdomen.

_____ 3. Angina should first be considered a sign of a heart-related problem that requires immediate help.

_____ 4. A heart attack, or myocardial infarction (MI), occurs when blood flow to part of the heart muscle is blocked.

_____ 5. Plaque rupturing within the coronary artery can cause a thrombus to form, leading to blockage.

_____ 6. As a result of increased blood flow, the heart muscle becomes severely damaged and dies, which can cause cardiac arrest.

_____ 7. Many heart attacks begin with hardly noticeable symptoms, such as discomfort or pain that comes and goes.

_____ 8. The mild, spreading pain characteristic of MI will improve through rest or sleep.

_____ 9. In women, MI can cause different symptoms, including generalized chest pain; pain in the arms, back, or jaw; sweating; nausea; or fatigue.

_____ 10. All heart attacks have clear, noticeable symptoms.

_____ 11. Symptoms of MI include discomfort or pain, sweating, nausea, dizziness, rapid or irregular heartbeats, and anxiety, but not indigestion or a feeling of fullness.

_____ 12. If possible, it is best to call 9-1-1 within five minutes of experiencing symptoms of MI.

_____ 13. Chewing and swallowing one noncoated 325 mg aspirin will slow down the activity of platelets and inhibit the growth of a blood clot.

_____ 14. Tightening a person's clothing and having a person stand up and lower his or her head will help with breathing.

_____ 15. If the person stops breathing, it is important to start CPR based on one's level of training.

Stroke

Complete the following sentences.

1. A stroke, or _____ accident, is the fifth leading cause of death in the United States and is also a leading cause of disability.

2. A stroke occurs when a blood vessel carrying oxygen and nutrients to the _____ becomes blocked by a clot or ruptures.

3. There are three types of strokes: _____ strokes, hemorrhagic strokes, and transient ischemic attacks (TIAs).

4. Symptoms of a stroke include a severe _____, weakness and tingling, paralysis on one side, difficulty walking, and sudden confusion.

5. Slurred speech, facial _____, drooling, changes in vision and vital signs, and difficulty speaking are all symptoms of a stroke.

6. If a person shows signs of a stroke, one should seek immediate help by calling _____ or transporting the person to the emergency department.

Anaphylaxis

Identify whether each statement is true or false.

_____ 1. Many people have allergies to medications, foods, and insect stings.

_____ 2. Anaphylaxis is a mild allergic reaction that can affect the whole body.

_____ 3. An allergic reaction usually occurs within several days of exposure to an allergen.

_____ 4. Anaphylaxis cannot occur 30 or more minutes after exposure to an allergen.

_____ 5. Symptoms of an allergic reaction include skin reactions; swelling of the face, eyes, lips, or throat; a feeling of warmth; the sensation of a lump in the throat; constriction of airways; a weak, rapid pulse; nausea, vomiting, or diarrhea; and dizziness, fainting, or unconsciousness.

_____ 6. If someone is experiencing moderate-to-severe symptoms of an allergic reaction or anaphylaxis, emergency treatment should be sought the next day.

_____ 7. In severe cases, untreated anaphylaxis can lead to death within 30 minutes.

_____ 8. Oral antihistamines are medications that reduce inflammation and work fast enough to treat anaphylaxis.

_____ 9. Symptoms of anaphylaxis must be acted on immediately.

_____ 10. Epinephrine auto-injectors can be used to treat allergic reactions.

Burns

Complete the following sentences.

1. A burn is a break in the body's _____ line of defense.

2. Burns can be classified as first degree, _____ degree, or third degree.

3. _____ burns are superficial, meaning they exist only on the surface or outer layer of the skin.

4. First-degree burns should be held under _____, running water until the pain eases.

5. If a first-degree burn affects a large portion of the hands, feet, face, groin, buttocks, or a major _____, emergency medical attention should be sought.

6. _____ burns, also called *partial-thickness burns*, are more serious than first-degree burns because they are deeper and may cause permanent injury and scarring.

7. Second-degree burns usually take two to three _____ to heal and are characterized by red, white, or splotchy skin; swelling; pain; and blistering.

8. If fewer than 3 inches in diameter, a second-degree burn should be treated the same as a(n) _____ burn.

9. If a second-degree burn is large or covers the hands, feet, face, groin, buttocks, or a major joint, it should be treated like a(n) _____ burn.

10. If a second-degree burn shows signs of _____, such as oozing from the burned area, increased pain, redness, and swelling, medical help should be sought.

11. The most serious burn is a third-degree burn, also called a(n) _____ burn.

12. Third-degree burns often result in permanent injury such as _____ and scarring.

13. Third-degree burns appear charred _____ or white and become leathery.

14. Jewelry, belts, and other restrictive items should be removed from a person with a third-degree burn, especially from around burned areas and the _____.

15. Using cold water for large, severe burns can cause _____, or loss of body heat.

Rule of Nines

Apply the appropriate percentages to the image.

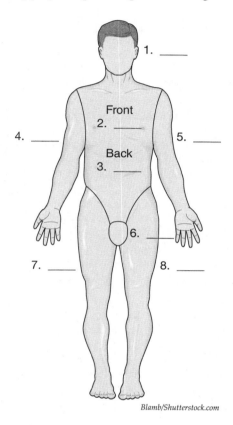

Blamb/Shutterstock.com

Poisoning

Identify whether each statement is true or false.

_____ 1. People with dementia are at increased risk for dying as a result of poisoning.

_____ 2. Most poisons are ingested, but poisons can also enter the body through the skin, by inhalation, intravenously, through radiation exposure, or through the consumption of food.

_____ 3. Poisoning can be unintentional or intentional.

_____ 4. A person can be poisoned and not show symptoms for hours, days, or even months.

_____ 5. Signs and symptoms of poisoning are unlike those of common illnesses such as strokes, seizures, and head injuries.

_____ 6. Signs and symptoms of poisoning include abnormal skin color, burns or redness around the mouth and lips, breath that smells like chemicals, nausea and vomiting, difficulty breathing, restlessness and agitation, seizure, and confusion or disorientation.

_____ 7. If someone has been poisoned, it is important to look for clues about the poisoning, such as empty pill bottles, scattered pills, burns, stains, or odors.

_____ 8. It is not appropriate to call 9-1-1 or go to a local emergency department if a person displays signs of poisoning.

_____ 9. Checking a person's mouth and carefully removing any poison that remains can help a person who has swallowed poison.

_____ 10. Household cleaners and other chemicals often show instructions for accidental poisoning.

_____ 11. Removing contaminated clothing and rinsing the skin for 15 to 20 minutes can help a person with poison in the lungs.

_____ 12. If poison is in a person's eye, the eye should be gently flushed with hot water for 20 minutes or until help arrives.

_____ 13. If a person has inhaled poison, he or she should be moved into an interior room as soon as possible.

_____ 14. Turning the head backward can help prevent choking if a poisoned person is vomiting.

_____ 15. Before trained healthcare providers arrive to help the poisoned person, one should gather any pill or vitamin bottles, packages or containers with labels, plants, or other information about the suspected poison.

Choking

Complete the following sentences.

1. Choking is a medical emergency that blocks the flow of air containing _____ to the lungs and the rest of the body.

2. Lack of oxygen causes_____, a condition in which the body is deprived of oxygen.

3. For adults, the most common cause of choking is the _____ of a piece of food.

4. Older adults who have a weakened _____ reflex are at increased risk for choking.

5. With a(n) _____ blockage, a person is coughing vigorously, can speak, and can breathe.

6. A person with a partial blockage should be encouraged to continue_____.

7. If a person is coughing, it is not appropriate to strike the person on the _____ or perform abdominal thrusts.

8. With a complete blockage, the person cannot _____ and makes high-pitched sounds or clutches at the throat.

9. Quick action using abdominal _____ can save the life of a person with a complete blockage.

Responding to Choking

Relieving choking can prevent injury or death. The following steps are part of the procedure for responding to choking using the Heimlich maneuver. For each set of steps, identify the proper order in which they should be completed by numbering them 1 through 5.

1. _____ Call for help or have someone else call for help. If you are in a healthcare facility, use the emergency call light. Otherwise, call 9-1-1.

   _____ Follow first aid guidelines and remain calm.

   _____ If coughing does not dislodge the object, stand or kneel behind the person. Wrap your arms around the person's waist.

   _____ If the person is coughing, wait to see if coughing dislodges the object.

   _____ Reassure the choking person that you are there to help. Check the person's ability to breathe.

2. _____ Perform five abdominal thrusts and then check to see if the object is visible or has been expelled.

   _____ Press forcefully into the abdomen with the thumb side of your fist. Use quick, inward and upward thrusts to dislodge the object.

   _____ Make a fist with one hand.

   _____ Place the thumb side of your fist against the person's abdomen, slightly above the navel and well below the sternum.

   _____ Grasp your clenched fist with your other hand. Do not tuck your thumb inside your fist. Avoid pressing on the person's ribs with your forearms.

3. _____ If the object is not visible or has not been expelled, keep performing abdominal thrusts until the object is expelled or the person loses consciousness.

   _____ If there is a pulse, open the airway by tilting the head back and lifting the chin. Deliver one breath and see if the chest rises. If the chest does not rise, try one more time.

   _____ Remove the foreign object only if you see it. To open the person's airway, tilt the head back and lift the chin. Look into the person's mouth for the object. Grasp and remove the object if it is within reach.

   _____ If a choking person loses consciousness, put on disposable gloves, if available. Turn the person so he or she is lying in the supine position

   _____ Check for a pulse.

4. _____ If you are not in a healthcare facility, report your observations and actions to the trained healthcare providers when they arrive. If you are in a healthcare facility, take the person's vital signs once the object has been expelled and alert the licensed nursing staff.

   _____ If rescue breaths do not cause the chest to rise, begin conventional or Hands-Only™ CPR depending on your level of training.

   _____ Every 30 compressions, open the person's airway and look for the foreign object in his or her mouth.

   _____ If you can see the foreign object in the person's mouth, remove it, but do not push it farther down into the throat.

   _____ Continue performing CPR and checking for the object until the object is expelled or until trained healthcare providers arrive.

Fainting

Complete the following sentences.

1. Fainting is a brief loss of _____ and is considered a medical emergency.

2. Fainting is also called _____ or passing out.

3. Fainting is caused by a drop in blood flow to the _____.

4. Reasons for fainting include fatigue, _____, certain medications, dehydration, heart conditions, age, or the temperature or ventilation in a room.

5. Warning signs that a person may faint include a pale face, skin that feels cold and _____, perspiration, a weak pulse, shallow breathing, trembling and shaking, and dizziness or blurred vision.

6. To help prevent fainting, a resident can sit on the side of the bed for a few minutes, _____ the legs, and breathe deeply before standing.

7. Residents who are dizzy or faint should not be allowed to _____.

8. A sitting person who feels faint should bend forward and place the head between the _____ for at least 5 minutes.

9. A person who is lying down and feels faint should lie in a supine position and elevate the legs approximately 12 inches so they are above the _____.

10. If fainting occurs when a person is not lying down, a nursing assistant should slowly lower the person to the floor using his or her _____ as an incline.

Seizures

Identify whether each statement is true or false.

_____ 1. Seizures are sudden changes in the brain's normal blood flow that cause an altered or loss of consciousness.

_____ 2. Seizures often result from a disease (such as epilepsy, tumors, or nervous system disorders) and head injury.

_____ 3. Seizures can occur at any age and generally last from a few seconds to several days.

_____ 4. There are two different types of seizures: incomplete seizures and stiff seizures.

_____ 5. Partial seizures include motor seizures, sensory seizures, and autonomic seizures.

_____ 6. Motor seizures occur in the muscles and cause the hands and fingers to fracture.

_____ 7. Motor seizures cause tingling sensations.

_____ 8. Autonomic seizures cause changes in respiratory rate, sweating, and heart rate.

_____ 9. Generalized seizures include petit mal seizures and grand mal seizures.

_____ 10. A person experiencing a petit mal seizure will have heightened awareness and responsiveness, may stare, and may have facial or body twitches.

_____ 11. A person having a petit mal seizure will experience tonic and clonic phases.

_____ 12. In the tonic phase, muscles stiffen, and air is forced out of the lungs. A person usually groans, loses consciousness, and may also fall to the floor, turn blue, and bite his or her tongue.

_____ 13. In the clonic phase, muscles contract and relax, which causes jerking and rhythmic movements of the arms and legs.

_____ 14. Consciousness returns quickly in a few seconds after a grand mal seizure.

_____ 15. If someone has a seizure, one should call for help or have someone else call for help and note the time the seizure started.

_____ 16. A person having a seizure should be lowered to the floor to protect against falling.

_____ 17. A person having a seizure should be turned onto his or her back to maintain an open airway.

_____ 18. Placing something soft under the head of a person having a seizure helps prevent the head from striking the floor.

_____ 19. When responding to a seizure, one should force the person's mouth open and put objects between the person's teeth.

_____ 20. After a seizure ends, a person should be placed in a recovery position lying on the back.

Hemorrhage

Complete the following sentences.

1. A hemorrhage is excessive _____ loss over a short period and is a medical emergency.

2. _____ hemorrhages cannot be seen, and external hemorrhages can be seen.

3. Internal hemorrhages occur inside the body's tissues and _____.

4. Signs of an internal hemorrhage are pain, shock, vomiting, coughing up _____, and loss of consciousness.

5. In _____ hemorrhage, blood may spurt from an artery or flow steadily from a vein out of the body.

6. When a person loses a large amount of blood, he or she may go into _____, in which there is not enough oxygen available to the organs and tissues of the body.

7. When a person is in shock, blood _____ drops; the pulse is rapid and weak; the skin is cool, clammy, and pale; and the person may lose consciousness.

8. Signs and symptoms of a hemorrhage include a pale or _____ face; low blood pressure; increased, weak heart rate; rapid, shallow respirations; feelings of weakness and helplessness; restlessness; complaints of thirst; and coldness, shaking, or trembling.

9. Direct _____ applied to the bleeding wound or indirect pressure applied to a pressure point near or on top of the wound can help control bleeding.

10. Pressure _____ exist where blood vessels are located close to the surface of the skin.

11. When responding to a hemorrhage, one should not remove _____ that may have caused the hemorrhage.

12. It is best to put on _____ gloves before applying direct pressure to a bleeding wound.

13. _____ dressings should be placed over wounds to help control bleeding.

14. _____ the affected area of the body will help minimize blood flow to that area and reduce bleeding.

15. A person experiencing a hemorrhage should not be given any _____.

Identifying Pressure Points

Apply the appropriate callouts to the image.

A. Femoral artery
B. Dorsalis pedis artery
C. Temporal artery
D. Brachial artery
E. Popliteal artery
F. Carotid artery
G. Radial artery

© Body Scientific International

Disasters, Terrorism, and Bioterrorism

Identify whether each statement is true or false.

_____ 1. According to the World Health Organization (WHO), a disaster causes human, material, economic, and environmental loss, but does not limit a community's ability to function.

_____ 2. Disasters include natural disasters, aircraft crashes, arson fires, explosions, and epidemics.

_____ 3. Terrorism is violence that is not politically motivated.

_____ 4. Terrorism and violent attacks cause significant casualties, damage to buildings, the need for heavy law enforcement, extensive media coverage, work and school closures, travel restrictions, and possible evacuation.

_____ 5. Bioterrorism is the intentional use of pathogens to cause illness or death in people, animals, or plants.

_____ 6. Bioterrorism agents can be spread by air, through water, or in food.

_____ 7. Nursing assistants receive specific training and practice to ensure they are ready for a disaster.

_____ 8. Outside a healthcare facility, people should create a supply kit and disaster and communication plan.

_____ 9. Disaster and communication plans include responsibilities, emergency contacts, pet safety guidelines, procedures, safe spots for different types of emergencies, evacuation routes, and a shelter location.

_____ 10. Disaster and communication plans should be practiced once every two years.

_____ 11. It is important to be familiar with emergency plans for schools, faith organizations, and sporting events.

_____ 12. Children should not be taught how and when to call 9-1-1 for help.

_____ 13. In the event of a disaster, it is important to remain calm, follow the advice of local emergency officials, and ignore instructions on the radio or television.

_____ 14. Agencies and organizations in the United States collaborate and coordinate their efforts to prepare for and respond to disasters.

_____ 15. The American Red Cross is responsible for mass care, including food, shelter, bulk distribution of disaster relief supplies, first aid, and disaster welfare information.

Disaster Preparedness

To learn more about disaster preparedness, explore disaster preparedness resources on the websites for the following US agencies: The American Red Cross, Centers for Disease Control and Prevention (CDC), US Department of Homeland Security, Federal Emergency Management Agency (FEMA), US Department of Homeland Security, Food and Drug Administration (FDA), and the Environmental Protection Agency (EPA). Then, create your own emergency supply kit and personal checklist for a disaster.

Name: _____ Date: _____

Matching Chapter 27 Key Terms
Match each definition with the key term.

A. advance directives
B. Cheyne-Stokes respiration
C. coroner
D. cremation
E. crypt
F. dignity
G. do-not-resuscitate (DNR) order
H. forensic
I. grief
J. incapacitation
K. living will
L. mausoleum
M. moribund
N. mourn
O. palliative care
P. pathologist
Q. postmortem care
R. power of attorney
S. rigor mortis
T. transplants

_____ 1. a freestanding building in which a person is buried

_____ 2. an advance directive that gives a designated person the authority to make healthcare decisions on behalf of another person; authority only takes effect if the person who writes the power of attorney becomes unable to make his or her own decisions

_____ 3. written legal documents that are signed by a living, competent person and describe that person's medical and healthcare instructions

_____ 4. the stiffening of the body's muscles several hours after death

_____ 5. related to the methods used for investigating and solving crimes

_____ 6. surgeries in which organs or body tissues are removed from one person and transferred into another

_____ 7. value or worth

_____ 8. about to die

_____ 9. a pattern of breathing that indicates death is near; characterized by rapid breathing followed by a period of no breathing

_____ 10. a medical and legal request that lifesaving measures such as CPR not be administered if a person's heart or breathing stops

_____ 11. to express feelings and behaviors that signify grief

_____ 12. a vault or chamber used for burial

_____ 13. care performed shortly after death; prepares the body for burial or cremation, puts the body in alignment, and prevents skin damage

_____ 14. an emotional response to or distress about a physical or personal loss

_____ 15. lack of ability to make decisions

_____ 16. a government official who can certify death and order an autopsy

_____ 17. an advance directive that details the life-prolonging treatments a person desires in the event of incapacitation during a terminal illness or permanent unconsciousness

_____ 18. care that provides relief from the symptoms of a disease or condition

_____ 19. a process in which a dead person's body is subjected to extreme heat for two or more hours, yielding 3–9 pounds of ashes

_____ 20. a doctor who specializes in studying diseases; conducts autopsies to determine causes of death

Dying, Death, and Grief
Complete the following sentences.

1. Death may come after an extended _____, after a long life, or suddenly.

2. When death is impending, a person is considered _____ ill.

3. A person with a terminal illness can be reasonably expected to die in _____ month(s) or less.

4. Examples of terminal illnesses include end-stage cancer or _____ disease, heart failure, stroke, or chronic respiratory problems.

5. It is important to reflect on personal feelings about dying and death, as strong feelings can _____ to those in a nursing assistant's care.

6. Nursing assistants can resolve feelings of fear and anger about death by _____ about them with a friend or other healthcare staff member.

7. One way to resolve negative feelings is to _____ more about the death-related beliefs and traditional practices of others.

8. Cultural _____ and sensitivity are especially important during end-of-life care.

9. Each family has unique _____ surrounding dying and death.

10. Some families do not discuss bad things such as death because they believe that _____ about bad things makes them happen.

11. Some families believe that one should _____ intensely until death arrives.

12. Some families believe that people who die move to a different _____ of life.

13. In some families, a strong sense of _____ accompanies loss, and extended family members gather at the time of death.

14. In some families, _____ typically provide the majority of care for a person who is terminally ill.

15. Some families believe that an older family member must be _____ at the time of death.

16. Some families resist _____ a loved one in a healthcare facility and prefer that the person die at home with family members close.

17. Many people rely on spirituality to understand death and believe that the _____ of the dead pass into a spirit world, an afterlife, or a life after death.

18. For people who embrace spirituality, death is part of _____, is not to be feared, and is a journey to another world.

19. Some people believe they need to ensure the soul of the deceased travels safely, with adequate _____, to the afterlife.

20. Spiritual beliefs and religious practices influence perspectives about burial, cremation, _____ donation, and autopsy.

21. Some religions teach _____, or the rebirth of the soul in another body, and may find comfort in thinking a person will continue to live in some capacity after death.

22. Residents who are dying may seek comfort from prayers or a(n) _____ leader, complete specific predeath rituals, or find solace in knowing loved ones will perform specific tasks after death.

23. If a nursing assistant's beliefs conflict with what he or she is asked to do, the nursing assistant must discuss this with a licensed _____ staff member.

Identifying the Stages of Grief

Identify the stages of grief in the illustration.

Stages of Grief

Stage 1
1. _____

Stage 2
2. _____

Stage 3
3. _____

Stage 4
4. _____

Stage 5
5. _____

Stage 6
6. _____

Stage 7
7. _____

Expressions of Loss and Grief

Match each description with the appropriate stage of grief.

A. anger and bargaining
B. reconstruction and working through
C. depression
D. acceptance or hope
E. pain and guilt
F. shock and denial
G. upward turn

_____ 1. The grieving person is initially numbed by shock and may deny the reality of the situation by temporarily blocking it out.

_____ 2. The grieving person feels emotional or physical pain and has guilty feelings about what they have or should have done.

_____ 3. Pain is expressed as anger with feelings of helplessness and vulnerability as the person tries to find a way to regain control.

_____ 4. The true extent of the loss is understood, which brings feelings of sadness, despair, or regret.

_____ 5. Depression lessens, a feeling of calmness develops, pain and depression become more manageable, and one's "spirits have lifted."

_____ 6. Depression continues to lift, acceptance becomes more of a reality, and things left undone or unsaid are more readily addressed.

_____ 7. The grieving person feels peace; a person may never reach this stage.

Holistic Care for Grieving Residents

Identify whether each statement is true or false.

_____ 1. Holistic nursing assistants provide support through the stages of grief by first recognizing that residents' reactions are not normal responses.

_____ 2. Nursing assistants should reject and detach from residents coping with the reality of the end of life.

_____ 3. If a resident expresses anger, a nursing assistant should take that anger personally.

_____ 4. Communication techniques such as mindfulness, active listening, open-ended questions, and reflection are helpful for giving holistic care to grieving residents.

_____ 5. Nursing assistants can help by using gentle touch and silence to provide a sense of calmness and comfort, particularly during the depression stage.

_____ 6. Prolonged grief is a reaction to impending loss as a person faces his or her own death or the death of a loved one.

_____ 7. Anticipatory grief is related to feelings of guilt and typically lasts more than one year after the death of a loved one.

Advance Directives

Match each description with the legal term.

A. living will
B. Patient Self-Determination Act (PSDA)
C. incapacitation
D. Five Wishes
E. do-not-resuscitate order (DNR)
F. power of attorney
G. advance directive
H. do-not-intubate order

_____ 1. a legal document containing medical and healthcare instructions that will take effect if a person is no longer able to make decisions

_____ 2. lack of ability to make decisions

_____ 3. an advance directive that instructs healthcare providers not to attempt resuscitation if a person's heart and breathing stop

_____ 4. an advance directive detailing the life-prolonging medical treatments a person desires in the event of incapacitation

_____ 5. an advance directive that instructs healthcare providers not to create an airway if a person's breathing stops

_____ 6. an advance directive that gives a designated person the authority to make healthcare decisions on behalf of another person in the event of incapacitation

_____ 7. a law that gives people the control and autonomy to make decisions about end-of-life care

_____ 8. an advance directive that addresses how a person wants to be treated medically, personally, emotionally, and spiritually at the end of life

Care for People Who Are Dying

Select the *best* answer.

_____ 1. Palliative care
A. aims to cure a disease or condition
B. improves the quality of life for a person who is dying, but not for his or her family
C. relieves symptoms such as pain, nausea, fatigue, breathing problems, and anxiety
D. aims to cure a condition that is caused by the family

_____ 2. What is hospice?
A. care provided at any time during a person's illness
B. care provided during the last six months of a person's life
C. a model and philosophy for the quality, compassionate care of people with acute illnesses
D. specialized care for people with terminal illnesses who are not covered by Medicare benefits

_____ 3. The hospice team
A. provides social services and spiritual resources
B. does not help family members deal with emotional and practical issues related to death
C. provides respite care for pets
D. prepares three daily meals and runs errands for the family

_____ 4. The Dying Patient's Bill of Rights
A. is identical to the Patient Bill of Rights
B. must be signed by the resident
C. is billed by the doctor for services rendered
D. is a useful guide to the expectations of those near death

_____ 5. Which of the following is a right of the dying patient?
A. the reality of dying alone
B. the right to cede individuality
C. the right to expect the sanctity of the human body will not be respected
D. the right not to be deceived

_____ 6. A nursing assistant honors a dying patient's rights when he or she
A. rejects the patient's spiritual experience
B. invites the patient to participate in decisions
C. denies the patient's sense of hopefulness
D. stops giving care

Meeting the Needs of Those Who Are Dying

Complete the following sentences.

1. Before death, breathing will become more difficult and rapid, and _____ may cause a rattling sound and cough.

2. Oxygen therapy may be used to improve breathlessness, and a(n) _____ position can be helpful to lower the risk of aspirating phlegm.

3. Due to slowed blood circulation, the nose, lips, fingers, nail beds, and extremities may become pale, gray, or _____.

4. Before death, the legs and ankles may _____, and wounds and infections may not heal well.

5. The _____ of a resident who is dying will be lower than normal, and pulse will be irregular.

6. As death approaches, body temperature often lowers by one degree or more and may be accompanied by _____.

7. Nursing assistants can help residents who are dying by maintaining a comfortable room temperature and using cold _____ on the forehead, if appropriate.

8. As the need for food declines, a resident may _____ meals and beverages or consume only small amounts.

9. A nursing assistant should offer a variety of _____ foods as long as the resident is conscious.

10. A resident who is dying will often have a(n) _____ mouth and nose, which can be alleviated with a moistened washcloth or lip balm.

11. Residents who are dying _____ more, so the eyes may not blink as often and may become dry with crusting.

12. A nursing assistant should use a warm, wet _____ to cleanse a resident's eyes and eyelids.

13. Residents who are dying have limited mobility, increasing their risk for _____ ulcers.

14. Nursing assistants should check the skin often, provide skin care, _____ the resident every two hours, and provide needed padding around bony parts of the body.

15. In residents who are dying, _____ is common due to immobility, poor diet, dehydration, and weakness.

16. During care, nursing assistants should observe for nonverbal cues of _____ and report to the licensed nursing staff.

17. Pain relief medications can make the resident more _____ during the process of dying.

18. Nursing assistants may provide a caring back _____, but should be careful not to jostle the resident.

19. It is important to remember that the sense of _____ continues even if a resident is not communicating.

20. During dying, physical changes in the body also affect a resident's _____ health.

21. Conscious residents may fear death, be worried about things they have not done or said, or want to start the process of saying _____.

22. Nursing assistants can help residents by listening _____ and carefully and encouraging residents to share their worries with their families or significant others.

23. Residents may feel restless, confused, or anxious due to an inability to _____ and due to staying in one position.

24. _____ or visions may occur due to medications, changes in metabolism, an infection, the disease itself, or brain metastases.

25. A holistic nursing assistant helps with communication between the _____ and resident, the doctor, and the healthcare staff by making sure concerns are addressed.

Empathizing with the Process of Dying

The sense of hearing continues during the process of dying, even if a resident is not communicating with others. Helping a resident through the process of death can be difficult, and facing one's own inevitable death can help the nursing assistant empathize with others. For this activity, imagine a peaceful, cozy, softly lit room. Create a list of 10 songs you would want played during the last stages of your death. Share your songs with a significant person in your life.

Self-Care

Identify whether each statement is true or false.

_____ 1. Ignoring emotions ensures they do not influence the care a nursing assistant gives.

_____ 2. If a nursing assistant is uncomfortable caring for a resident, he or she should tell the licensed nursing staff.

_____ 3. Talking with other appropriate staff can help a nursing assistant process feelings.

_____ 4. Nursing assistants should consult with the charge nurse about any care issues and ask for assistance from the palliative care team, if needed.

_____ 5. Understanding what is and is not within the scope of practice is not important when caring for a resident who is dying.

_____ 6. It is appropriate to spend extra time with a resident who is not part of work assignments.

_____ 7. Talking a lot about a resident when not at work is an example of maintaining professional boundaries.

_____ 8. A nursing assistant may be crossing boundaries if he or she takes sides with a resident against the resident's family members.

_____ 9. Accepting personal gifts from a resident or family is an example of crossing a boundary.

_____ 10. Nursing assistants should not act in verbally or physically abusive ways or use touch inappropriately.

_____ 11. Sharing inappropriate personal information is acceptable if a resident is dying.

Signs of Approaching Death
Select the *best* answer.

_____ 1. Death typically arrives
   A. on a resident's schedule
   B. after certain changes in the body signal death is imminent
   C. before a person is declared moribund by a doctor
   D. three days after the heart stops

_____ 2. The two phases of dying
   A. include the pre-active phase and the active phase
   B. collectively last fewer than two weeks
   C. last approximately three days
   D. do not affect the respiratory and cardiovascular systems

_____ 3. During the process of dying, the respiratory system
   A. functions effectively
   B. has periods of rapid breathing followed by periods of deep breathing
   C. is not affected by irregular and slow breaths
   D. develops a pattern of breathing called Cheyne-Stokes respiration

_____ 4. Which of the following is true of secretions?
   A. They improve periods of apnea and other abnormal breathing patterns.
   B. They improve if breathing is very fast.
   C. They collect in the throat, causing a loud, rattling sound during breathing.
   D. They cannot be avoided or treated with palliative care.

_____ 5. What changes occur in the cardiovascular system as a person dies?
   A. Blood circulation increases.
   B. Blood pressure rises.
   C. Skin becomes warm to the touch.
   D. Discoloration affects the hands, feet, lips, and nail beds.

_____ 6. During the process of dying,
   A. a person will drift in and out of consciousness
   B. the eyes will focus on surroundings
   C. a person will become more responsive
   D. agitation and restlessness are due to sadness

_____ 7. How does the process of dying affect the musculoskeletal system?
   A. The person who is dying will become more active.
   B. The jaw will droop to the side.
   C. The body will become less rigid.
   D. The person will move his or her extremities more often.

_____ 8. A person who is dying
   A. will eat regularly
   B. will not experience bowel incontinence
   C. eats less, which causes chemical changes that lead to a sense of well-being
   D. can swallow easily

_____ 9. As the body slows down,
   A. a person drinks more fluids
   B. urine becomes lighter
   C. dehydration causes distress
   D. urine output decreases

_____ 10. Which of the following happens at the time of death?
   A. The heart speeds up.
   B. The jaw closes.
   C. The muscles relax and then stiffen.
   D. The pupils constrict.

_____ 11. How can nursing assistants care for the family at the time of death?
   A. by rejecting family traditions
   B. by responding to angry complaints
   C. by not telling the family how the body will be prepared
   D. by ensuring privacy

Care After Death
Complete the following sentences.

1. When a person dies, the care a nursing assistant delivers will depend on decisions made regarding organ or tissue _____ and autopsy.

2. Donated organs and tissues are used for _____, or surgeries in which organs or body tissues are removed from one person and transferred into another.

3. A person can become an organ or tissue donor by registering with a state donor agency or placing the decision on a(n) _____ license.

4. It is important that a donor lets his or her _____ or a significant individual know about his or her decision.

5. If a person has not made a decision about organ donation before death, the _____ may be consulted.

6. Organ donation can only occur after a person has been declared dead by an approved healthcare provider who is not in any way connected to the donation or _____ recovery team.

7. Quick action ensures that organs are still _____ and smooths the way for the family to proceed with burial or cremation.

Name: _____   Date: _____

8. A(n) _____ is a specialized surgical procedure performed by a pathologist, or disease specialist, for legal or medical reasons.

9. Autopsies are forensic when the cause of death is suspected to be _____.

10. Autopsies are ordered by a(n) _____, a government official who certifies death.

11. In a(n) _____ autopsy, a person's body is fingerprinted and photographed, but not opened.

12. The family or a legally responsible party must sign a(n) _____ form for an internal autopsy.

13. A medical _____ can order an autopsy without the family's permission if the cause of death is unclear or suspicious.

14. A person and his or her family can select an in-ground or above-ground _____.

15. An in-ground burial may use a casket or a(n) _____.

16. An above-ground burial is burial inside a(n) _____ or crypt.

17. Burial arrangements are usually made with a(n) _____ home.

18. _____ exposes the deceased person's body to extreme heat, usually 1800–2000°F, for two or more hours to yield 3–9 pounds of remains.

19. Cremations are done in a special facility called a(n) _____.

20. The purposes of _____ care include preparing the resident's body for viewing by the family, providing appropriate care and disposition of belongings, and ensuring proper identification prior to transport to the morgue or funeral home.

Providing Postmortem Care

Postmortem care must be provided as soon as possible after death to keep the resident's body in proper alignment, prevent skin damage, and prepare the resident's body for family viewing and transport. The following steps are part of the procedure for providing postmortem care. For each set of steps, identify the proper order in which they should be completed by numbering them 1 through 5.

1. _____ Introduce yourself to the deceased resident's family using your full name and title. Explain that you work with the licensed nursing staff and will be providing care.

_____ Ask the licensed nursing staff how this procedure fits into the plan of care, if there are doctor's orders, and if there are any special instructions or precautions (such as organ donation or autopsy). A licensed nursing staff member will provide instructions about the maintenance or removal of equipment such as IV or urinary catheters.

_____ Knock before entering the room if the deceased resident's family is in the room.

_____ Check the deceased resident's identification bracelet.

_____ Wash your hands or use hand sanitizer before entering the room.

2. _____ Bring the necessary equipment into the room. Place the following items in an accessible location: a postmortem kit, an envelope or bag for personal belongings, several pairs of disposable gloves, several washcloths, several towels, a disposable protective pad, a bath blanket, cotton balls, gauze bandages and tape, a clean gown, a washbasin, and a labeled denture cup.

_____ Use Mr., Mrs., or Ms. and family members' last names when conversing.

_____ Determine if the family will be staying in the room for the procedure. If the family wants to stay, explain the procedure in simple terms.

_____ Lock the bed wheels and then raise the bed to hip level.

_____ Provide privacy by closing the curtains, using a screen, or closing the door to the room.

3. _____ Fanfold the linens to the foot of the bed.

_____ If there are side rails, raise and secure the rails on the opposite side of the bed from where you will be working. Lower the rail on the side you are working.

_____ Put on disposable gloves.

_____ Make sure the bed is flat. Place a pillow under the resident's head and shoulders to keep the body aligned.

_____ Wash your hands or use hand sanitizer to ensure infection control.

4. _____ Close the resident's mouth. If the mouth will not stay closed, request instructions from the charge nurse. A rolled washcloth under the chin can help keep the mouth closed.

_____ Straighten the resident's arms and legs and place the arms at the side of the body.

_____ If appropriate, clean and insert dentures into the resident's mouth. If dentures are not to be worn, clean and place them in a labeled denture cup.

_____ Gently close the resident's eyes if they are open by grasping the eyelashes and pulling the eyelids down. Hold the eyes shut for a few seconds. Place moistened cotton balls over the eyelids if the eyelids will not stay closed.

_____ Undress the resident and cover the resident with a bath blanket.

5. _____ Wash your hands or use hand sanitizer to ensure infection control.

_____ Remove and discard your gloves.

_____ Empty and replace any drainage bags. If instructed, remove tubing and appliances. Ask for guidance from the licensed nursing staff if the resident is wearing a prosthetic.

_____ Place the resident's jewelry and personal belongings into an envelope or bag designated for valuables. Attach an identification tag to the envelope or bag. All valuables should remain in the facility safe until they are claimed and signed for by an approved relative or person.

_____ Remove all jewelry, except for a wedding ring, unless instructed otherwise. If a ring is left in place, put a cotton ball over it and tape it in place.

6. _____ Fill the washbasin with warm water. Place the washbasin on the overbed table.

_____ Put on a new pair of disposable gloves.

_____ Change any wet or soiled linens on the bed.

_____ Wash the resident's body. Dry the body thoroughly. Place and tape gauze bandages on areas that may need drainage absorbed.

_____ Place a disposable protective pad under the resident's buttocks.

7. _____ Keep a pillow behind the resident's head and raise the bed to a supine or low Fowler's position. Cover the resident's body up to the shoulders with a sheet. *Never* cover the resident's face.

_____ Remove and discard your gloves.

_____ Before the family arrives, dispose of any soiled linens, dressings, and tubing. Straighten the room, lower the lights, and provide chairs for the family.

_____ Wash your hands or use hand sanitizer to ensure infection control. Maintain the family's privacy and provide sufficient time for the viewing.

_____ If the family will view the resident, put a clean gown on the resident's body. Comb or brush the hair as needed.

8. _____ If using a shroud, bring the top of the shroud over the resident's head and fold the bottom up over the resident's feet. Fold the sides of the shroud over the resident's body and pin or tape the shroud in place.

_____ When the family leaves, close the door and remove the sheet covering the resident's body.

_____ Put on disposable gloves.

_____ Fill out the identification tags. Tie one identification tag on the resident's ankle or right big toe.

_____ Position the shroud or body bag under the resident's body.

9. _____ Attach one identification tag to the shroud.

_____ Gather all personal belongings and the denture cup, if used. List and label these items, as they will stay with the resident's body.

_____ Remove, clean, and store equipment in the proper location. Remove soiled linens and discard disposable equipment.

_____ If the resident's body is still in the room, pull the privacy curtain around the bed or close the door.

_____ Ask the licensed nursing staff if the resident's body should stay in the room until transport to the funeral home or be moved to the morgue. If the resident's body should be transported to the morgue, check facility transport policy.

10. _____ Record information, along with the care provided, in the chart or EMR.

_____ Report to the licensed nursing staff and communicate the date and time the resident's body was transported to the funeral home or moved to the morgue. Report how the resident's personal belongings and valuables were handled and secured and if dentures and other artificial body parts accompanied the resident.

_____ After the resident's body has been removed from the room, follow the steps for cleaning a room after discharge.

_____ Wash your hands or use hand sanitizer before leaving the room.

_____ Remove and discard your gloves.

CHAPTER 28 Certification, Employment, and Lifelong Learning

Name: _____   Date: _____

Matching Chapter 28 Key Terms

Match each definition with the key term.

A. auditory
B. bullying
C. concentration
D. cover message
E. cramming
F. flash cards
G. job campaign
H. network
I. procrastination
J. résumé

_____ 1. studying large amounts of information in a short period of time

_____ 2. the act of purposely postponing a task

_____ 3. a set of cards used for studying; typically have a question on one side and an answer on the other

_____ 4. related to the sense of hearing

_____ 5. to communicate with an informal, interconnected group of people

_____ 6. repeated and harmful verbal, physical, social, or psychological behavior toward others

_____ 7. a formal, written representation of a person's experience, skills, and credentials

_____ 8. complete attention directed toward a particular object or task

_____ 9. organized activities needed to find a desired job

_____ 10. a formal, written introduction that outlines a person's capabilities and skills to a prospective employer

The Certification Competency Examination

Complete the following sentences.

1. The certification _____ examination is a test that nursing assistants must take and pass to become certified.

2. Each state is responsible for making sure nursing assistant education and training programs meet the Omnibus Budget Reconciliation Act, or _____, standards set by the federal government.

3. Each state has its own minimum _____ at which people can enter a nursing assistant education and training program.

4. Individual _____ determine how nursing assistant certification is granted, which certification competency examination is used, and when and where the exam occurs.

5. Each state has different fees for taking the certification competency _____, requirements for application, exam schedules, and regulations regarding how many times a person can attempt the exam.

6. The length of instruction in a nursing assistant training program ranges from a minimum of _____ hour(s) to more than 150 hours.

7. Requirements for supervised _____ training may be 24 hours or more in long-term care facilities and sometimes hospital and other related experiences.

8. Upon completion of a state-approved nursing assistant education and training program, graduates take the certification competency examination required by the states in which they _____.

9. The certification competency exam tests knowledge in a written or oral exam and skills in a hands-on _____.

10. The written exam may be completed _____ or by hand and consists of 50 or more multiple-choice questions.

11. Information about a state's exam can be found in a handbook on the state's board of nursing website, on the Department of Health and Human Services website, or through the state's exam _____.

12. The skills demonstration portion of the exam requires applicants to perform specified procedures on a(n) _____ in front of a test observer or evaluator.

13. In the skills demonstration, only skills that are _____, not verbalized or explained, count.

14. Generally, the _____ of required skills is provided ahead of time on the day of the exam.

15. Some states provide specific _____ for performing each skill, while other states randomly draw skills to test from the list of skills provided.

16. To become certified as a nursing assistant, a person must meet the exam application requirements, verify completion of a state-approved training program, pay the fees, schedule the exam, and _____ both parts with a state-determined score.

17. Requirements for becoming certified can include photo identification, documentation that shows legal presence in the United States, and a fingerprint _____ check.

18. It is best to take the exam right _____ completing the training program, as the knowledge and skills learned are most current at this time.

19. A nursing assistant candidate should check state _____ regarding test-taking requirements and time lines.

Preparing for the Certification Competency Exam

Identify whether each statement is true or false.

_____ 1. Knowing what to expect is an important part of successfully taking the certification competency exam.

_____ 2. Reviewing the certification competency exam handbook will provide information about what to prepare for and bring on the day of the exam.

_____ 3. To be successful on the certification competency exam, nursing assistant candidates should read their states' handbooks and review the end of each textbook chapter to find a list of topics that might be covered.

_____ 4. The way a person learns best is called his or her *learning style*.

_____ 5. Auditory learners see material to learn it best.

_____ 6. Visual learners prefer to listen to material to learn it best.

_____ 7. Kinesthetic learners feel or experience material to learn it best.

_____ 8. A good study space is quiet, well lit, and devoted to studying.

_____ 9. Setting a realistic daily study schedule that includes study time, breaks, and enjoyable activities can help increase motivation.

_____ 10. The time between the start of studying and the mind wandering is called *complication span* and ranges between 10 and 20 minutes.

_____ 11. People should not study beyond their concentration spans; instead, they should take a break.

_____ 12. Two types of memory are short-term memory and long-term memory.

_____ 13. Long-term memory allows a person to temporarily remember information for a brief period of time.

_____ 14. Short-term memories are formed through rehearsal, repetition, and association with information.

_____ 15. Long-term memory allows a person to readily retrieve information, such as the steps for performing nursing assistant skills.

_____ 16. Asking questions during reading can help improve long-term memory.

_____ 17. To form long-term memories, one should write everything down in notes taken.

_____ 18. Study groups are helpful for practicing skills.

_____ 19. Rewarding study efforts will not help improve long-term memory.

Studying the Nursing Assistant Certification Competency Exam Handbook

In this activity, you will practice skills identified in your state's nursing assistant certification competency exam handbook. To prepare for this activity, find your state's nursing assistant certification competency exam handbook online and print it for yourself. Study the handbook from cover to cover and memorize each skill by writing the number of steps on a blank piece of paper and then filling in the steps until you have memorized them.

Form a group of three and assign each person a role. One person will be the nursing assistant, another a resident, and the third person will serve as the evaluator. Then simulate each of the skills identified in your nursing assistant certification competency exam handbook. Time each simulation using the time limit established by your state and then exchange roles. The evaluator in the group will use the printed handbook to check off steps the nursing assistant completed successfully. If any steps are missed, the evaluator will discuss the omission after the time is complete.

Successful Test-Taking Strategies

Complete the following effective test-taking strategies.

1. Eat a healthy _____ and go to bed early before the exam.

2. Arrive at the exam early and use the _____ before the exam begins.

3. Be familiar with the specific instructions in your state's _____.

4. Make sure you have everything you _____ at hand.

5. _____ closely to verbal directions and read instructions slowly and carefully.

6. Ask for _____ of any instructions you do not understand.

7. Stay _____, and if you feel nervous, take two or three deep breaths to relax yourself.

8. Be _____ and visualize yourself completing the exam successfully.

9. If taking a paper test, quickly scan the _____ to determine how you will spend your time.

10. If taking a(n) _____ test, know how long you have to complete the exam and the number of test items.

11. _____ on your own test and on each question, do not let your mind wander, and don't be concerned if others finish before you do.

12. If possible, answer all of the questions you are sure about _____.

13. If you don't know the answer to a question, _____ it, and if you still cannot answer it, move on and come back to it later.

14. When answering multiple-choice questions, read the _____ question.

15. Think of the answer _____ looking at the options listed for a multiple-choice question.

16. Read all of the answer options and choose the one that most closely _____ your answer.

17. If you are unsure of the answer, _____ any answer options that appear totally wrong.

18. If you are forced to guess, choose the longest, most _____ answer.

19. Don't keep _____ your answer; your first choice is usually the correct answer.

20. If you finish with time left, _____ your answers.

21. Review questions you were not sure of, but only change an answer if you did not correctly _____ the question or misread it.

Finding a Nursing Assistant Position

Identify whether each statement is true or false.

_____ 1. To find a position, new nursing assistants should explore the facilities that most interest them.

_____ 2. Some nursing assistants secure positions in the facility where they completed clinical training.

_____ 3. A job campaign often includes visiting school or college job-placement centers; looking for open position ads in newspapers, online websites, or job boards; and networking.

_____ 4. It is not appropriate for a nursing assistant to talk with the human resources department of a facility.

Obtaining a Nursing Assistant Position

Complete the following sentences.

1. A(n) _____ message precedes a résumé and introduces a candidate's capabilities and skills to a prospective employer.

2. A cover message should specifically greet the person responsible for _____ by name and be to the point.

3. A great _____ quickly grabs the reader's attention, is one page and detailed, and sells the applicant's accomplishments and strengths.

4. _____ are typically furnished upon request, but never without advance permission.

5. A cover message, résumé, and application should always have correct _____, grammar, and sentence structure.

6. An employment candidate should answer all of the questions on a(n) _____, even if they seem repetitive.

7. The purpose of an interview is for the facility to find the right person, but an interview is also an opportunity for the applicant to determine if the position and facility are a good _____.

8. A(n) _____ interview is a screening tool that allows the hiring manager to determine which candidates to meet in person.

9. During a phone or in-person interview, it is important to speak _____ and confidently and answer questions about skills and experience.

10. A candidate should _____ a facility before the interview to know the facility's leadership, mission, and values.

11. For a(n) _____, a candidate should dress in clean, neat business attire; not wear cologne or perfume; remove body jewelry; cover body art; and not chew gum.

12. At the beginning of an interview, a candidate should politely greet the interviewer, offer a firm handshake, establish _____ contact, and smile.

13. During an interview, a candidate should actively _____, be friendly, not slouch, answer questions honestly, and ask questions.

14. At the close of an interview, it is important to emphasize one's _____.

15. After an interview, it is appropriate to send a(n) _____ message to the interviewer.

16. If a job is offered, it should be in _____ with salary, wages, benefits, and other requirements outlined.

17. If unsure about accepting a job offer, a candidate can ask for _____ hour(s) to think it over before accepting.

18. At the start of a new job, a nursing assistant will be oriented to the facility; learn what is expected; and be provided with on-the-job training, a(n) _____ handbook, and guidance from the licensed nursing staff.

Answering Interview Questions

Choose a partner and then review the interview questions listed in Figure 28.12 in the text. Add two other challenging questions of your choice and then perform a mock interview with your partner. Film the interview as you ask your partner the interview questions and answer the questions you are asked. Pay attention to and provide feedback about your partner's verbal and nonverbal communication. Then, review the video of the interview together. Discuss ways you can both improve.

Managing the Work Environment

Complete the following sentences.

1. The probationary period is typically between 60 and 90 _____.

2. When a nursing assistant starts a new position, he or she should pay attention to whether the position is a good _____.

3. Residents in a nursing assistant's care will have needs and demands that can create a great deal of _____.

4. Sometimes stress can lead patients, residents, family members, other healthcare providers, and coworkers to act _____.

5. One example of an aggressive act is _____, or repeated and harmful verbal, physical, social, or psychological behavior.

6. The Occupational Safety and Health Administration (OSHA) reports that incidents of serious workplace _____ that require days off work for the injured worker are four times more common in healthcare than in other industries.

7. To deal with workplace violence, nursing assistants can understand the facility's policy, immediately _____ incidents, recognize warning signs, use effective communication to resolve conflicts, use stress-management techniques, be aware of fatigue, and practice personal security measures.

Resignation and Advancement

Identify whether each statement is true or false.

_____ 1. Before resigning, it is helpful to talk with a supervisor to see if the same position is available in another facility.

_____ 2. If resigning, a nursing assistant should be professional and give at least a two-day notice by providing a letter of resignation devoid of negative comments about the experience.

_____ 3. Nursing assistants cannot advance their careers through further education, training, and experience.

_____ 4. Experience as a nursing assistant may lead to interest in becoming a registered nurse, dietitian, physical therapist, doctor, or other healthcare professional.

_____ 5. There are two stages in career planning for advancement.

_____ 6. In the first stage of career planning, the nursing assistant determines present values, skills, and abilities.

_____ 7. The second stage of career planning is exploration and preparation, in which careers of interest are researched.

_____ 8. The third stage of career planning is commitment to a career.

_____ 9. The final stage of career planning is transformation.

_____ 10. An action plan helps guide a person through all four stages of career planning and aids in identifying goals.

Becoming a Lifelong Learner

Select the *best* answer.

_____ 1. A lifelong learner
   A. does not read books or articles
   B. makes self-improvement a priority
   C. does not feel challenged
   D. does not reflect on his or her practice

_____ 2. Which of the following strategies strengthens lifelong learning?
   A. not being self-aware
   B. avoiding those with similar interests
   C. seeking easy tasks
   D. keeping a bucket list of things to learn

_____ 3. Lifelong learners are
   A. curious
   B. rigid and uncomfortable with change
   C. not creative
   D. reliant on others

_____ 4. Which of the following helps make a lifelong learner?
   A. lack of accountability
   B. education that promotes self-development
   C. lack of innovation
   D. workplaces that devalue lifelong learning

Name: _____ Date: _____

Procedure: Admission to a Healthcare Facility

Preparation

S U Comments

1. Practiced hand hygiene. _____ _____ _____
2. Assembled the necessary equipment. _____ _____ _____
3. Prepared the bed by pulling back linen, lowering the bed, and locking the wheels. _____ _____ _____
4. Ensured the call light is easily accessible. _____ _____ _____

The Procedure

5. Introduced yourself using your name and title. Explained that you worked with the licensed nursing staff and would be providing care. _____ _____ _____
6. Placed an identification bracelet on the patient's wrist if necessary. _____ _____ _____
7. Addressed the patient as Mr., Mrs., or Ms. and the last name. _____ _____ _____
8. Explained the procedure in simple terms. _____ _____ _____
9. Provided privacy to the patient. _____ _____ _____
10. Accessed the appropriate admissions forms. _____ _____ _____
11. Asked the patient any unanswered questions on the admissions forms. _____ _____ _____
12. Made introductions if the patient had a roommate. _____ _____ _____
13. Helped the patient change into a gown or pajamas, if appropriate. _____ _____ _____
14. Helped the patient into bed or a chair. _____ _____ _____
15. Assisted in the patient assessment by measuring vital signs, height, and weight. _____ _____ _____
16. Completed the patient's belongings list, labeled personal items, and placed valuables in the safe. _____ _____ _____
17. Put away the patient's clothing and belongings. _____ _____ _____
18. Orientated the patient to the room:

    A. identified and explained items in the bedside stand _____ _____ _____

    B. explained how to use the overbed table _____ _____ _____

    C. showed the patient how to use the call light, bed controls, TV, and light control _____ _____ _____

    D. explained how to make a telephone call and placed telephone in reach _____ _____ _____

    E. showed the patient the bathroom and instructed him or her on use of the bathroom call light _____ _____ _____
19. Explained the facility's policies and visiting hours, how to identify staff, and important locations in the facility. _____ _____ _____
20. Explained any ordered activity limitations. _____ _____ _____
21. Explained when meals were served and how to request snacks. _____ _____ _____
22. Filled the water pitcher and cup if fluids were allowed. _____ _____ _____
23. Provided a denture cup labeled with the patient's name, room number, and bed number, if dentures were used. _____ _____ _____

Date of Completion: _____ Instructor's Initials: _____

Name: _____   Date: _____

	S	U	Comments
Follow-Up			
24. Practiced hand hygiene.	_____	_____	_____
25. Ensured patient comfort and placed the call light and personal items within reach.	_____	_____	_____
26. Conducted a safety check before leaving the room.	_____	_____	_____
27. Practiced hand hygiene before leaving the room.	_____	_____	_____
Reporting and Documentation			
28. Reported the completion of admission and communicated any concerns to the licensed nursing staff.	_____	_____	_____
29. Documented care provided in the chart or EMR.	_____	_____	_____

Date of Completion: _____   Instructor's Initials: _____

Name: _____ Date: _____

Procedure: Transfer Within or to Another Facility

Preparation

		S	U	Comments
1.	Consulted the licensed nursing staff or plan of care for special instructions and precautions.			
2.	Obtained the transfer forms.			
3.	Practiced hand hygiene before entering the room.			
4.	Knocked before entering the room.			
5.	Introduced yourself using your name and title. Explained that you worked with the licensed nursing staff and would be providing care.			
6.	Greeted the patient and confirmed the patient's identification.			
7.	Addressed the patient as Mr., Mrs., or Ms. and the last name.			
8.	Explained the procedure in simple terms and asked permission to perform the procedure.			

The Procedure

		S	U	Comments
9.	Provided privacy to the patient.			
10.	Assisted in moving or packing belongings.			
11.	Safely transferred the patient from the bed to a wheelchair, if needed.			
12.	Assisted the patient in changing clothing.			
13.	Transferred the patient's chart to the new unit or transport vehicle.			
14.	Monitored the patient's vital signs during transfer.			
15.	Ensured safety during the transfer process.			
16.	If transferring within the same facility:			
	A. alerted the destination unit's charge nurse that the patient arrived			
	B. ensured patient comfort in the new room			
17.	If transferring to a new facility:			
	A. ensured the patient moved safely into the transport vehicle			

Follow-Up

		S	U	Comments
18.	Practiced hand hygiene.			

Reporting and Documentation

		S	U	Comments
19.	Reported completion of the transfer to the licensed nursing staff.			
20.	Communicated any concerns to the licensed nursing staff.			

Date of Completion: _____ Instructor's Initials: _____

Procedure: Discharge from a Healthcare Facility

	S	U	Comments
Preparation			
1. Consulted the licensed nursing staff or plan of care for special instructions and precautions.	_____	_____	_____
2. Obtained discharge forms.	_____	_____	_____
3. Practiced hand hygiene before entering the room.	_____	_____	_____
4. Knocked before entering the room.	_____	_____	_____
5. Introduced yourself using your name and title. Explained that you worked with the licensed nursing staff and would be providing care.	_____	_____	_____
6. Greeted the patient and confirmed the patient's identification.	_____	_____	_____
7. Addressed the patient as Mr., Mrs., or Ms. and the last name.	_____	_____	_____
8. Explained the procedure in simple terms.	_____	_____	_____
The Procedure			
9. Provided privacy to the patient.	_____	_____	_____
10. Helped the patient get dressed and packed.	_____	_____	_____
11. Returned any valuables from the facility's safe.	_____	_____	_____
12. Checked the belongings against the list created during admission.	_____	_____	_____
13. Observed and reported any issues regarding the patient's ADLs and concerns.	_____	_____	_____
14. Notified licensed nursing staff that patient was ready for discharge instructions.	_____	_____	_____
15. Helped escort the patient in a wheelchair to the transport vehicle.	_____	_____	_____
16. Locked the wheelchair and assisted the patient into the transport vehicle.	_____	_____	_____
17. Helped move the patient's belongings into the transport vehicle.	_____	_____	_____
Follow-Up			
18. Returned the wheelchair and cart to storage.	_____	_____	_____
19. Put on disposable gloves.	_____	_____	_____
20. Prepared the room for a new occupant:			
A. stripped the bedding and cleaned the room	_____	_____	_____
B. disposed of dirty linen	_____	_____	_____
C. made the bed using clean linen	_____	_____	_____
21. Practiced hand hygiene.	_____	_____	_____
Reporting and Documentation			
22. Reported the completion of the discharge to the licensed nursing staff.	_____	_____	_____
23. Documented care provided in the chart or EMR.	_____	_____	_____

Date of Completion: _____ Instructor's Initials: _____

Procedure: Hand Washing ▶️ Video

Preparation	S	U	Comments
1. Located a nearby sink.			
2. Pushed up long sleeves using a paper towel.	_____	_____	_____
3. Removed any watches or rings, or pushed up a watch using a paper towel.	_____	_____	_____

The Procedure

	S	U	Comments
4. Turned on the faucet using a paper towel.	_____	_____	_____
5. Thoroughly wet your hands, wrists, and 1–2 inches of skin above your wrists.	_____	_____	_____
6. Applied soap and worked it into a thick lather.	_____	_____	_____
7. Rubbed palms together in a circular, counterclockwise motion.	_____	_____	_____
8. Pushed the fingers of the right hand between the fingers of the left hand and rubbed up and down.	_____	_____	_____
9. Pushed the fingers of the left hand between the fingers of the right hand and rubbed up and down.	_____	_____	_____
10. Rubbed palms together with the fingers interlaced.	_____	_____	_____
11. Interlocked fingers and rubbed side to side.	_____	_____	_____
12. Held the left thumb in the palm of the right hand and rubbed in a circular, counterclockwise motion.	_____	_____	_____
13. Held the right thumb in the palm of the left hand and rubbed in a circular, counterclockwise motion.	_____	_____	_____
14. Held the fingers of the right hand in the middle of the left palm and rubbed in a circular, counterclockwise motion.	_____	_____	_____
15. Held the fingers of the left hand in the middle of the right palm and rubbed in a circular, counterclockwise motion.	_____	_____	_____
16. Washed your hands for a minimum of 20 seconds.	_____	_____	_____
17. Rinsed your hands thoroughly, fingers pointing downward.	_____	_____	_____
18. Dried your hands using a paper towel. Avoided touching the dispenser or shaking water from your hands.	_____	_____	_____
19. Discarded the paper towel in the waste container.	_____	_____	_____

Follow-Up

	S	U	Comments
20. Turned off the faucet using a paper towel.	_____	_____	_____
21. Discarded the paper towel in the waste container.	_____	_____	_____

Date of Completion: _____ Instructor's Initials:_____

Name: _____   Date: _____

Procedure: Using Hand Sanitizer

	S	U	Comments

Preparation

1. Located hand sanitizer dispenser. _____ _____ _____
2. Pushed up long sleeves using a paper towel. _____ _____ _____
3. Removed any watches or rings, or pushed up a watch using a paper towel. _____ _____ _____

The Procedure

4. Used enough hand sanitizer to cover all surfaces of the palms and fingers. _____ _____ _____
5. Rubbed your hands together in a circular, counterclockwise motion. _____ _____ _____
6. Pushed the fingers of the right hand between the fingers of the left hand and rubbed up and down. _____ _____ _____
7. Pushed the fingers of the left hand between the fingers of the right hand and rubbed up and down. _____ _____ _____
8. Rubbed palms together with fingers interlaced. _____ _____ _____
9. With bent, interlocked fingers, rubbed your palms together. _____ _____ _____
10. Held the left thumb in the palm of the right hand and rubbed in a circular, counterclockwise motion. _____ _____ _____
11. Held the right thumb in the palm of the left hand and rubbed in a circular, counterclockwise motion. _____ _____ _____
12. Held the fingers of the right hand together in the middle of the left palm and rubbed in a circular, counterclockwise motion. _____ _____ _____
13. Held the fingers of the left hand together in the middle of the right palm and rubbed in a circular, counterclockwise motion. _____ _____ _____
14. Rubbed hands together for 20 seconds. _____ _____ _____

Follow-Up

15. Completed the procedure when the hands felt dry. _____ _____ _____

Date of Completion: _____   Instructor's Initials: _____

Name: _____ Date: _____

	S	U	Comments

Preparation

1. Identified gloves of the correct size.

2. Inspected the gloves for cracks, holes, tears, or discoloration.

The Procedure: Putting on Disposable Gloves

3. Practiced hand hygiene.

4. Waited until hands were dry before putting on gloves.

5. Picked up the first glove by its cuff.

6. Pulled the first glove onto your hand.

7. Picked up the second glove by its cuff.

8. Pulled the second glove onto your hand.

9. Interlaced your fingers to adjust the gloves on your hands.

The Procedure: Removing Disposable Gloves

10. Grasped the gloved hand just below the cuff of the glove.

11. Pulled the cuff of the glove down, drawing it over your hand and turning it inside out.

12. Pulled the glove off your hand and held it in the palm of the other hand.

13. Inserted the fingers of the ungloved hand under the cuff of the glove remaining on the other hand.

14. Slowly pulled the glove off, turning it inside out and drawing it over the first glove.

15. Discarded both gloves in the waste container.

Follow-Up

16. Practiced hand hygiene.

Date of Completion: _____ Instructor's Initials: _____

Procedure: Putting On and Removing Gowns ▶ Video

Preparation	S	U	Comments
1. Selected the appropriate gown.	_____	_____	_____
2. Removed any jewelry or watches.	_____	_____	_____
3. Rolled long sleeves up over the elbows.	_____	_____	_____

The Procedure: Putting On a Gown

	S	U	Comments
4. Practiced hand hygiene.	_____	_____	_____
5. Held the gown by the shoulders out in front of you with the back of the gown facing you.	_____	_____	_____
6. Unfolded the gown carefully, without shaking.	_____	_____	_____
7. Slid your hands and arms in each of the gown sleeves.	_____	_____	_____
8. Pulled the top of the gown around your neck to cover your scrubs.	_____	_____	_____
9. Tied the neck ties using a simple shoelace bow.	_____	_____	_____
10. Reached behind the gown and pulled the edges so they overlap, completely covering your clothing.	_____	_____	_____
11. Tied the waist ties in the back using a simple shoelace bow.	_____	_____	_____
12. Put on disposable gloves and pulled the glove cuffs over the sleeves of the gown.	_____	_____	_____

The Procedure: Removing a Gown

	S	U	Comments
13. Removed and discarded your gloves before removing your gown.	_____	_____	_____
14. Reached behind the gown and untied the neck and waist ties.	_____	_____	_____
15. Slid your hands inside the sleeves of the gown. Used one hand to hold the cuff of the opposite sleeve and pulled your arm out of that sleeve.	_____	_____	_____
16. Pulled the opposite arm out of the sleeve and the gown down off of your shoulders.	_____	_____	_____
17. Avoided touching the outside of the gown.	_____	_____	_____
18. Turned the gown inside out as you removed it.	_____	_____	_____
19. Held the gown away from your clothing.	_____	_____	_____
20. Rolled the gown so the contaminated outside faces inward toward the gown.	_____	_____	_____
21. Disposed of the gown in the appropriate container.	_____	_____	_____

Follow-Up

	S	U	Comments
22. Practiced hand hygiene.	_____	_____	_____

Date of Completion: _____   Instructor's Initials: _____

Procedure: Wearing Face Protection

Preparation	S	U	Comments
1. Assembled the necessary equipment.			
2. Practiced hand hygiene.	____	____	_____

The Procedure: Putting On a Mask or Respirator

	S	U	Comments
3. Picked up the mask or respirator by the ties or elastic band.	____	____	_____
4. Placed the mask or respirator over your nose, face, and chin.	____	____	_____
5. Secured the ties or elastic bands behind your head and neck.	____	____	_____
6. Avoided touching the portion of the mask or respirator that would cover your face.	____	____	_____
7. Adjusted the mask or respirator over your nose, mouth, and chin by pinching the portion covering the bridge of the nose.	____	____	_____
8. Ensured the mask or respirator fits properly and is sealed tightly.	____	____	_____
9. Replaced the mask or respirator if it became moist, contaminated, or damaged.	____	____	_____
10. Avoided letting the mask or respirator hang around your neck when not in use.	____	____	_____

The Procedure: Removing a Mask or Respirator

	S	U	Comments
11. Removed and discarded your gloves.	____	____	_____
12. Practiced hand hygiene before removing the mask or respirator.	____	____	_____
13. Untied the bottom ties of the mask or respirator before untying the top ties.	____	____	_____
14. Held the mask or respirator by the ties and pulled it away from your face.	____	____	_____
15. Disposed of the contaminated mask or respirator.	____	____	_____

The Procedure: Putting On Goggles or a Face Shield

	S	U	Comments
16. Placed the goggles or face shield on face and eyes.	____	____	_____
17. Replaced goggles or face shield if it became moist, contaminated, or damaged.	____	____	_____
18. Avoided letting the goggles or face shield dangle around your neck when not in use.	____	____	_____

The Procedure: Removing Goggles or a Face Shield

	S	U	Comments
19. Removed and discarded your gloves.	____	____	_____
20. Practiced hand hygiene.	____	____	_____
21. Removed goggles or face shield by grasping earpiece with both hands and lifting away from your face.	____	____	_____
22. Discarded the goggles or face shield.	____	____	_____

Follow-Up

	S	U	Comments
24. Practiced hand hygiene.	____	____	_____

Date of Completion: _____   Instructor's Initials:_____

Name: _____ Date: _____

Procedure: Double-Bagging

	S	U	Comments

Preparation

1. Assembled the necessary equipment.

The Procedure: Inside the Isolation Room

2. Wore disposable gloves and other appropriate PPE.

3. Stood in room by the doorway with bag of waste, making sure the biohazard bag was closed tightly.

4. Waited until the staff member outside the room folded a clean biohazard bag into a cuff.

5. Placed contaminated bag inside clean bag.

The Procedure: Outside the Isolation Room

6. Wore disposable gloves.

7. Stood outside doorway with a clean biohazard waste bag.

8. Folded a clean biohazard waste bag into a cuff.

9. Held the clean bag open wide while staff member inside the room placed the contaminated bag into the clean bag.

10. Tied the clean waste bag.

11. Took the biohazard waste bag to the appropriate department for disposal, disinfection, or sterilization.

Follow-Up: Inside the Isolation Room

12. Removed PPE before leaving the room.

13. Practiced hand hygiene.

Follow-Up: Outside the Isolation Room

14. Removed and discarded your gloves.

15. Practiced hand hygiene.

Date of Completion: _____ Instructor's Initials: _____

Name: _____ Date: _____

Procedure: Cleaning a Room After Discharge

	S	U	Comments
Preparation			
1. Assembled the necessary equipment.	___	___	_____
The Procedure			
2. Put on disposable gloves.			
3. Placed all disposable materials in plastic bags and discarded.	___	___	_____
4. Bagged, labeled, and made a list of any personal items that were left behind.	___	___	_____
5. Removed, cleaned, disinfected, and sterilized all items from the bedside stand.	___	___	_____
6. Removed all linens from the room and placed in appropriate laundry container.	___	___	_____
7. Washed any special equipment with a disinfectant solution and returned to proper storage location.	___	___	_____
8. Washed the following items with a disinfectant solution:	___	___	_____
A. plastic mattress and pillow covers	___	___	_____
B. bed frame	___	___	_____
C. bedside table and stand	___	___	_____
D. bedside chair	___	___	_____
10. Cleaned the light fixture, call light, telephone, and windows.	___	___	_____
11. Removed and discarded your gloves.	___	___	_____
12. Practiced hand hygiene.	___	___	_____
13. Restocked room with necessary supplies.	___	___	_____
14. Made bed.	___	___	_____
15. Checked that call light, light fixture, and telephone were in working order.	___	___	_____
16. Placed a new bag liner in the waste container.	___	___	_____
17. Checked bed's side rails.	___	___	_____
Follow-Up			
18. Returned cleaning supplies to storage.	___	___	_____
19. Practiced hand hygiene.	___	___	_____
Reporting and Documentation			
20. Alerted appropriate staff that room is ready for admission.	___	___	_____

Date of Completion: _____ Instructor's Initials: _____

Procedure: Transporting to and from Isolation

Preparation	S	U	Comments
1. Consulted the licensed nursing staff or plan of care for special instructions and precautions.			
2. Notified the department that will receive the patient.	_____	_____	_____
3. Practiced hand hygiene.	_____	_____	_____
4. Put on required PPE.	_____	_____	_____
5. Knocked before entering the room.	_____	_____	_____
6. Introduced yourself using your name and title. Explained that you worked with the licensed nursing staff and would be providing care.	_____	_____	_____
7. Greeted the patient and confirmed the patient's identification.	_____	_____	_____
8. Addressed the patient as Mr., Mrs., or Ms. and the last name.	_____	_____	_____
9. Explained the procedure in simple terms and asked permission to perform the procedure.	_____	_____	_____
10. Assembled the necessary equipment.	_____	_____	_____
11. Asked for assistance from a coworker.	_____	_____	_____
12. Covered the stretcher or wheelchair with a clean sheet.	_____	_____	_____

The Procedure	S	U	Comments
13. Provided privacy to the patient.	_____	_____	_____
14. Raised or lowered the bed to the appropriate position for the transport vehicle.	_____	_____	_____
15. Locked the wheels on both the bed and the transport vehicle.	_____	_____	_____
16. Raised and secured the side rails on the opposite side of the bed from where you would be working.	_____	_____	_____
17. Put a mask on the patient, if instructed.	_____	_____	_____
18. Helped the patient onto the transport vehicle.	_____	_____	_____
19. Wrapped or covered the patient with a sheet or bath blanket.	_____	_____	_____
20. Removed PPE and practiced hand hygiene, if appropriate.	_____	_____	_____
21. Moved the patient out of the isolation unit.	_____	_____	_____
22. Placed the transport vehicle holding the patient near the door of the room and put on PPE before entering, if returning patient to isolation.	_____	_____	_____
23. Unwrapped the patient and removed his or her mask after entering the room.	_____	_____	_____
24. Discarded the mask in the biohazard waste container.	_____	_____	_____
25. Assisted the patient from the transport vehicle to the bed.	_____	_____	_____
26. Checked that the bed wheels were locked.	_____	_____	_____
27. Repositioned the patient, lowered the bed, and raised or lowered side rails according to the plan of care.	_____	_____	_____
28. Removed, cleaned, and stored equipment properly.	_____	_____	_____
29. Removed soiled linens and discarded disposable equipment.	_____	_____	_____

Date of Completion: _____ Instructor's Initials:_____

Name: _____   Date: _____

Follow-Up

		S	U	Comments

Follow-Up

30. Ensured patient comfort and placed the call light and personal items within reach.

31. Conducted a safety check before leaving the room.   _____ _____ _____

32. Removed your PPE before leaving the room.   _____ _____ _____

33. Practiced hand hygiene.

34. Removed and stored the transport vehicle.   _____ _____ _____

Reporting and Documentation

35. Communicated any concerns to the licensed nursing staff.   _____ _____ _____

36. Documented care provided in the chart or EMR.   _____ _____ _____

Date of Completion: _____   Instructor's Initials: _____

Name: _____   Date: _____

Procedure: Assisting with Nonsterile Dressing Changes

	S	U	Comments

Preparation

1. Consulted the licensed nursing staff or plan of care for special instructions and precautions.
2. Practiced hand hygiene.
3. Knocked before entering the room.
4. Introduced yourself using your name and title. Explained that you worked with the licensed nursing staff and would be providing care.
5. Greeted the patient and confirmed the patient's identification.
6. Addressed the patient as Mr., Mrs., or Ms. and the last name.
7. Explained the procedure in simple terms and asked permission to perform the procedure.
8. Assembled the necessary equipment.

The Procedure

9. Provided privacy to the patient.
10. Raised the bed to hip height and locked the wheels.
11. Raised and secured side rails on the opposite side of the bed from where you would be working.
12. Assisted the patient into a comfortable position.
13. Placed a bath blanket over the top linens and fanfolded the linens underneath to prevent patient exposure.
14. Placed the waterproof drape around the exposed affected area.
15. Made a cuff at the top of the plastic bag and placed it within reach.
16. Practiced hand hygiene.
17. Put on disposable gloves and PPE, as required.
18. Removed tape or Montgomery straps to expose existing dressing.
19. Wet a 4x4 dressing with tape-adhesive remover and cleaned around the tape, wiping away from the dressing.
20. Removed each layer of the existing dressing and placed it in the plastic bag.
21. Removed the dressing covering the wound and placed it in the plastic bag.
22. Observed the wound, wound drainage, and wound site.
23. Removed and discarded your gloves.
24. Practiced hand hygiene.
25. Put on a new pair of disposable gloves.
26. Opened new dressings and cut the length of tape needed.
27. Cleaned wound by stroking outward and placed soiled gauze in the plastic bag.
28. Applied clean dressings.
29. Secured the dressings using tape or Montgomery straps.
30. Removed and discarded your gloves.
31. Practiced hand hygiene.
32. Put on a new pair of disposable gloves.

Date of Completion: _____   Instructor's Initials:_____

	S	U	Comments

33. Covered the patient with top linens and removed the bath blanket by rolling it with the patient side facing inward.

34. Discarded used supplies in the plastic bag.

35. Removed and discarded your gloves.

36. Practiced hand hygiene.

37. Put on a new pair of disposable gloves.

38. Checked that the bed wheels were locked.

39. Repositioned the patient, lowered the bed, and raised or lowered side rails according to the plan of care.

40. Removed, cleaned, and stored equipment properly.

41. Removed soiled linens and discarded disposable equipment.

Follow-Up

42. Removed and discarded your gloves.

43. Practiced hand hygiene.

44. Ensured patient comfort and placed the call light and personal items within reach.

45. Conducted a safety check before leaving the room.

46. Practiced hand hygiene.

Reporting and Documentation

47. Communicated any concerns to the licensed nursing staff.

48. Documented care provided in the chart or EMR.

Date of Completion: _____   Instructor's Initials: _____

Procedure: Putting On and Removing Sterile Gloves

	S	U	Comments
Preparation			
1. Located a package of sterile gloves in the correct size.	_____	_____	_____
2. Arranged the area and ensured enough room to maintain the sterile field.	_____	_____	_____
3. Prepared the work surface at waist level.	_____	_____	_____
4. Cleaned and dried the work surface.	_____	_____	_____
5. Practiced hand hygiene.	_____	_____	_____
The Procedure: Putting On Sterile Gloves			
6. Opened the outer packaging of the gloves.	_____	_____	_____
7. Removed the inner package and read the manufacturer's instructions.	_____	_____	_____
8. Arranged the inner package on the work surface so that the left and right gloves are on their respective sides, the cuffs of the gloves lie near you, and the fingers of the gloves point away.	_____	_____	_____
9. Folded back the inner package using the thumb and index finger of each hand.	_____	_____	_____
10. Picked up glove by its cuff using your thumb, index finger, and middle finger.	_____	_____	_____
11. Put glove on dominant hand first.	_____	_____	_____
12. Reached under the cuff of the second glove using the four fingers of your gloved hand.	_____	_____	_____
13. Put on the second glove with your fingers still under the cuff.	_____	_____	_____
14. Adjusted each glove for comfort with the opposite hand.	_____	_____	_____
15. Slid your fingers under the cuffs to pull them up.	_____	_____	_____
16. Only touched sterile items while wearing sterile gloves.	_____	_____	_____
The Procedure: Removing Sterile Gloves			
17. Grasped one gloved hand just below the cuff with the fingers of the opposite hand.	_____	_____	_____
18. Pulled cuff of the glove down over your hand and turned it inside out.	_____	_____	_____
19. Pulled glove off of your hand and held it in the palm of the gloved hand.	_____	_____	_____
20. Inserted ungloved fingers under the cuff of the remaining glove, slowly pulling it off and drawing it over the first glove.	_____	_____	_____
21. Disposed of both gloves in the appropriate waste container.	_____	_____	_____
Follow-Up			
22. Practiced hand hygiene.	_____	_____	_____

Date of Completion: _____ Instructor's Initials: _____

Name: _____ Date: _____

Procedure: Positioning in Bed

Preparation

		S	U	Comments

Preparation

1. Consulted the licensed nursing staff or plan of care for special instructions and precautions.
2. Asked for assistance from a coworker.
3. Practiced hand hygiene.
4. Knocked before entering the room.
5. Introduced yourself using your name and title. Explained that you worked with the licensed nursing staff and would be providing care.
6. Greeted the patient and confirmed the patient's identification.
7. Addressed the patient as Mr., Mrs., or Ms. and the last name.
8. Explained the procedure in simple terms and asked permission to perform the procedure.
9. Assembled the necessary equipment.

The Procedure

10. Provided privacy to the patient.
11. Raised the bed to hip height and locked the wheels.
12. Raised and secured side rails on the opposite side of the bed from where you would be working.
13. Asked the patient about personal comfort preferences, if appropriate.
14. Checked that all tubing was not dislodged or kinked.
15. Placed pillows under the head and against the headboard for safety.
16. Grasped each side of the draw sheet and slid the patient up in the bed in unison with a coworker, if the patient was immobile.
17. Put one arm under a mobile patient's shoulders and the other under the patient's hips.
18. Asked the patient to bend his or her knees and push toward the foot of the bed with his or her hands and feet.
19. Slid the patient while still supporting his or her shoulders and hips.
20. Used proper body mechanics.
21. Supported the appropriate body areas with pillows, rolled towels, trochanter rolls, or blankets.
22. Supported the knees and calves before raising the patient's ankles.
23. Supported flexed knees and feet, if appropriate.
24. Properly aligned the patient's body and straightened the bed linens.
25. Raised the head of the bed, locked the bed wheels, lowered the bed, and raised or lowered side rails according to the plan of care.
26. Rechecked all tubing for security and placement.
27. Removed, cleaned, and stored equipment properly.
28. Removed soiled linens and discarded disposable equipment.

Date of Completion: _____ Instructor's Initials: _____

Follow-Up	S	U	Comments
29. Practiced hand hygiene.	_____	_____	_____
30. Ensured patient comfort and placed the call light and personal items within reach.	_____	_____	_____
31. Conducted a safety check before leaving the room.	_____	_____	_____
32. Practiced hand hygiene.	_____	_____	_____

Reporting and Documentation

	S	U	Comments
33. Communicated any concerns to the licensed nursing staff.	_____	_____	_____
34. Documented care provided in the chart or EMR.	_____	_____	_____

Date of Completion: _____ Instructor's Initials:_____

Procedure: Turning a Patient in Bed ▶ Video

Preparation

	S	U	Comments
1. Consulted the licensed nursing staff or plan of care for special instructions and precautions.	___	___	_____
2. Asked for assistance from a coworker.	___	___	_____
3. Practiced hand hygiene.	___	___	_____
4. Knocked before entering the room.	___	___	_____
5. Introduced yourself using your name and title. Explained that you worked with the licensed nursing staff and would be providing care.	___	___	_____
6. Greeted the patient and confirmed the patient's identification.	___	___	_____
7. Addressed the patient as Mr., Mrs., or Ms. and the last name.	___	___	_____
8. Explained the procedure in simple terms and asked permission to perform the procedure.	___	___	_____
9. Assembled the necessary equipment.	___	___	_____

The Procedure

	S	U	Comments
10. Provided privacy to the patient.	___	___	_____
11. Asked patient about any concerns.	___	___	_____
12. Raised the bed to hip height and locked the wheels.	___	___	_____
13. Raised and secured side rails on the opposite side of the bed from where you would be working.	___	___	_____
14. Checked that all tubing was not dislodged or kinked.	___	___	_____
15. Placed pillow against the headboard for safety.	___	___	_____
16. Untucked farthest side of draw sheet or placed a draw sheet below the patient's hips and shoulders.	___	___	_____
17. Asked patient to bend the knees.	___	___	_____
18. Crossed patient's arms over the chest and crossed the patient's legs.	___	___	_____
19. Supported the shoulders and hip while rolling the patient.	___	___	_____
20. Positioned the patient comfortably, using pillows for support and proper alignment.	___	___	_____
21. Locked the bed wheels, lowered the bed, and raised or lowered side rails according to the plan of care.	___	___	_____
22. Rechecked all tubing for security and placement.	___	___	_____
23. Removed, cleaned, and stored equipment properly.	___	___	_____
24. Removed soiled linens and discarded disposable equipment.	___	___	_____

Follow-Up

	S	U	Comments
25. Practiced hand hygiene.	___	___	_____
26. Ensured patient comfort and placed the call light and personal items within reach.	___	___	_____
27. Conducted a safety check before leaving the room.	___	___	_____
28. Practiced hand hygiene.	___	___	_____

Reporting and Documentation

	S	U	Comments
29. Communicated any concerns to the licensed nursing staff.	___	___	_____
30. Documented care provided in the chart or EMR.	___	___	_____

Date of Completion: _____ Instructor's Initials: _____

Name: _____   Date: _____

Procedure: Logrolling

	S	U	Comments

Preparation

1. Consulted the licensed nursing staff or plan of care for special instructions and precautions.
2. Asked for assistance from a coworker.
3. Practiced hand hygiene.
4. Knocked before entering the room.
5. Introduced yourself using your name and title. Explained that you worked with the licensed nursing staff and would be providing care.
6. Greeted the patient and confirmed the patient's identification.
7. Addressed the patient as Mr., Mrs., or Ms. and the last name.
8. Explained the procedure in simple terms and asked permission to perform the procedure.
9. Assembled the necessary equipment.

The Procedure

10. Provided privacy to the patient.
11. Raised the bed to hip height and locked the wheels.
12. Raised and secured side rails on the opposite side of the bed from where you would be working.
13. Checked that all tubing was not dislodged or kinked.
14. Checked that the bed was flat and the patient was in the supine position with no pillow beneath the head.
15. Stood with one leg in front of the other with knees slightly bent while moving the patient's entire body to the side of the bed nearest you.
16. Crossed the patient's arms across the chest and placed a pillow lengthwise between the legs.
17. Raised the side rail on the side of the bed where you worked before moving to the opposite side and lowering the opposite side rail.
18. Stood near the patient's shoulders and chest with a coworker standing near the patient's hips and thighs.
19. Stood with feet apart and one foot in front of the other while you and your coworker rolled the patient toward you in a single movement.
20. Kept the patient's head, spine, and legs aligned during rolling.
21. Repositioned the pillow under the patient's head and positioned the patient to maintain good alignment, using additional pillows as instructed.
22. Straightened the patient's bed linens, clothing, and tubing.
23. Locked the bed wheels, lowered the bed, and raised or lowered side rails according to the plan of care.
24. Straightened the patient's bed linens and clothing and rechecked tubing.
25. Placed soiled linens in appropriate hamper.

Date of Completion: _____   Instructor's Initials: _____

Follow-Up	**S**	**U**	**Comments**
26. Practiced hand hygiene.			
27. Ensured patient comfort and placed the call light and personal items within reach.	_____	_____	_____
28. Conducted a safety check before leaving the room.	_____	_____	_____
29. Practiced hand hygiene.	_____	_____	_____
Reporting and Documentation	_____	_____	_____
30. Communicated any concerns to the licensed nursing staff.			
31. Documented care provided in the chart or EMR.	_____	_____	_____
	_____	_____	_____

Date of Completion: _____   Instructor's Initials:_____

Name: _____ Date: _____

Procedure: Dangling at the Edge of the Bed

	S	U	Comments
Preparation			
1. Consulted the licensed nursing staff or plan of care for special instructions and precautions.	____	____	_____
2. Practiced hand hygiene.	____	____	_____
3. Knocked before entering the room.	____	____	_____
4. Introduced yourself using your name and title. Explained that you worked with the licensed nursing staff and would be providing care.	____	____	_____
5. Greeted the patient and confirmed the patient's identification.	____	____	_____
6. Addressed the patient as Mr., Mrs., or Ms. and the last name.	____	____	_____
7. Explained the procedure in simple terms and asked permission to perform the procedure.	____	____	_____
8. Cleared the area of obstacles and placed the patient's robe and shoes nearby.	____	____	_____
The Procedure			
9. Provided privacy to the patient.	____	____	_____
10. Raised the bed to hip height and locked the wheels.	____	____	_____
11. Raised and secured side rails on the opposite side of the bed from where you would be working.	____	____	_____
12. Fanfolded the linens to the foot of the bed.	____	____	_____
13. Asked the patient to move to the edge of the bed and raised the head of the bed slowly so the patient was in a sitting position.	____	____	_____
14. Stood facing the patient at the bedside with your feet apart and knees slightly bent.	____	____	_____
15. Slipped one arm under the patient's shoulders and the other arm under the knees.	____	____	_____
16. Slid the patient's legs over the side of the bed and moved the shoulders upward in a single, pivoting movement.	____	____	_____
17. Instructed the patient to hold onto the bed for support, and blocked from falling forward.	____	____	_____
18. Provided support and did not leave the patient.	____	____	_____
19. Observed the patient for dizziness, lightheadedness, change in pulse, difficult respirations, and cyanosis.	____	____	_____
20. Made sure the patient was stable and felt well enough to get out of bed if doing so.	____	____	_____
21. Reversed this procedure to return the patient to a lying position.	____	____	_____
22. Positioned the patient using proper body alignment.	____	____	_____
Follow-Up			
23. Practiced hand hygiene.	____	____	_____
24. Ensured patient comfort and placed the call light and personal items within reach.	____	____	_____
25. Conducted a safety check before leaving the room.	____	____	_____
26. Practiced hand hygiene.	____	____	_____
Reporting and Documentation			
27. Communicated any concerns to the licensed nursing staff.	____	____	_____
28. Documented care provided in the chart or EMR.	____	____	_____

Date of Completion: _____   Instructor's Initials: _____

Procedure: Transferring from a Bed to a Chair or Wheelchair ▶ Video

Preparation

		S	U	Comments
1.	Consulted the licensed nursing staff or plan of care for special instructions and precautions.	_____	_____	_____
2.	Practiced hand hygiene.	_____	_____	_____
3.	Knocked before entering the room.	_____	_____	_____
4.	Introduced yourself using your name and title. Explained that you worked with the licensed nursing staff and would be providing care.	_____	_____	_____
5.	Greeted the patient and confirmed the patient's identification.	_____	_____	_____
6.	Addressed the patient as Mr., Mrs., or Ms. and the last name.	_____	_____	_____
7.	Explained the procedure in simple terms and asked permission to perform the procedure.	_____	_____	_____
8.	Assembled the necessary equipment.	_____	_____	_____

The Procedure

		S	U	Comments
9.	Provided privacy to the patient.	_____	_____	_____
10.	Raised the bed to hip height and locked the wheels.	_____	_____	_____
11.	Raised and secured side rails on the opposite side of the bed from where you would be working.	_____	_____	_____
12.	Positioned the chair or wheelchair next to the bed so that the patient could transfer using the stronger side.	_____	_____	_____
13.	Stabilized the chair for safety, locking the wheels and raising the footboards of the wheelchair if using one.	_____	_____	_____
14.	Assisted the patient into a dangling position and applied a gait belt around the waist.	_____	_____	_____
15.	Checked that the gait belt was snug but that there was still enough room to place your fingers under it.	_____	_____	_____
16.	Stood with one foot between and one outside of the patient's feet, with enough room to pivot your feet toward the chair.	_____	_____	_____
17.	Faced the patient and held the gait belt with an underhand grip.	_____	_____	_____
18.	Instructed the patient to hold onto your shoulders or arms.	_____	_____	_____
19.	Used the gait belt to assist the patient into a standing position using your arm and leg muscles and without twisting your body.	_____	_____	_____
20.	Held the gait belt while the patient gained balance.	_____	_____	_____
21.	Led the patient toward the chair or wheelchair slowly.	_____	_____	_____
22.	Ensured the patient felt the chair or wheelchair on the back of the legs and instructed the patient to place both hands on the armrests.	_____	_____	_____
23.	Assisted the patient into a seated position using proper body mechanics.	_____	_____	_____
24.	Positioned the patient in the chair or wheelchair with proper back, buttocks, feet, and leg support.	_____	_____	_____
25.	Arranged the patient's robe and clothing and covered the patient's legs with a bath blanket.	_____	_____	_____
26.	Observed for signs of discomfort or dizziness.	_____	_____	_____
27.	Pushed wheelchair from behind and pulled it into the elevator backward if transporting.	_____	_____	_____

Date of Completion: _____ Instructor's Initials: _____

Follow-Up	**S**	**U**	**Comments**
28. Ensured patient comfort and placed the call light and personal items within reach.	_____	_____	_____
29. Conducted a safety check before leaving the room.	_____	_____	_____
30. Practiced hand hygiene.	_____	_____	_____

Reporting and Documentation

	S	**U**	**Comments**
31. Communicated any concerns to the licensed nursing staff.	_____	_____	_____
32. Documented care provided in the chart or EMR.	_____	_____	_____

Date of Completion: _____ Instructor's Initials:_____

Name: _____ Date: _____

Procedure: Transferring to a Chair or Wheelchair Using a Lift

	S	U	Comments

Preparation

1. Consulted the licensed nursing staff or plan of care for special instructions and precautions.
2. Asked for assistance from a coworker.
3. Practiced hand hygiene.
4. Knocked before entering the room.
5. Introduced yourself using your name and title. Explained that you worked with the licensed nursing staff and would be providing care.
6. Greeted the patient and confirmed the patient's identification.
7. Addressed the patient as Mr., Mrs., or Ms. and the last name.
8. Explained the procedure in simple terms and asked permission to perform the procedure.
9. Assembled the necessary equipment.

The Procedure

10. Provided privacy to the patient.
11. Positioned the chair or wheelchair next to the bed and stabilized for safety, locking the wheels and raising the footboards of the wheelchair if using one.
12. Raised and secured side rails on the opposite side of the bed from where you would be working.
13. Rolled the patient toward you and positioned the sling under the patient, with the lower part resting behind the knees and the upper part beneath the upper shoulders.
14. Positioned the lift bar and frame over the bed in an open position and locked the wheels.
15. Attached the sling to the lift, making sure the open ends of the lift's hooks faced away from the patient.
16. Asked the patient to fold both arms across the chest.
17. Moved the patient away from the bed once the lift held the patient freely and stably.
18. Positioned the patient above the chair or wheelchair, as your coworker held the patient's legs.
19. Lowered the patient gently, as your coworker guided the patient's body into the seat.
20. Ensured comfortable positioning of the patient's hands and feet.
21. Lowered the lift bar to unhook the sling.
22. Consulted facility policy to determine if the sling could be left beneath the patient.
23. Covered the patient with a blanket.
24. Removed, cleaned, and stored equipment properly.
25. Removed soiled linens and discarded disposable equipment.

Follow-Up

26. Practiced hand hygiene.
27. Ensured patient comfort and placed the call light and personal items within reach.
28. Conducted a safety check before leaving the room.
29. Practiced hand hygiene.

Reporting and Documentation

30. Communicated any concerns to the licensed nursing staff.
31. Documented care provided in the chart or EMR.

Date of Completion: _____ Instructor's Initials: _____

Name: _____ Date: _____

Procedure: Transferring from a Bed to a Stretcher

Preparation	S	U	Comments
1. Consulted the licensed nursing staff or plan of care for special instructions and precautions.	_____	_____	_____
2. Asked for assistance from a coworker.	_____	_____	_____
3. Practiced hand hygiene.	_____	_____	_____
4. Knocked before entering the room.	_____	_____	_____
5. Introduced yourself using your name and title. Explained that you worked with the licensed nursing staff and would be providing care.	_____	_____	_____
6. Greeted the patient and confirmed the patient's identification.	_____	_____	_____
7. Addressed the patient as Mr., Mrs., or Ms. and the last name.	_____	_____	_____
8. Explained the procedure in simple terms and asked permission to perform the procedure.	_____	_____	_____
9. Assembled the necessary equipment.	_____	_____	_____

The Procedure

	S	U	Comments
10. Provided privacy to the patient.	_____	_____	_____
11. Raised the bed to hip height and locked the wheels.	_____	_____	_____
12. Raised and secured side rails on the opposite side of the bed from where you would be working.	_____	_____	_____
13. Positioned the stretcher next to the bed and locked the wheels.	_____	_____	_____
14. Lowered the head of the bed until flat and raised the bed to stretcher height.	_____	_____	_____
15. Stood with the stretcher between your body and the patient's bed, with a coworker on the opposite side of the bed to assist.	_____	_____	_____
16. Placed a draw sheet under the patient or untucked the draw sheet already on the bed, adjusting to support the patient's head.	_____	_____	_____
17. Asked the patient to move closer to the stretcher, if able, or instructed the patient to cross both arms and tuck in the chin if too weak to assist with transfer.	_____	_____	_____
18. Moved the patient gently and smoothly onto the stretcher using a draw sheet or slide board, starting with the lower body.	_____	_____	_____
19. Covered the patient and fastened safety straps.	_____	_____	_____
20. Raised the side rails of the stretcher and released the brake.	_____	_____	_____
21. Pushed stretcher from the head with patient's feet forward and your body close to the stretcher.	_____	_____	_____

Follow-Up

	S	U	Comments
22. Ensured patient comfort and placed the call light and personal items within reach.	_____	_____	_____
23. Conducted a safety check before leaving the room.	_____	_____	_____
24. Practiced hand hygiene.	_____	_____	_____

Reporting and Documentation

	S	U	Comments
25. Communicated any concerns to the licensed nursing staff.	_____	_____	_____
26. Documented care provided in the chart or EMR.	_____	_____	_____

Date of Completion: _____ Instructor's Initials: _____

Name: _____ Date: _____

	S	U	Comments
Preparation			
1. Consulted the licensed nursing staff or plan of care for special instructions and precautions.			
2. Practiced hand hygiene.			
3. Knocked before entering the room.			
4. Introduced yourself using your name and title. Explained that you worked with the licensed nursing staff and would be providing care.			
5. Greeted the patient and confirmed the patient's identification.			
6. Addressed the patient as Mr., Mrs., or Ms. and the last name.			
7. Explained the procedure in simple terms and asked permission to perform the procedure.			
8. Assembled the necessary equipment.			
The Procedure			
9. Provided privacy to the patient.			
10. Lowered the bed to its lowest position and locked the wheels.			
11. Raised and secured side rails on the opposite side of the bed from where you would be working.			
12. Assisted the patient into a dangling position and helped put on shoes and a robe, if needed.			
13. Applied the gait belt snugly around the waist over clothing.			
14. Faced the patient and held the gait belt with an underhand grip.			
15. Used the gait belt to assist the patient into a standing position using your arm and leg muscles and without twisting your body.			
16. Held the gait belt while the patient gained balance.			
17. Walked behind and to one side of the patient during ambulation.			
18. Held the gait belt from behind and watched for signs of collapse.			
19. Did not attempt to catch a falling patient and eased the patient to the floor using your body as an incline instead.			
20. Determined if the patient had a weak side and positioned yourself accordingly.			
21. Let the patient set the pace and encouraged the patient to ambulate the ordered distance.			
22. Observed for signs of fatigue.			
23. Helped the patient back to the room or bed and removed robe and shoes.			
24. Ensured the bed wheels were locked and bed was in low position before repositioning the patient.			
25. Raised or lowered bed side rails according to plan of care.			
26. Removed, cleaned, and stored equipment properly.			
27. Removed soiled linens and discarded disposable equipment.			
Follow-Up			
28. Practiced hand hygiene.			
29. Ensured patient comfort and placed the call light and personal items within reach.			
30. Conducted a safety check before leaving the room.			
31. Practiced hand hygiene.			
Reporting and Documentation			
32. Communicated any concerns to the licensed nursing staff.			
33. Documented care provided in the chart or EMR.			

Date of Completion: _____ Instructor's Initials: _____

Name: _____ Date: _____

Procedure: Providing Assistance with a Cane

Preparation	S	U	Comments
1. Consulted the licensed nursing staff or plan of care for special instructions and precautions.	___	___	_____
2. Practiced hand hygiene.	___	___	_____
3. Knocked before entering the room.	___	___	_____
4. Introduced yourself using your name and title. Explained that you worked with the licensed nursing staff and would be providing care.	___	___	_____
5. Greeted the patient and confirmed the patient's identification.	___	___	_____
6. Addressed the patient as Mr., Mrs., or Ms. and the last name.	___	___	_____
7. Explained the procedure in simple terms and asked permission to perform the procedure.	___	___	_____
8. Assembled the necessary equipment.	___	___	_____

The Procedure

	S	U	Comments
9. Provided privacy to the patient.	___	___	_____
10. Lowered the bed to its lowest position and locked the wheels.	___	___	_____
11. Raised and secured side rails on the opposite side of the bed from where you would be working.	___	___	_____
12. Assisted the patient into a dangling position and helped put on shoes and a robe, if needed.	___	___	_____
13. Applied the gait belt snugly around the waist over clothing, if needed.	___	___	_____
14. Faced the patient and held the gait belt with an underhand grip.	___	___	_____
15. Used the gait belt to assist the patient into a standing position using your arm and leg muscles and without twisting your body.	___	___	_____
16. Held the gait belt while the patient gained balance.	___	___	_____
17. Positioned the cane and stabilized the patient before ambulation.	___	___	_____
18. Stood slightly behind and on the weaker side of the patient to provide additional support.	___	___	_____
19. Held the gait belt from behind and encouraged the patient to use the handrails, if available.	___	___	_____
20. Let the patient set the pace and encouraged the patient to ambulate the ordered distance.	___	___	_____
21. Assisted the patient with climbing stairs, if permissible.	___	___	_____
22. Reminded the patient to face forward and "go up with the good, down with the bad" when climbing stairs.	___	___	_____
23. Helped patient back to room or bed and removed robe, cane, and shoes.	___	___	_____
24. Ensured the bed wheels were locked and bed was in low position before repositioning the patient.	___	___	_____
25. Raised or lowered bed side rails according to plan of care.	___	___	_____
26. Removed, cleaned, and stored equipment properly.	___	___	_____
27. Removed soiled linens and discarded disposable equipment.	___	___	_____

Date of Completion: _____ Instructor's Initials: _____

	S	U	Comments
Follow-Up			
28. Practiced hand hygiene.			
29. Ensured patient comfort and placed the call light and personal items within reach.	_____	_____	_____
30. Conducted a safety check before leaving the room.	_____	_____	_____
31. Practiced hand hygiene.	_____	_____	_____
Reporting and Documentation	_____	_____	_____
32. Communicated any concerns to the licensed nursing staff.			
33. Documented care provided in the chart or EMR.	_____	_____	_____
	_____	_____	_____

Date of Completion: _____   Instructor's Initials: _____

Name: _____   Date: _____

Procedure: Providing Assistance with a Walker

Preparation   S   U   Comments

1. Consulted the licensed nursing staff or plan of care for special
   instructions and precautions.   _____   _____   _____
2. Practiced hand hygiene.   _____   _____   _____
3. Knocked before entering the room.   _____   _____   _____
4. Introduced yourself using your name and title. Explained
   that you worked with the licensed nursing staff and would be
   providing care.   _____   _____   _____
5. Greeted the patient and confirmed the patient's identification.   _____   _____   _____
6. Addressed the patient as Mr., Mrs., or Ms. and the last name.   _____   _____   _____
7. Explained the procedure in simple terms and asked permission to
   perform the procedure.   _____   _____   _____
8. Assembled the necessary equipment.   _____   _____   _____

The Procedure

9. Provided privacy to the patient.   _____   _____   _____
10. Lowered the bed to its lowest position and locked the wheels.   _____   _____   _____
11. Raised and secured side rails on the opposite side of the bed from
    where you would be working.   _____   _____   _____
12. Assisted the patient into a dangling position and helped put on
    shoes and a robe, if needed.   _____   _____   _____
13. Applied the gait belt snugly around the waist over clothing,
    if needed.   _____   _____   _____
14. Positioned the seated patient centered in front of and inside the
    frame of the walker.   _____   _____   _____
15. Placed the walker one step ahead of the patient, with its legs level
    on the ground and stable.   _____   _____   _____
16. Instructed the patient to grip the top of the walker with both hands,
    stand, and walk forward leading with the weaker leg.   _____   _____   _____
17. Positioned yourself behind and slightly to the side of the patient
    during ambulation.   _____   _____   _____
18. Ensured the patient took small steps without rushing.   _____   _____   _____
19. Let the patient set the pace and encouraged the patient to ambulate
    the ordered distance.   _____   _____   _____
20. Held the gait belt from behind and watched for signs of fatigue or
    possible collapse.   _____   _____   _____
21. Did not attempt to catch a falling patient and eased the patient to
    the floor using your body as an incline instead.   _____   _____   _____
22. Assisted the patient to a sitting position in a stable chair.   _____   _____   _____
23. Assisted the patient to a standing position using the walker for
    balance before continuing ambulation.   _____   _____   _____
24. Helped patient back to room or bed and removed robe, walker,
    and shoes.   _____   _____   _____
25. Ensured the bed wheels were locked and bed was in low position
    before repositioning the patient.   _____   _____   _____
26. Raised or lowered bed side rails according to plan of care.   _____   _____   _____
27. Removed, cleaned, and stored equipment properly.   _____   _____   _____
28. Removed soiled linens and discarded disposable equipment.   _____   _____   _____

Date of Completion: _____   Instructor's Initials: _____

Name: _____ Date: _____

Follow-Up

	S	U	Comments
29. Practiced hand hygiene.			
30. Ensured patient comfort and placed the call light and personal items within reach.	___	___	_____
31. Conducted a safety check before leaving the room.	___	___	_____
32. Practiced hand hygiene.	___	___	_____

Reporting and Documentation

33. Communicated any concerns to the licensed nursing staff.	___	___	_____
34. Documented care provided in the chart or EMR.	___	___	_____

Date of Completion: _____ Instructor's Initials: _____

Name: _____ Date: _____

Procedure: Providing Assistance with Crutches

	S	U	Comments
Preparation			
1. Consulted the licensed nursing staff or plan of care for special instructions and precautions.	_____	_____	_____
2. Practiced hand hygiene.	_____	_____	_____
3. Knocked before entering the room.	_____	_____	_____
4. Introduced yourself using your name and title. Explained that you worked with the licensed nursing staff and would be providing care.	_____	_____	_____
5. Greeted the patient and confirmed the patient's identification.	_____	_____	_____
6. Addressed the patient as Mr., Mrs., or Ms. and the last name.	_____	_____	_____
7. Explained the procedure in simple terms and asked permission to perform the procedure.	_____	_____	_____
8. Assembled the necessary equipment.	_____	_____	_____
The Procedure			
9. Provided privacy to the patient.	_____	_____	_____
10. Lowered the bed to its lowest position and locked the wheels.	_____	_____	_____
11. Raised and secured side rails on the opposite side of the bed from where you would be working.	_____	_____	_____
12. Assisted the patient into a dangling position and helped put on shoes and a robe, if needed.	_____	_____	_____
13. Applied the gait belt snugly around the waist over clothing, if needed.	_____	_____	_____
14. Checked that the crutches fit properly and were in the tripod position.	_____	_____	_____
15. Determined the gait ordered by the doctor and instructed patient to follow its sequence while using the handholds to absorb weight.	_____	_____	_____
16. Ensured patient kept an erect posture and focused straight ahead.	_____	_____	_____
17. Walked at the patient's side.	_____	_____	_____
18. Let the patient set the pace and encouraged the patient to ambulate the ordered distance.	_____	_____	_____
19. Held the gait belt from behind and watched for signs of fatigue or possible collapse.	_____	_____	_____
20. Did not attempt to catch a falling patient, and eased the patient to the floor using your body as an incline instead.	_____	_____	_____
21. Assisted the patient with climbing stairs using proper form, if permissible.	_____	_____	_____
22. Helped patient back to room or bed and removed robe, crutches, and shoes.	_____	_____	_____
23. Ensured the bed wheels were locked and bed was in low position before repositioning the patient.	_____	_____	_____
24. Raised or lowered bed side rails according to plan of care.	_____	_____	_____
25. Removed, cleaned, and stored equipment properly.	_____	_____	_____
26. Removed soiled linens and discarded disposable equipment.	_____	_____	_____

Date of Completion: _____ Instructor's Initials: _____

	S	U	Comments

Follow-Up

27. Practiced hand hygiene.

28. Ensured patient comfort and placed the call light and personal items within reach.

29. Conducted a safety check before leaving the room.

30. Practiced hand hygiene.

Reporting and Documentation

31. Communicated any concerns to the licensed nursing staff.

32. Documented care provided in the chart or EMR.

Name: _____ Date: _____

Procedure: Performing Range-of-Motion Exercises ▶ Video

	S	U	Comments

Preparation

1. Consulted the licensed nursing staff or plan of care for special instructions and precautions. _____ _____ _____

2. Practiced hand hygiene. _____ _____ _____

3. Knocked before entering the room. _____ _____ _____

4. Introduced yourself using your name and title. Explained that you worked with the licensed nursing staff and would be providing care. _____ _____ _____

5. Greeted the patient and confirmed the patient's identification. _____ _____ _____

6. Addressed the patient as Mr., Mrs., or Ms. and the last name. _____ _____ _____

7. Explained the procedure in simple terms and asked permission to perform the procedure. _____ _____ _____

8. Assembled the necessary equipment. _____ _____ _____

The Procedure

9. Provided privacy to the patient. _____ _____ _____

10. Lowered the bed to its lowest position and locked the wheels. _____ _____ _____

11. Raised and secured side rails on the opposite side of the bed from where you would be working. _____ _____ _____

12. Helped the patient into the supine position and fanfolded the linens to the foot of the bed. _____ _____ _____

13. Exposed only the body part being exercised. _____ _____ _____

The Procedure: Exercising the Neck

14. Consulted facility policy or the licensed nursing staff before exercising this body part. _____ _____ _____

15. Supported the patient's head and jaw with both hands. _____ _____ _____

16. Brought head forward until the chin touched the chest. _____ _____ _____

17. Brought the head back without hyperextending. _____ _____ _____

18. Turned the head from side to side. _____ _____ _____

19. Tilted the patient's head to the left and right. _____ _____ _____

The Procedure: Exercising the Shoulder

20. Grasped and supported the patient's wrist with one hand and elbow with the other. _____ _____ _____

21. Raised the arm straight out in front of the patient and over the head before bringing it down to the side. _____ _____ _____

22. Moved the straight arm away from and back toward the side of the body. _____ _____ _____

23. Bent the elbow at the same level as the shoulder and moved the forearm down toward the body. _____ _____ _____

24. Moved the forearm toward the head. _____ _____ _____

The Procedure: Exercising the Elbow

25. Grasped and supported the patient's wrist with one hand and elbow with the other. _____ _____ _____

26. Bent the arm to touch the same-side shoulder before straightening the arm. _____ _____ _____

Date of Completion: _____ Instructor's Initials:_____

Name: _____   Date: _____

The Procedure: Exercising the Forearm	S	U	Comments

The Procedure: Exercising the Forearm

27. Grasped and supported the patient's wrist with one hand and elbow with the other.

28. Rotated the hand so the palm faced downward and then upward.

The Procedure: Exercising the Wrist

29. Held the wrist with both hands.

30. Bent the hand downward and straightened it.

31. Turned the upward hand toward the thumb before rotating back toward the little finger, as if waving.

The Procedure: Exercising the Thumb

32. Grasped the patient's hand with one of your hands and thumb with the other.

33. Moved thumb outward and inward.

34. Touched each of the patient's fingertips with the thumb.

35. Bent the thumb into the hand and back outward.

The Procedure: Exercising the Fingers

36. Spread the fingers and thumbs apart and brought them back together.

37. Curled and straightened the fingers.

The Procedure: Exercising the Hip

38. Supported the hip with one hand on the patient's thigh and the other on the calf.

39. Raised the leg before bending and straightening the knee.

40. Moved the leg away from and back toward the body.

41. Rotated the leg inward and outward.

The Procedure: Exercising the Knee

42. Supported the knee by placing one hand under the patient's knee and the other under the ankle.

43. Bent and straightened the knee.

The Procedure: Exercising the Ankle

44. Supported the foot and ankle by placing one hand under the patient's foot and one under the ankle.

45. Pulled the foot forward while pushing down on the heel.

46. Turned the foot down or pointed the toes.

The Procedure: Exercising the Foot

47. Supported the foot and ankle by placing one hand under the patient's foot and one under the ankle.

48. Rotated the inside and outside of the foot up and down.

The Procedure: Exercising the Toes

49. Curled and straightened the toes.

50. Spread and reunited the toes.

The Procedure: Repeating and Concluding Range-of-Motion Exercises

51. Covered the exposed patient and raised the side rail.

52. Lowered the side rail on the opposite side of the bed.

53. Repeated the exercises on the opposite side of the body.

Date of Completion: _____   Instructor's Initials:_____

	S	U	Comments
54. Ensured the bed wheels were locked and bed was in low position before repositioning the patient.	_____	_____	_____
55. Raised or lowered bed side rails according to plan of care.	_____	_____	_____
56. Removed, cleaned, and stored equipment properly.	_____	_____	_____
57. Removed soiled linens and discarded disposable equipment.	_____	_____	_____

Follow-Up

58. Practiced hand hygiene.	_____	_____	_____
59. Ensured patient comfort and placed the call light and personal items within reach.	_____	_____	_____
60. Conducted a safety check before leaving the room.	_____	_____	_____
61. Practiced hand hygiene.	_____	_____	_____

Reporting and Documentation

62. Communicated any concerns to the licensed nursing staff.	_____	_____	_____
63. Documented care provided in the chart or EMR.	_____	_____	_____

Date of Completion: _____   Instructor's Initials: _____

Name: _____   Date: _____

	S	U	Comments

Preparation

1. Consulted the licensed nursing staff or plan of care for special instructions and precautions.

2. Practiced hand hygiene.

3. Knocked before entering the room.

4. Introduced yourself using your name and title. Explained that you worked with the licensed nursing staff and would be providing care.

5. Greeted the patient and confirmed the patient's identification.

6. Addressed the patient as Mr., Mrs., or Ms. and the last name.

7. Explained the procedure in simple terms and asked permission to perform the procedure.

8. Assembled the necessary equipment.

9. Ensured the patient had not eaten, drank, smoked, or chewed gum for at least 15 minutes prior to the procedure.

The Procedure

10. Provided privacy to the patient.

11. Lowered the bed to its lowest position and locked the wheels.

12. Raised and secured side rails on the opposite side of the bed from where you would be working.

13. Positioned the patient comfortably.

14. Placed a disposable cover over the blue probe and waited until the thermometer was ready.

15. Inserted the covered probe under and to one side of the patient's tongue.

16. Held the probe in place in the patient's closed mouth under the lowered tongue until you heard or saw the signal that the reading was complete.

17. Removed the thermometer from the patient's mouth before reading the temperature on the display screen.

18. Disposed of the used probe cover appropriately, without touching it with your bare hands.

19. Ensured the bed wheels were locked and bed was in low position before repositioning the patient.

20. Raised or lowered bed side rails according to plan of care.

21. Cleaned the probe and returned it to its storage compartment.

22. Practiced hand hygiene.

23. Recorded the temperature on a pad, form, or the EMR.

24. Returned the thermometer to a charging location.

Follow-Up

25. Ensured patient comfort and placed the call light and personal items within reach.

26. Conducted a safety check before leaving the room.

27. Practiced hand hygiene.

Reporting and Documentation

28. Communicated any concerns to the licensed nursing staff.

Date of Completion: _____   Instructor's Initials: _____

Name: _____ Date: _____

Procedure: Using a Rectal Thermometer—Digital

		S	U	Comments

Preparation

1. Consulted the licensed nursing staff or plan of care for special instructions and precautions.

2. Practiced hand hygiene.

3. Knocked before entering the room.

4. Introduced yourself using your name and title. Explained that you worked with the licensed nursing staff and would be providing care.

5. Greeted the patient and confirmed the patient's identification.

6. Addressed the patient as Mr., Mrs., or Ms. and the last name.

7. Explained the procedure in simple terms and asked permission to perform the procedure.

8. Assembled the necessary equipment.

The Procedure

9. Provided privacy to the patient.

10. Lowered the bed to its lowest position and locked the wheels.

11. Raised and secured side rails on the opposite side of the bed from where you would be working.

12. Practiced hand hygiene and put on disposable gloves.

13. Placed a disposable cover over the red probe and waited until the thermometer was ready.

14. Assisted the patient into a side-lying or lateral position with the upper leg bent up to the stomach as far as possible.

15. Folded back any coverings to expose only the buttocks.

16. Applied water-soluble lubricating gel.

17. Used one hand to raise the upper buttock to expose the anal area and the other to gently insert the probe 1 inch or less into the anus.

18. Held the probe in place until you heard or saw the signal that the reading was complete.

19. Removed the thermometer before reading the temperature on the display screen.

20. Disposed of the probe cover appropriately.

21. Wiped the lubricant off the patient and discarded the tissue or paper towel.

22. Cleaned the probe with alcohol before returning it to its storage compartment.

23. Removed gloves and practiced hand hygiene.

24. Recorded the temperature on a pad, form, or the EMR.

25. Ensured the bed wheels were locked and bed was in low position before repositioning the patient.

26. Raised or lowered bed side rails according to plan of care.

27. Returned the thermometer to a charging location.

Follow-Up

28. Ensured patient comfort and placed the call light and personal items within reach.

29. Conducted a safety check before leaving the room.

30. Practiced hand hygiene.

Reporting and Documentation

31. Communicated any concerns to the licensed nursing staff.

Date of Completion: _____ Instructor's Initials: _____

Name: _____ Date: _____

Procedure: Using an Axillary Thermometer—Digital

	S	U	Comments
Preparation			
1. Consulted the licensed nursing staff or plan of care for special instructions and precautions.	_____	_____	_____
2. Practiced hand hygiene.	_____	_____	_____
3. Knocked before entering the room.	_____	_____	_____
4. Introduced yourself using your name and title. Explained that you worked with the licensed nursing staff and would be providing care.	_____	_____	_____
5. Greeted the patient and confirmed the patient's identification.	_____	_____	_____
6. Addressed the patient as Mr., Mrs., or Ms. and the last name.	_____	_____	_____
7. Explained the procedure in simple terms and asked permission to perform the procedure.	_____	_____	_____
8. Assembled the necessary equipment.	_____	_____	_____
The Procedure			
9. Provided privacy to the patient.	_____	_____	_____
10. Lowered the bed to its lowest position and locked the wheels.	_____	_____	_____
11. Raised and secured side rails on the opposite side of the bed from where you would be working.	_____	_____	_____
12. Dried the axilla with a towel.	_____	_____	_____
13. Placed the covered probe in the center of the axilla and crossed the patient's arm across his or her chest.	_____	_____	_____
14. Held the probe in place until you heard or saw the signal that the reading was complete.	_____	_____	_____
15. Removed the thermometer from the axilla before reading the temperature on the display screen.	_____	_____	_____
16. Disposed of the probe cover safely and cleaned the probe with alcohol before returning the probe to its storage compartment.	_____	_____	_____
17. Practiced hand hygiene.	_____	_____	_____
18. Recorded temperature on a pad, form, or the EMR.	_____	_____	_____
19. Assisted the patient in replacing and securing clothing.	_____	_____	_____
20. Ensured the bed wheels were locked and bed was in low position before repositioning the patient.	_____	_____	_____
21. Raised or lowered bed side rails according to plan of care.	_____	_____	_____
22. Returned the thermometer to a charging location.	_____	_____	_____
Follow-Up			
23. Ensured patient comfort and placed the call light and personal items within reach.	_____	_____	_____
24. Conducted a safety check before leaving the room.	_____	_____	_____
25. Practiced hand hygiene.	_____	_____	_____
Reporting and Documentation			
26. Communicated any concerns to the licensed nursing staff.	_____	_____	_____

Date of Completion: _____ Instructor's Initials:_____

Procedure: Using a Tympanic Thermometer—Digital

Preparation

		S	U	Comments

Preparation

1. Consulted the licensed nursing staff or plan of care for special instructions and precautions.
2. Practiced hand hygiene.
3. Knocked before entering the room.
4. Introduced yourself using your name and title. Explained that you worked with the licensed nursing staff and would be providing care.
5. Greeted the patient and confirmed the patient's identification.
6. Addressed the patient as Mr., Mrs., or Ms. and the last name.
7. Explained the procedure in simple terms and asked permission to perform the procedure.
8. Assembled the necessary equipment.

The Procedure

9. Provided privacy to the patient.
10. Lowered the bed to its lowest position and locked the wheels.
11. Raised and secured side rails on the opposite side of the bed from where you would be working.
12. Checked the lens of the tympanic thermometer.
13. Positioned the patient's head with the ear being used directly in front of you.
14. Placed a disposable plastic cover on the thermometer.
15. Pulled the patient's ear up and back before gently inserting the covered thermometer into the ear canal.
16. Held the probe in place until you heard or saw the signal that the reading was complete.
17. Removed the thermometer from the ear before reading the temperature on the display screen.
18. Disposed of the plastic cover safely and cleaned the thermometer with alcohol.
19. Practiced hand hygiene.
20. Recorded temperature on a pad, form, or the EMR.
21. Ensured the bed wheels were locked and bed was in low position before repositioning the patient.
22. Raised or lowered bed side rails according to plan of care.
23. Returned the thermometer to a charging location.

Follow-Up

24. Ensured patient comfort and placed the call light and personal items within reach.
25. Conducted a safety check before leaving the room.
26. Practiced hand hygiene.

Reporting and Documentation

27. Communicated any concerns to the licensed nursing staff.

Date of Completion: _____   Instructor's Initials:_____

Name: _____ Date: _____

Procedure: Using a Temporal Artery Thermometer—Digital

Preparation   S   U   Comments

1. Consulted the licensed nursing staff or plan of care for special instructions and precautions.
2. Practiced hand hygiene.
3. Knocked before entering the room.
4. Introduced yourself using your name and title. Explained that you worked with the licensed nursing staff and would be providing care.
5. Greeted the patient and confirmed the patient's identification.
6. Addressed the patient as Mr., Mrs., or Ms. and the last name.
7. Explained the procedure in simple terms and asked permission to perform the procedure.
8. Assembled the necessary equipment.

The Procedure

9. Provided privacy to the patient.
10. Lowered the bed to its lowest position and locked the wheels.
11. Raised and secured side rails on the opposite side of the bed from where you would be working.
12. Positioned the patient comfortably and turned the patient so the forehead faced you.
13. Waited until the thermometer showed it was ready before placing the probe in the middle of the patient's forehead, moving slowly across the forehead and stopping in front of the ear.
14. Waited until you saw or heard the signal that the temperature reading was complete.
15. Practiced hand hygiene.
16. Recorded temperature on a pad, form, or the EMR.
17. Ensured the bed wheels were locked and bed was in low position before repositioning the patient.
18. Raised or lowered bed side rails according to plan of care.
19. Cleaned and stored the thermometer appropriately.

Follow-Up

20. Ensured patient comfort and placed the call light and personal items within reach.
21. Conducted a safety check before leaving the room.
22. Practiced hand hygiene.

Reporting and Documentation

23. Communicated any concerns to the licensed nursing staff.

Date of Completion: _____ Instructor's Initials:_____

Name: _____ Date: _____

Procedure: Measuring a Radial Pulse ▶ Video

Preparation

		S	U	Comments
1.	Consulted the licensed nursing staff or plan of care for special instructions and precautions.	___	___	_____
2.	Practiced hand hygiene.	___	___	_____
3.	Knocked before entering the room.	___	___	_____
4.	Introduced yourself using your name and title. Explained that you worked with the licensed nursing staff and would be providing care.	___	___	_____
5.	Greeted the patient and confirmed the patient's identification.	___	___	_____
6.	Addressed the patient as Mr., Mrs., or Ms. and the last name.	___	___	_____
7.	Explained the procedure in simple terms and asked permission to perform the procedure.	___	___	_____
8.	Assembled the necessary equipment.	___	___	_____

The Procedure

		S	U	Comments
9.	Provided privacy to the patient.	___	___	_____
10.	Lowered the bed to its lowest position and locked the wheels.	___	___	_____
11.	Raised and secured side rails on the opposite side of the bed from where you would be working.	___	___	_____
12.	Positioned the patient in a sitting or lying position with the arm or hand you selected for the pulse measurement supported comfortably.	___	___	_____
13.	Located the radial artery on the inside of the patient's wrist using your middle and index fingers.	___	___	_____
14.	Pressed your fingers gently on the bare skin until you felt the pulse, noting its rhythm and quality.	___	___	_____
15.	Counted pulse beats according to facility policy.	___	___	_____
16.	Recorded temperature on a pad, form, or the EMR.	___	___	_____
17.	Ensured the bed wheels were locked and bed was in low position before repositioning the patient.	___	___	_____
18.	Raised or lowered bed side rails according to plan of care.	___	___	_____

Follow-Up

		S	U	Comments
19.	Practiced hand hygiene.	___	___	_____
20.	Ensured patient comfort and placed the call light and personal items within reach.	___	___	_____
21.	Conducted a safety check before leaving the room.	___	___	_____
22.	Practiced hand hygiene.	___	___	_____

Reporting and Documentation

		S	U	Comments
23.	Communicated any concerns to the licensed nursing staff.	___	___	_____

Date of Completion: _____ Instructor's Initials: _____

Name: _____ Date: _____

Procedure: Measuring an Apical Pulse

Preparation	S	U	Comments
1. Consulted the licensed nursing staff or plan of care for special instructions and precautions.			
2. Practiced hand hygiene.	_____	_____	_____
3. Knocked before entering the room.	_____	_____	_____
4. Introduced yourself using your name and title. Explained that you worked with the licensed nursing staff and would be providing care.			
5. Greeted the patient and confirmed the patient's identification.	_____	_____	_____
6. Addressed the patient as Mr., Mrs., or Ms. and the last name.	_____	_____	_____
7. Explained the procedure in simple terms and asked permission to perform the procedure.			
8. Assembled the necessary equipment.	_____	_____	_____

The Procedure

	S	U	Comments
9. Provided privacy to the patient.	_____	_____	_____
10. Lowered the bed to its lowest position and locked the wheels.	_____	_____	_____
11. Raised and secured side rails on the opposite side of the bed from where you would be working.			
12. Positioned the patient in a sitting or lying position.	_____	_____	_____
13. Cleaned the earpieces and diaphragm of the stethoscope with an antiseptic wipe, and warmed the diaphragm by rubbing it with your palms.			
14. Placed the earpieces in your ears.	_____	_____	_____
15. Uncovered the left side of the patient's chest and placed the diaphragm of the stethoscope under the breast or just below the left nipple.			
16. Counted the patient's heartbeats for one full minute, noting the rhythm and quality.			
17. Covered the patient's chest.	_____	_____	_____
18. Recorded pulse on a pad, form, or the EMR.	_____	_____	_____
19. Ensured the bed wheels were locked and bed was in low position before repositioning the patient.			
20. Raised or lowered bed side rails according to plan of care.	_____	_____	_____

Follow-Up

	S	U	Comments
21. Practiced hand hygiene.	_____	_____	_____
22. Ensured patient comfort and placed the call light and personal items within reach.			
23. Conducted a safety check before leaving the room.	_____	_____	_____
24. Practiced hand hygiene.	_____	_____	_____

Reporting and Documentation

	S	U	Comments
25. Communicated any concerns to the licensed nursing staff.	_____	_____	_____

Date of Completion: _____ Instructor's Initials: _____

Name: _____ Date: _____

Procedure: Counting Respirations ▶ Video

Preparation	S	U	Comments
1. Consulted the licensed nursing staff or plan of care for special instructions and precautions.	_____	_____	_____
2. Practiced hand hygiene.	_____	_____	_____
3. Knocked before entering the room.	_____	_____	_____
4. Introduced yourself using your name and title. Explained that you worked with the licensed nursing staff and would be providing care.	_____	_____	_____
5. Greeted the patient and confirmed the patient's identification.	_____	_____	_____
6. Addressed the patient as Mr., Mrs., or Ms. and the last name.	_____	_____	_____
7. Explained the procedure in simple terms and asked permission to perform the procedure.	_____	_____	_____
8. Assembled the necessary equipment.	_____	_____	_____

The Procedure

	S	U	Comments
9. Provided privacy to the patient.	_____	_____	_____
10. Lowered the bed to its lowest position and locked the wheels.	_____	_____	_____
11. Raised and secured side rails on the opposite side of the bed from where you would be working.	_____	_____	_____
12. Positioned the patient in a sitting or lying position.	_____	_____	_____
13. Counted respirations immediately after counting pulse rate, without notifying the patient.	_____	_____	_____
14. Counted each rise and fall of the chest as one respiration, noting the regularity and depth, the chest expansion, and any pain or difficulty.	_____	_____	_____
15. Counted respirations for the length of time required by facility policy.	_____	_____	_____
16. Notified the licensed nursing staff of any patient complaints of pain or difficulty breathing.	_____	_____	_____
17. Recorded respirations on a pad, form, or the EMR.	_____	_____	_____
18. Ensured the bed wheels were locked and bed was in low position before repositioning the patient.	_____	_____	_____
19. Raised or lowered bed side rails according to plan of care.	_____	_____	_____

Follow-Up

	S	U	Comments
20. Practiced hand hygiene.	_____	_____	_____
21. Ensured patient comfort and placed the call light and personal items within reach.	_____	_____	_____
22. Conducted a safety check before leaving the room.	_____	_____	_____
23. Practiced hand hygiene.	_____	_____	_____

Reporting and Documentation

	S	U	Comments
24. Communicated any concerns to the licensed nursing staff.	_____	_____	_____

Date of Completion: _____ Instructor's Initials:_____

Name: _____ Date: _____

Preparation   S   U   Comments

1. Consulted the licensed nursing staff or plan of care for special instructions and precautions. _____ _____ _____

2. Practiced hand hygiene. _____ _____ _____

3. Knocked before entering the room. _____ _____ _____

4. Introduced yourself using your name and title. Explained that you worked with the licensed nursing staff and would be providing care. _____ _____ _____

5. Greeted the patient and confirmed the patient's identification. _____ _____ _____

6. Addressed the patient as Mr., Mrs., or Ms. and the last name. _____ _____ _____

7. Explained the procedure in simple terms and asked permission to perform the procedure. _____ _____ _____

8. Assembled the necessary equipment. _____ _____ _____

The Procedure

9. Provided privacy to the patient. _____ _____ _____

10. Lowered the bed to its lowest position and locked the wheels. _____ _____ _____

11. Raised and secured side rails on the opposite side of the bed from where you would be working. _____ _____ _____

12. Positioned the patient in a sitting or lying position according to preference and allowed the patient to choose which arm would be used. _____ _____ _____

13. Cleaned the cuff, the diaphragm, and the earpieces with an antiseptic wipe and warmed the diaphragm by rubbing it with your palms. _____ _____ _____

14. Positioned the patient's arm so it rested level with the heart and turned the palm upward. _____ _____ _____

15. Unrolled the cuff, squeezed it to expel any remaining air, and loosened the bulb of the sphygmomanometer by turning it counterclockwise. _____ _____ _____

16. Located the brachial artery. _____ _____ _____

17. Wrapped the cuff smoothly and snugly around the exposed arm about 1 inch above the elbow with the center of the cuff above the brachial artery. _____ _____ _____

18. Closed the valve on the bulb of the sphygmomanometer by turning it counterclockwise. _____ _____ _____

19. Placed the earpieces of the stethoscope in your ears. _____ _____ _____

20. Placed the warmed diaphragm over the brachial artery. _____ _____ _____

21. Kept the measuring scale at eye level, if using a manual aneroid sphygmomanometer. _____ _____ _____

22. Inflated the cuff to 180 mmHg, or 200 mmHg if able to hear the patient's pulse. _____ _____ _____

23. Deflated the cuff slowly by turning the bulb counterclockwise at a rate of 2–4 millimeters per second. _____ _____ _____

24. Noted the dial reading for the systolic blood pressure when you heard the first beat. _____ _____ _____

25. Continued deflating the cuff slowly and evenly until the sound disappeared, noting the dial reading as the diastolic blood pressure. _____ _____ _____

26. Removed the earpieces from your ears and removed the deflated cuff from the patient's arm. _____ _____ _____

_____

Date of Completion: _____ Instructor's Initials:_____

	S	U	Comments
27. Recorded blood pressure on a pad, form, or the EMR.	_____	_____	_____
28. Reported any abnormal findings to the licensed nursing staff immediately.	_____	_____	_____
29. Returned the cuff to its case or wall mount.	_____	_____	_____
30. Cleaned the earpieces and diaphragm with an antiseptic wipe before returning the stethoscope and cuff case (if appropriate) to their storage locations.	_____	_____	_____
31. Ensured the bed wheels were locked and bed was in low position before repositioning the patient.	_____	_____	_____
32. Raised or lowered bed side rails according to plan of care.	_____	_____	_____

Follow-Up

33. Practiced hand hygiene.	_____	_____	_____
34. Ensured patient comfort and placed the call light and personal items within reach.	_____	_____	_____
35. Conducted a safety check before leaving the room.	_____	_____	_____
36. Practiced hand hygiene.	_____	_____	_____

Reporting and Documentation

37. Communicated any concerns to the licensed nursing staff.	_____	_____	_____

Date of Completion: _____ Instructor's Initials:_____

Name: _____ Date: _____

Procedure: Taking a Blood Pressure Using an Electronic Device

Preparation   S   U   Comments

1. Consulted the licensed nursing staff or plan of care for special
   instructions and precautions.

2. Practiced hand hygiene.

3. Knocked before entering the room.

4. Introduced yourself using your name and title. Explained
   that you worked with the licensed nursing staff and would be
   providing care.

5. Greeted the patient and confirmed the patient's identification.

6. Addressed the patient as Mr., Mrs., or Ms. and the last name.

7. Explained the procedure in simple terms and asked permission
   to perform the procedure.

8. Assembled the necessary equipment.

The Procedure

9. Provided privacy to the patient.

10. Lowered the bed to its lowest position and locked the wheels.

11. Raised and secured side rails on the opposite side of the bed from
    where you would be working.

12. Positioned the patient in a sitting or lying position according
    to preference and allowed the patient to choose which arm would
    be used.

13. Removed any restrictive clothing from the patient's arm.

14. Brought the electronic blood pressure unit near the patient, plugged
    it into an electricity source, and turned on the *Power* switch.

15. Cleaned the cuff with an antiseptic wipe or covered with a disposable
    paper cover, squeezed any excess air out of the cuff, and connected
    it to the connector hose.

16. Wrapped the cuff smoothly and snugly around the exposed arm
    with the arrow on the outside of the cuff over the brachial artery.

17. Ensured the connector hose was not kinked.

18. Pressed the *Start* button and waited to hear or see the signal
    indicating the reading was complete.

19. Set the machine for the frequency of blood pressure measurements
    designated by facility policy, if taking periodic, automatic
    measurements.

20. Recorded blood pressure on a pad, form, or the EMR.

21. Reported any abnormal findings to the licensed nursing staff
    immediately.

22. Cleaned the tubing and cuff with an antiseptic wipe or discarded
    the disposable sleeve.

23. Removed the machine and stored it properly.

24. Loosened the cuff and rotated it every two hours, observing for
    redness or irritation, if the cuff is left on the arm.

25. Ensured the bed wheels were locked and bed was in low position
    before repositioning the patient.

26. Raised or lowered bed side rails according to plan of care.

Date of Completion: _____ Instructor's Initials: _____

	S	U	Comments
Follow-Up			
27. Practiced hand hygiene.	_____	_____	_____
28. Ensured patient comfort and placed the call light and personal items within reach.	_____	_____	_____
29. Conducted a safety check before leaving the room.	_____	_____	_____
30. Practiced hand hygiene.	_____	_____	_____
Reporting and Documentation			
31. Communicated any concerns to the licensed nursing staff.	_____	_____	_____

Date of Completion: _____   Instructor's Initials: _____

Name: _____ Date: _____

Procedure: Measuring the Height and Weight of Ambulatory Patients

▶ Video

Preparation	S	U	Comments
1. Consulted the licensed nursing staff or plan of care for special instructions and precautions.			
2. Practiced hand hygiene.			
3. Knocked before entering the room.			
4. Introduced yourself using your name and title. Explained that you worked with the licensed nursing staff and would be providing care.			
5. Greeted the patient and confirmed the patient's identification.			
6. Addressed the patient as Mr., Mrs., or Ms. and the last name.			
7. Explained the procedure in simple terms and asked permission to perform the procedure.			
8. Assembled the necessary equipment.			

The Procedure

	S	U	Comments
9. Provided privacy to the patient.			
10. Placed a paper towel on the scale platform.			
11. Raised the height bar above the patient's head.			
12. Helped the patient remove footwear.			
13. Assisted the patient onto the center of the scale platform and instructed the patient to stand straight with arms and hands at the sides.			
14. Lifted the height bar, extended the arm, and lowered the arm until it rested atop the patient's head.			
15. Read the height at the movable part of the ruler.			
16. Recorded the patient's height on a pad, form, or the EMR.			
17. Raised the height bar above the head to a safe height before lowering the arm and returning the height bar to its starting point.			
18. Asked the patient to stand straight with arms and hands at the sides.			
19. Moved the weights on the balance scale bar to zero.			
20. Moved the lower and upper weights until the balance point was in the middle.			
21. Added the amounts shown on both bars to determine weight.			
22. Recorded the patient's weight on a pad, form, or the EMR.			
23. Assisted the patient with stepping down and replacing footwear.			
24. Removed and discarded the paper towel from the scale.			
25. Assisted the patient back to the room or bed.			
26. Ensured the bed wheels were locked and bed was in low position before repositioning the patient.			
27. Raised or lowered bed side rails according to plan of care.			

Date of Completion: _____ Instructor's Initials: _____

	S	U	Comments
Follow-Up			
28. Practiced hand hygiene.	_____	_____	_____
29. Ensured patient comfort and placed the call light and personal items within reach.	_____	_____	_____
30. Conducted a safety check before leaving the room.	_____	_____	_____
31. Practiced hand hygiene.	_____	_____	_____
Reporting and Documentation			
32. Communicated any concerns to the licensed nursing staff.	_____	_____	_____

Date of Completion: _____   Instructor's Initials:_____

Name: _____   Date: _____

Procedure: Measuring the Height of Bedridden Patients

	S	U	Comments

Preparation

1. Consulted the licensed nursing staff or plan of care for special instructions and precautions.

2. Practiced hand hygiene.

3. Knocked before entering the room.

4. Introduced yourself using your name and title. Explained that you worked with the licensed nursing staff and would be providing care.

5. Greeted the patient and confirmed the patient's identification.

6. Addressed the patient as Mr., Mrs., or Ms. and the last name.

7. Explained the procedure in simple terms and asked permission to perform the procedure.

8. Assembled the necessary equipment.

9. Asked for assistance from a coworker.

The Procedure

10. Provided privacy to the patient.

11. Lowered the bed to its lowest position and locked the wheels.

12. Raised and secured side rails on the opposite side of the bed from where you would be working.

13. Positioned the patient in a lying position on the back with both arms against the sides as straight as possible.

14. Extended the tape measure along the patient's side from the top of the head to the bottom of the heel, measuring the distance between.

15. Recorded the patient's height on a pad, form, or the EMR.

16. Ensured the bed wheels were locked and bed was in low position before repositioning the patient.

17. Raised or lowered bed side rails according to plan of care.

Follow-Up

18. Practiced hand hygiene.

19. Ensured patient comfort and placed the call light and personal items within reach.

20. Conducted a safety check before leaving the room.

21. Practiced hand hygiene.

Reporting and Documentation

22. Communicated any concerns to the licensed nursing staff.

Date of Completion: _____   Instructor's Initials: _____

Name: _____ Date: _____

Procedure: Weighing Bedridden Patients Using a Hydraulic Digital Lift or Sling Bed Scale

	S	U	Comments

Preparation

1. Consulted the licensed nursing staff or plan of care for special instructions and precautions.

2. Practiced hand hygiene.

3. Knocked before entering the room.

4. Introduced yourself using your name and title. Explained that you worked with the licensed nursing staff and would be providing care.

5. Greeted the patient and confirmed the patient's identification.

6. Addressed the patient as Mr., Mrs., or Ms. and the last name.

7. Explained the procedure in simple terms and asked permission to perform the procedure.

8. Assembled the necessary equipment.

9. Asked for assistance from a coworker.

The Procedure

10. Provided privacy to the patient.

11. Lowered the bed to its lowest position and locked the wheels.

12. Raised and secured side rails on the opposite side of the bed from where you would be working.

13. Balanced the bed scale.

14. Helped the patient roll to one side and positioned the sling lengthwise beneath the patient's shoulders, thighs, and buttocks.

15. Rolled the patient back onto the sling and ensured the sling was smooth and correctly positioned.

16. Centered the scale over the bed, lowered the weighting arms, and attached them securely to the sling bars.

17. Instructed the patient to keep both arms at the sides.

18. Raised the sling until it and the patient's body hung freely over the bed.

19. Adjusted the weights until the balance bar hung freely or read the digital display screen.

20. Recorded the patient's weight on a pad, form, or the EMR.

21. Lowered the patient onto the bed and removed the sling.

22. Ensured the bed wheels were locked and bed was in low position before repositioning the patient.

23. Raised or lowered bed side rails according to plan of care.

Follow-Up

24. Practiced hand hygiene.

25. Ensured patient comfort and placed the call light and personal items within reach.

26. Conducted a safety check before leaving the room.

27. Practiced hand hygiene.

Reporting and Documentation

28. Communicated any concerns to the licensed nursing staff.

Date of Completion: _____ Instructor's Initials: _____

Name: _____ Date: _____

Procedure: Preparing for an Examination

	S	U	Comments

Preparation

1. Consulted the licensed nursing staff or plan of care for special instructions and precautions.   _____ _____ _____
2. Practiced hand hygiene.   _____ _____ _____
3. Prepared the necessary paperwork, chart, or EMR.   _____ _____ _____
4. Covered the examination table with a disposable sheet.   _____ _____ _____
5. Assembled the necessary equipment.   _____ _____ _____
6. Prepared the necessary drapes.   _____ _____ _____
7. Introduced yourself using your name and title. Explained that you worked with the licensed nursing staff and would be providing care.   _____ _____ _____
8. Escorted the patient to the examining room.   _____ _____ _____
9. Encouraged the patient to use the bathroom before the examination.   _____ _____ _____
10. Measured the patient's height and weight, if scales were outside the examining room.   _____ _____ _____

The Procedure

11. Provided privacy to the patient.   _____ _____ _____
12. Instructed the patient to remove only the clothes required by the examination.   _____ _____ _____
13. Asked the patient to put on a gown and left the room until the patient was ready.   _____ _____ _____
14. Ensured there was adequate lighting.   _____ _____ _____
15. Measured vital signs and height and weight, if scales were in the examining room.   _____ _____ _____
16. Assisted the patient onto the examining table and into any necessary special positions.   _____ _____ _____
17. Ensured patient safety and did not leave the patient alone once positioned.   _____ _____ _____
18. Draped the patient for examination, being mindful of warmth and the patient's privacy.   _____ _____ _____

Follow-Up

19. Provided assistance during the examination as requested.   _____ _____ _____
20. Provided the patient with tissues to clean off any lubricant used during an examination of the vagina or rectum.   _____ _____ _____
21. Assisted with dressing and ensured the patient's safety and comfort.   _____ _____ _____
22. Removed, cleaned, and stored equipment properly.   _____ _____ _____
23. Removed soiled linens and discarded disposable equipment.   _____ _____ _____
24. Sent a speculum or other equipment to the supply area for sterilization.   _____ _____ _____
25. Practiced hand hygiene.   _____ _____ _____

Reporting and Documentation

26. Communicated any concerns to the licensed nursing staff.   _____ _____ _____

Date of Completion: _____   Instructor's Initials: _____

Name: _____ Date: _____

Procedure: Collecting a Sputum Specimen

	S	U	Comments
Preparation			
1. Consulted the licensed nursing staff or plan of care for special instructions and precautions.	_____	_____	_____
2. Practiced hand hygiene.	_____	_____	_____
3. Knocked before entering the room.	_____	_____	_____
4. Introduced yourself using your name and title. Explained that you worked with the licensed nursing staff and would be providing care.	_____	_____	_____
5. Greeted the patient and confirmed the patient's identification.	_____	_____	_____
6. Addressed the patient as Mr., Mrs., or Ms. and the last name.	_____	_____	_____
7. Explained the procedure in simple terms and asked permission to perform the procedure.	_____	_____	_____
8. Assembled the necessary equipment.	_____	_____	_____
9. Asked the licensed nursing staff if PPE should be worn and put on appropriate PPE.	_____	_____	_____
10. Completed the label with the necessary information before placing the label on the specimen container.	_____	_____	_____
The Procedure			
11. Provided privacy to the patient.	_____	_____	_____
12. Lowered the bed to its lowest position and locked the wheels.	_____	_____	_____
13. Raised and secured side rails on the opposite side of the bed from where you would be working.	_____	_____	_____
14. Practiced hand hygiene.	_____	_____	_____
15. Put on disposable gloves and any other necessary PPE.	_____	_____	_____
16. Positioned the patient in either a Fowler's or sitting position.	_____	_____	_____
17. Asked the patient to rinse the mouth with water and spit into the emesis basin.	_____	_____	_____
18. Gave the patient the specimen container, instructed the patient not to touch the inside of the container or lid, and placed the lid on a paper towel on the overbed table.	_____	_____	_____
19. Instructed the patient to take three, deep, open-mouth breaths and cough deeply, covering the mouth with a tissue.	_____	_____	_____
20. Collected 1–2 tablespoons of sputum, unless otherwise instructed.	_____	_____	_____
21. Covered the container with its lid immediately.	_____	_____	_____
22. Removed and discarded your gloves.	_____	_____	_____
23. Practiced hand hygiene.	_____	_____	_____
24. Put on a new pair of disposable gloves.	_____	_____	_____
25. Ensured that the specimen label matched the specimen collected.	_____	_____	_____
26. Attached the requisition form and ensured the lid was tightly placed on the container.	_____	_____	_____
27. Placed the specimen container in a transport bag, using a biohazard bag or label if necessary.	_____	_____	_____
28. Ensured the bed wheels were locked and bed was in low position before repositioning the patient.	_____	_____	_____

Date of Completion: _____ Instructor's Initials: _____

	S	U	Comments
29. Raised or lowered bed side rails according to plan of care.			
30. Offered the patient a glass of water and emesis basin to clean the mouth.	_____	_____	_____
31. Removed, cleaned, and stored equipment properly.	_____	_____	_____
32. Removed soiled linens and discarded disposable equipment.	_____	_____	_____

Follow-Up

33. Removed and discarded your gloves.	_____	_____	_____
34. Practiced hand hygiene.	_____	_____	_____
35. Ensured patient comfort and placed the call light and personal items within reach.	_____	_____	_____
36. Conducted a safety check before leaving the room.	_____	_____	_____
37. Practiced hand hygiene.	_____	_____	_____
38. Sent or took labeled specimen container to the appropriate location with the requisition form.	_____	_____	_____

Reporting and Documentation

39. Communicated any concerns to the licensed nursing staff.	_____	_____	_____
40. Documented care provided in the chart or EMR.	_____	_____	_____

Date of Completion: _____ Instructor's Initials: _____

Name: _____ Date: _____

Procedure: Collecting a Routine Urine Specimen

	S	U	Comments

Preparation

1. Consulted the licensed nursing staff or plan of care for special instructions and precautions. _____ _____ _____
2. Practiced hand hygiene. _____ _____ _____
3. Knocked before entering the room. _____ _____ _____
4. Introduced yourself using your name and title. Explained that you worked with the licensed nursing staff and would be providing care. _____ _____ _____
5. Greeted the patient and confirmed the patient's identification. _____ _____ _____
6. Addressed the patient as Mr., Mrs., or Ms. and the last name. _____ _____ _____
7. Explained the procedure in simple terms and asked permission to perform the procedure. _____ _____ _____

The Procedure

8. Assembled the necessary equipment. _____ _____ _____
9. Completed the label with the necessary information before placing the label on the specimen container. _____ _____ _____
10. Provided privacy to the patient. _____ _____ _____
11. Practiced hand hygiene and put on disposable gloves. _____ _____ _____
12. Had the patient urinate into a urinary hat, bedpan, or urinal. _____ _____ _____
13. Asked the patient not to have a bowel movement or put toilet paper into the urine specimen; instead, provided a bag or waste container for toilet paper. _____ _____ _____
14. Covered the urinal or bedpan before taking it to the bathroom and measured I&O with a clean graduate. _____ _____ _____
15. Removed and discarded your gloves. _____ _____ _____
16. Practiced hand hygiene. _____ _____ _____
17. Put on a new pair of gloves. _____ _____ _____
18. Noted the total urine output amount and recorded it on the I&O form. _____ _____ _____
19. Placed a paper towel on a flat surface, and placed the lid from the urine specimen container facing upward on top of the towel. _____ _____ _____
20. Poured about 120 mL of urine from the graduate into the specimen container or poured directly from the urinal. _____ _____ _____
21. Replaced the lid on the specimen container tightly and ensured that the specimen label matched the specimen collected. _____ _____ _____
22. Attached the requisition form. _____ _____ _____
23. Placed the specimen container in a transport bag, using a biohazard bag or label if necessary. _____ _____ _____
24. Emptied the rest of the urine into the toilet. _____ _____ _____
25. Removed, cleaned, and stored equipment properly. _____ _____ _____
26. Removed soiled linens and discarded disposable equipment. _____ _____ _____
27. Removed and discarded your gloves. _____ _____ _____
28. Practiced hand hygiene and put on a new pair of gloves. _____ _____ _____
29. Assisted the patient with hygiene, as needed. _____ _____ _____
30. Ensured the bed wheels were locked and bed was in low position before repositioning the patient. _____ _____ _____
31. Raised or lowered bed side rails according to plan of care. _____ _____ _____

Date of Completion: _____ Instructor's Initials: _____

Follow-Up	**S**	**U**	**Comments**
32. Removed and discarded your gloves.			
33. Practiced hand hygiene.	_____	_____	_____
34. Ensured patient comfort and placed the call light and personal items within reach.	_____	_____	_____
35. Conducted a safety check before leaving the room.	_____	_____	_____
36. Practiced hand hygiene.	_____	_____	_____
37. Sent or took labeled specimen container to the appropriate location with the requisition form.	_____	_____	_____
Reporting and Documentation			
38. Communicated any concerns to the licensed nursing staff.	_____	_____	_____
39. Documented care provided in the chart or EMR.	_____	_____	_____

Date of Completion: _____   Instructor's Initials: _____

Name: _____ Date: _____

Procedure: Collecting a Midstream Urine Specimen

	S	U	Comments

Preparation

1. Consulted the licensed nursing staff or plan of care for special instructions and precautions.

2. Practiced hand hygiene.

3. Knocked before entering the room.

4. Introduced yourself using your name and title. Explained that you worked with the licensed nursing staff and would be providing care.

5. Greeted the patient and confirmed the patient's identification.

6. Addressed the patient as Mr., Mrs., or Ms. and the last name.

7. Explained the procedure in simple terms and asked permission to perform the procedure.

The Procedure

8. Assembled the necessary equipment.

9. Completed the label with the necessary information before placing the label on the specimen container.

10. Provided privacy to the patient.

11. Practiced hand hygiene and put on disposable gloves.

12. Assisted the patient to the bathroom or provided a bedside commode, bedpan, or urinal.

13. Had the patient cleanse the perineal area, assisting if needed:

    A. Used one hand to separate the labia with a wipe and cleaned down the urethral area from front to back using a clean wipe each time, if the patient was female.

    B. Used one hand to hold the penis and pull back the foreskin and cleaned the penis in a circular motion starting at the urethral opening and working outward using a new wipe each time, if the patient was male.

14. Removed and discarded your gloves.

15. Practiced hand hygiene.

16. Opened the midstream specimen kit and kept the contents on top of the sterile wrapper.

17. Put on a new pair of gloves.

18. Opened the specimen container and the wipes in the kit, removed the container lid, and placed facing up on the sterile wrapper.

19. Ensured the specimen container and toilet paper were reachable.

20. Instructed the patient to begin urinating and stop after a few seconds.

21. Had the patient hold the container to catch the stream of urine or held the container yourself if the patient was unable.

22. Removed the container once the specimen was obtained and before the flow of urine stopped.

23. Placed the lid on the specimen container tightly and without touching the inside of the container.

24. Ensured that the specimen label matched the specimen collected.

25. Attached the requisition form.

26. Placed the specimen container in a transport bag, using a biohazard bag or label if necessary.

27. Removed, cleaned, and stored equipment properly.

Date of Completion: _____ Instructor's Initials:_____

Name: _____   Date: _____

	S	U	Comments

28. Removed soiled linens and discarded disposable equipment.

29. Removed and discarded your gloves.

30. Practiced hand hygiene and put on a new pair of gloves.

31. Assisted the patient with hygiene, as needed.

32. Ensured the bed wheels were locked and bed was in low position before repositioning the patient.

33. Raised or lowered bed side rails according to plan of care.

Follow-Up

34. Removed and discarded your gloves.

35. Practiced hand hygiene.

36. Ensured patient comfort and placed the call light and personal items within reach.

37. Conducted a safety check before leaving the room.

38. Practiced hand hygiene.

39. Sent or took labeled specimen container to the appropriate location with the requisition form.

Reporting and Documentation

40. Communicated any concerns to the licensed nursing staff.

41. Documented care provided in the chart or EMR.

Date of Completion: _____   Instructor's Initials: _____

Name: _____   Date: _____

Procedure: Collecting a 24-Hour Urine Specimen

	S	U	Comments

Preparation

1. Consulted the licensed nursing staff or plan of care for special instructions and precautions.   _____ _____ _____
2. Practiced hand hygiene.   _____ _____ _____
3. Knocked before entering the room.   _____ _____ _____
4. Introduced yourself using your name and title. Explained that you worked with the licensed nursing staff and would be providing care.   _____ _____ _____
5. Greeted the patient and confirmed the patient's identification.   _____ _____ _____
6. Addressed the patient as Mr., Mrs., or Ms. and the last name.   _____ _____ _____
7. Explained the procedure in simple terms and asked permission to perform the procedure.   _____ _____ _____

The Procedure

8. Assembled the necessary equipment.   _____ _____ _____
9. Completed the label with the necessary information before placing the label on the specimen container.   _____ _____ _____
10. Placed the 24-hour urine collection container in the bathroom in a pan of ice.   _____ _____ _____
11. Posted a sign over the bed or in the bathroom about the specimen collection.   _____ _____ _____
12. Provided privacy to the patient.   _____ _____ _____
13. Practiced hand hygiene and put on disposable gloves.   _____ _____ _____
14. Ensured the patient understood how to save and pour all urine into the designated container for the next 24 hours.   _____ _____ _____
15. Had the patient empty his or her bladder to begin the 24-hour collection period and noted the date and time.   _____ _____ _____
16. Instructed the patient to urinate into the urinary hat, to refrain from putting toilet paper into the pan, and to notify you when finished. Collected the urine from the bedside commode, bedpan, or urinal if the patient was not ambulatory.   _____ _____ _____
17. Measured and recorded all urine before pouring it into the 24-hour collection container.   _____ _____ _____
18. Maintained fresh ice in the pan.   _____ _____ _____
19. Instructed the patient to urinate one final time at the end of the 24 hours and poured the urine into the container.   _____ _____ _____
20. Replaced the lid on the specimen container tightly and ensured that the specimen label matched the specimen collected.   _____ _____ _____
21. Attached the requisition form.   _____ _____ _____
22. Removed the sign about the 24-hour collection.   _____ _____ _____
23. Removed and discarded your gloves.   _____ _____ _____
24. Performed hand hygiene and put on a new pair of gloves.   _____ _____ _____
25. Assisted the patient with hygiene, as needed.   _____ _____ _____
26. Ensured the bed wheels were locked and bed was in low position before repositioning the patient.   _____ _____ _____
27. Raised or lowered bed side rails according to plan of care.   _____ _____ _____
28. Removed, cleaned, and stored equipment properly.   _____ _____ _____
29. Removed soiled linens and discarded disposable equipment.   _____ _____ _____

Date of Completion: _____   Instructor's Initials:_____

	S	U	Comments

Follow-Up

30. Removed and discarded your gloves.

31. Practiced hand hygiene.

32. Ensured patient comfort and placed the call light and personal items within reach.

33. Conducted a safety check before leaving the room.

34. Practiced hand hygiene.

35. Sent or took labeled specimen container to the appropriate location with the requisition form.

Reporting and Documentation

36. Communicated any concerns to the licensed nursing staff.

37. Documented care provided in the chart or EMR.

Procedure: Collecting a Stool Specimen

	S	U	Comments
Preparation			
1. Consulted the licensed nursing staff or plan of care for special instructions and precautions.	_____	_____	_____
2. Practiced hand hygiene.	_____	_____	_____
3. Knocked before entering the room.	_____	_____	_____
4. Introduced yourself using your name and title. Explained that you worked with the licensed nursing staff and would be providing care.	_____	_____	_____
5. Greeted the patient and confirmed the patient's identification.	_____	_____	_____
6. Addressed the patient as Mr., Mrs., or Ms. and the last name.	_____	_____	_____
7. Explained the procedure in simple terms and asked permission to perform the procedure.	_____	_____	_____
8. Assembled the necessary equipment.	_____	_____	_____
9. Completed the label with the necessary information before placing the label on the specimen container.	_____	_____	_____
The Procedure			
10. Provided privacy to the patient.	_____	_____	_____
11. Practiced hand hygiene and put on disposable gloves.	_____	_____	_____
12. Had the patient urinate into the toilet, a urinary hat, bedpan, or urinal depending on ambulation, and discarded the urine.	_____	_____	_____
13. Placed a disposable specimen container:			
A. at the back of the toilet for ambulatory patients	_____	_____	_____
B. inside the back half of the bedside commode for nonambulatory patients	_____	_____	_____
14. Instructed the patient to have a bowel movement into the specimen container and provided a plastic bag or waste container for toilet paper.	_____	_____	_____
15. Covered the specimen pan and took it into the bathroom.	_____	_____	_____
16. Removed 2 teaspoons of stool from the pan with a wooden tongue blade and observed for color; amount; quality; and any pus, mucus, or blood.	_____	_____	_____
17. Replaced the lid on the specimen container tightly and ensured that the specimen label matched the specimen collected.	_____	_____	_____
18. Attached the requisition form.	_____	_____	_____
19. Placed the specimen container in a transport bag, using a biohazard bag or label if necessary.	_____	_____	_____
20. Wrapped the wooden tongue blade in toilet paper, discarded it, and emptied the remaining stool into the toilet.	_____	_____	_____
21. Removed and discarded your gloves.	_____	_____	_____
22. Practiced hand hygiene and put on a new pair of gloves.	_____	_____	_____
23. Assisted the patient with hygiene, as needed.	_____	_____	_____
24. Ensured the bed wheels were locked and bed was in low position before repositioning the patient.	_____	_____	_____
25. Raised or lowered bed side rails according to plan of care.	_____	_____	_____
26. Removed, cleaned, and stored equipment properly.	_____	_____	_____
27. Removed soiled linens and discarded disposable equipment.	_____	_____	_____

Date of Completion: _____   Instructor's Initials: _____

	S	U	Comments

Follow-Up

28. Removed and discarded your gloves.

29. Practiced hand hygiene.

30. Ensured patient comfort and placed the call light and personal items within reach.

31. Conducted a safety check before leaving the room.

32. Practiced hand hygiene.

33. Sent or took labeled specimen container to the appropriate location with the requisition form.

Reporting and Documentation

34. Communicated any concerns to the licensed nursing staff.

35. Documented care provided in the chart or EMR.

Date of Completion: _____   Instructor's Initials: _____

Name: _____ Date: _____

	S	U	Comments

Preparation

1. Consulted the licensed nursing staff or plan of care for special instructions and precautions.

2. Practiced hand hygiene.

3. Knocked before entering the room.

4. Introduced yourself using your name and title. Explained that you worked with the licensed nursing staff and would be providing care.

5. Greeted the patient and confirmed the patient's identification.

6. Addressed the patient as Mr., Mrs., or Ms. and the last name.

7. Explained the procedure in simple terms and asked permission to perform the procedure.

8. Assembled the necessary equipment.

The Procedure

9. Provided privacy to the patient.

10. Raised the bed to hip height and locked the wheels.

11. Raised and secured side rails on the opposite side of the bed from where you would be working.

12. Arranged the clean linens in the order they would be used.

13. Removed the call light and flattened the bed.

14. Loosened the top linens from the foot of the bed and placed the bath blanket over the top linens.

15. Removed the top linens from under the bath blanket carefully without exposing the patient and placed the top linens in the laundry hamper.

16. Asked the patient to hold the top edge of the bath blanket or tucked it under the shoulders.

17. Made the bed one side at a time, replacing the mattress with the help of a coworker if it has slipped out of place.

18. Asked the patient to turn toward the furthest side of the bed and to grasp the side rail.

19. Kept the patient covered, moved the pillow with the patient, and adjusted for comfort.

20. Started at the head of the bed, loosened the soiled bottom linens, and discarded the disposable protective pad, if used.

21. Rolled the soiled bottom linens and tucked them against the patient's back.

22. Placed a clean bottom sheet on top of the mattress, tucked the corners and edges tightly and smoothly, and made a mitered corner.

23. Positioned the draw sheet with the center fold next to the patient and tucked it under the mattress.

24. Asked the patient to roll toward you over the soiled linens and moved the pillow and bath blanket.

25. Raised and secured the side rail before moving to the opposite side of the bed and lowering its side rail.

26. Removed the soiled bottom linens by rolling the edges inward toward you and put the soiled linens in the laundry hamper.

Date of Completion: _____ Instructor's Initials: _____

	S	U	Comments
27. Pulled the clean bottom sheet into place quickly, tightly, smoothly, and securely.	____	____	_____
28. Pulled and tucked the draw sheet tightly and placed a disposable protective pad on top of the draw sheet under the patient's buttocks.	____	____	_____
29. Asked the patient to lie on the back in the center of the bed.	____	____	_____
30. Changed the pillowcases, replaced the pillows under the patient's head, and discarded the used pillowcases in the laundry hamper.	____	____	_____
31. Placed a clean top sheet over the patient.	____	____	_____
32. Removed the bath blanket and discarded it in the laundry hamper.	____	____	_____
33. Placed the blanket and bedspread on the patient and tucked these into mitered corners.	____	____	_____
34. Made toe pleats in the top linens, if needed.	____	____	_____
35. Ensured the bed wheels were locked and bed was in low position before repositioning the patient.	____	____	_____
36. Raised or lowered bed side rails according to plan of care.	____	____	_____

Follow-Up

	S	U	Comments
37. Practiced hand hygiene.	____	____	_____
38. Ensured patient comfort and placed the call light and personal items within reach.	____	____	_____
39. Conducted a safety check before leaving the room.	____	____	_____
40. Practiced hand hygiene.	____	____	_____

Reporting and Documentation

	S	U	Comments
41. Communicated any concerns to the licensed nursing staff.	____	____	_____
42. Documented care provided in the chart or EMR.	____	____	_____

Date of Completion: _____   Instructor's Initials: _____

Name: _____ Date: _____

Procedure: Making an Unoccupied Bed

	S	U	Comments

Preparation

1. Practiced hand hygiene. _____ _____ _____
2. Knocked before entering the room. _____ _____ _____
3. Introduced yourself using your name and title. Explained that you worked with the licensed nursing staff and would be providing care. _____ _____ _____
4. Greeted the patient and confirmed the patient's identification. _____ _____ _____
5. Addressed the patient as Mr., Mrs., or Ms. and the last name. _____ _____ _____
6. Explained the procedure in simple terms and asked permission to perform the procedure. _____ _____ _____
7. Assembled the necessary equipment. _____ _____ _____

The Procedure

8. Raised the bed to hip height or a comfortable working level, locked the wheels, and lowered the side rails. _____ _____ _____
9. Arranged the clean linens in the order they would be used. _____ _____ _____
10. Removed the soiled linens by rolling the edges inward and deposited them in the laundry hamper. _____ _____ _____
11. Replaced the mattress if it slid down. _____ _____ _____
12. Worked on one side of the bed at a time. _____ _____ _____
13. Placed the mattress pad even with the top of the mattress and pulled the corners tightly and smoothly over the corners of the mattress. _____ _____ _____
14. Unfolded the bottom sheet lengthwise on top of the mattress pad with the center fold in the middle of the bed, the hem stitching facing the mattress pad, and the small hem at the foot of the bed. _____ _____ _____
15. Placed a bottom sheet on top of the mattress, tucked the corners and edges tightly and smoothly, and made a mitered corner. _____ _____ _____
16. Placed a draw sheet on the bed, tucked it under the mattress, and placed a disposable protective pad on top of and in the center of it. _____ _____ _____
17. Unfolded and applied the top sheet with the wrong side up, the hem even with the upper edge of the mattress, and the center fold in the center of the bed. _____ _____ _____
18. Spread the blanket and bedspread over the top sheet and foot of the mattress. _____ _____ _____
19. Tucked the top sheet, blanket, and bedspread under the mattress at the foot of the bed. _____ _____ _____
20. Made a mitered corner at the foot of the bed, folded the top sheet back over the blanket to form an 8-inch cuff, and tucked in the sides of the linens if making a closed bed. _____ _____ _____
21. Did not tuck the linens, but instead fanfolded them to the foot of the bed if making an open bed. _____ _____ _____
22. Inserted the pillows into the pillowcases and placed the pillows at the head of the bed with the open ends facing away from the door. _____ _____ _____
23. Ensured the bed wheels were locked and bed was in its lowest position. _____ _____ _____

Date of Completion: _____ Instructor's Initials: _____

Follow-Up   S   U   **Comments**

24. Practiced hand hygiene.

25. Placed call light on the bed.   _____   _____   _____

26. Placed the chair in its assigned location.   _____   _____   _____

27. Positioned the overbed table over the foot of the bed, opposite   _____   _____   _____
    the chair.

28. Took the laundry hamper to the proper location.   _____   _____   _____

29. Conducted a safety check before leaving the room.   _____   _____   _____

30. Practiced hand hygiene.   _____   _____   _____

                                                          _____   _____   _____

Date of Completion: _____   Instructor's Initials:_____

Name: _____   Date: _____

Procedure: Making a Surgical Bed

	S	U	Comments

Preparation

1. Practiced hand hygiene.   _____ _____ _____
2. Assembled the necessary equipment.   _____ _____ _____

The Procedure

3. Raised the bed to hip height or a comfortable working level and
   locked the wheels.   _____ _____ _____
4. Arranged the clean linens in the order they would be used.   _____ _____ _____
5. Stripped the bed and deposited used linens in the laundry hamper.   _____ _____ _____
6. Practiced hand hygiene.   _____ _____ _____
7. Placed the mattress pad even with the top of the mattress
   and pulled the corners tightly and smoothly over the corners
   of the mattress.   _____ _____ _____
8. Unfolded the bottom sheet lengthwise on top of the mattress pad
   with the center fold in the middle of the bed, the hem stitching
   facing the mattress pad, and the small hem at the foot of the bed.   _____ _____ _____
9. Placed a bottom sheet on top of the mattress, tucked the corners
   and edges tightly and smoothly, and made a mitered corner.   _____ _____ _____
10. Placed a draw sheet on the bed, tucked it under the mattress, and
    placed a disposable protective pad on top of and in the center of it. _____ _____ _____
11. Unfolded and applied the top sheet with the wrong side up, the
    hem even with the upper edge of the mattress, and the center fold
    in the center of the bed.   _____ _____ _____
12. Spread the blanket and bedspread over the top sheet and foot
    of the mattress.   _____ _____ _____
13. Did not tuck the linens, but instead fanfolded them to the foot
    of the bed.   _____ _____ _____
14. Inserted the pillows into the pillowcases and placed the pillows
    upright against the headboard.   _____ _____ _____
15. Ensured the bed wheels were locked and bed was in its highest
    position.   _____ _____ _____
16. Left both side rails down.   _____ _____ _____
17. Moved furniture away from the bed to make room for the
    stretcher.   _____ _____ _____

Follow-Up

18. Placed the call light on the bedside stand or under the pillow.   _____ _____ _____
19. Took the laundry hamper to the proper location.   _____ _____ _____
20. Conducted a safety check before leaving the room.   _____ _____ _____
21. Practiced hand hygiene.   _____ _____ _____

Date of Completion: _____   Instructor's Initials:_____

Name: _____ Date: _____

Procedure: Giving a Back Rub

Preparation

	S	U	Comments
1. Consulted the licensed nursing staff or plan of care for special instructions and precautions.			
2. Practiced hand hygiene.			
3. Knocked before entering the room.			
4. Introduced yourself using your name and title. Explained that you worked with the licensed nursing staff and would be providing care.			
5. Greeted the patient and confirmed the patient's identification.			
6. Addressed the patient as Mr., Mrs., or Ms. and the last name.			
7. Explained the procedure in simple terms and asked permission to perform the procedure.			
8. Assembled the necessary equipment.			

The Procedure

	S	U	Comments
9. Provided privacy to the patient.			
10. Raised the bed to hip height and locked the wheels.			
11. Raised and secured side rails on the opposite side of the bed from where you would be working.			
12. Placed the lotion bottle in a basin of warm water.			
13. Ensured the room was a comfortable temperature and dimmed the lights.			
14. Covered the patient with a bath blanket and asked the patient to hold it in place while you fanfolded the bed linens at the foot of the bed.			
15. Moved the patient into the prone or a side-lying position.			
16. Exposed the patient's back, but kept the rest of the body covered.			
17. Checked the skin for signs of redness, paying special attention to the coccyx and bony areas.			
18. Poured a small amount of lotion into your palm and rubbed your hands together, using friction to warm the lotion.			
19. Stood with knees slightly bent and back straight while applying the warm lotion to the patient's back.			
20. Made small circular motions with your palms, stroked upward on both sides of the spine, applied pressure away from the spine, and moved your hands from the sacral area up to the back of the neck.			
21. Used firm, smooth strokes across and around the shoulders before moving down the upper arms.			
22. Moved hands from the shoulders down the sides of the back to the buttocks using a circular motion.			
23. Repeated the procedure for three to five minutes, using more lotion as needed.			
24. Completed the back rub by providing long, gentle strokes up from the lower back to the base of the neck and down again several times.			
25. Removed any excess lotion and patted the patient's skin dry with a bath towel.			
26. Closed or changed the patient's clothing, removed the bath blanket, and straightened the linens.			

Date of Completion: _____ Instructor's Initials: _____

	S	U	Comments
27. Ensured the bed wheels were locked and bed was in low position before repositioning the patient.	_____	_____	_____
28. Raised or lowered bed side rails according to plan of care.	_____	_____	_____
29. Removed, cleaned, and stored equipment properly.	_____	_____	_____
30. Removed soiled linens and discarded disposable equipment.	_____	_____	_____

Follow-Up

31. Practiced hand hygiene.	_____	_____	_____
32. Ensured patient comfort and placed the call light and personal items within reach.	_____	_____	_____
33. Conducted a safety check before leaving the room.	_____	_____	_____
34. Practiced hand hygiene.	_____	_____	_____

Reporting and Documentation

35. Communicated any concerns to the licensed nursing staff.	_____	_____	_____
36. Documented care provided in the chart or EMR.	_____	_____	_____

Date of Completion: _____ Instructor's Initials: _____

Name: _____ Date: _____

Preparation	S	U	Comments
1. Consulted the licensed nursing staff or plan of care for special instructions and precautions.			
2. Practiced hand hygiene.	___	___	___
3. Knocked before entering the room.	___	___	___
4. Introduced yourself using your name and title. Explained that you worked with the licensed nursing staff and would be providing care.	___	___	___
5. Greeted the patient and confirmed the patient's identification.	___	___	___
6. Addressed the patient as Mr., Mrs., or Ms. and the last name.	___	___	___
7. Explained the procedure in simple terms and asked permission to perform the procedure.	___	___	___
8. Assembled the necessary equipment.	___	___	___

The Procedure	S	U	Comments
9. Provided privacy to the patient.	___	___	___
10. Raised the bed to hip height and locked the wheels.	___	___	___
11. Raised and secured side rails on the opposite side of the bed from where you would be working.	___	___	___
12. Practiced hand hygiene and put on disposable gloves.	___	___	___
13. Loosened and pulled the bed linens from under the mattress, letting them hang.	___	___	___
14. Fanfolded the bedspread and blanket to the foot of the bed, but left the top sheet covering the patient.	___	___	___
15. Placed the bath blanket over the top sheet, had the patient hold it while you pulled the top sheet out from under the bath blanket, and:			
A. fanfolded the top sheet to the foot of the bed if you would not be changing the bed linens	___	___	___
B. placed the soiled top sheet in the laundry hamper if you would be changing the bed linens	___	___	___
16. Kept the patient covered as you removed the gown and put it in the laundry basket.	___	___	___
17. Filled the washbasin with warm water and ensured the water was a suitable temperature.	___	___	___
18. Covered the overbed table with a hand towel and placed the washbasin atop it with the washcloths and towels in reach.	___	___	___
19. Positioned the patient on the side of the bed closest to you in Fowler's position with a dry towel across the chest, under the chin, and under the head.	___	___	___
20. Made a bath mitt with a washcloth and wet it using only water unless the patient requested soap.	___	___	___
21. Washed each eye from the inner to outer corner using a different, clean part of the mitt for each swipe and kept soap away from the patient's eyes.	___	___	___
21. Wiped the entire face, ears, and neck with a new bath mitt, rinsed off any soap used, and patted dry with a towel.	___	___	___
22. Supported the farther arm while washing the shoulder, axilla, arm, hand, and fingers with a clean bath mitt; washed the axilla thoroughly; rinsed; and dried well.	___	___	___

Date of Completion: _____ Instructor's Initials:_____

	S	U	Comments
23. Applied deodorant unless otherwise directed.	_____	_____	_____
24. Applied and gently massaged lotion onto the patient's arm and hand, unless otherwise directed.	_____	_____	_____
25. Covered the bath towel with a bath blanket before removing the towel.	_____	_____	_____
26. Lowered the bed, raised the side rails, and gave the patient the call light.	_____	_____	_____
27. Emptied, rinsed, and refilled the washbasin two-thirds full of warm water and ensured the water temperature was suitable before placing the washbasin on the overbed table.	_____	_____	_____
28. Placed a dry towel under the leg farthest from you and ensured the genitalia were not exposed.	_____	_____	_____
29. Supported the leg and thigh while you washed, rinsed, and dried them.	_____	_____	_____
30. Applied lotion according to plan of care using gentle, circular motions.	_____	_____	_____
31. Washed, rinsed, dried, and applied lotion to the leg nearest you, covering both legs afterward.	_____	_____	_____
32. Exposed the foot and thigh nearest you, bent the knee, and placed the washbasin on top of a towel near the exposed foot.	_____	_____	_____
33. Supported the knee, placed the patient's foot in the washbasin, used a bath mitt to wash and clean the toes and toenails, rinsed, and dried the foot well.	_____	_____	_____
34. Applied lotion accordion to plan of care using gentle, circular motions and avoided the space between the toes.	_____	_____	_____
35. Washed, rinsed, dried, and applied lotion to the other foot.	_____	_____	_____
36. Removed the washbasin and towel and covered the patient with the bath blanket.	_____	_____	_____
37. Lowered the bed, raised the side rails, and gave the patient the call light.	_____	_____	_____
38. Placed any soiled linens in the laundry hamper.	_____	_____	_____
39. Emptied, rinsed, and refilled the washbasin two-thirds full of warm water and ensured the water temperature was suitable.	_____	_____	_____
40. Assisted the patient into a side-lying position with back and buttocks exposed, placing a towel lengthwise next to the patient's back.	_____	_____	_____
41. Washed, rinsed, and dried the back of the neck, back, and buttocks.	_____	_____	_____
42. Gave the patient a back rub following proper procedure.	_____	_____	_____
43. Assisted the patient onto the back with a towel under the buttocks and upper legs.	_____	_____	_____
44. Lowered the bed, raised the side rails, and gave the patient the call light.	_____	_____	_____
45. Emptied, rinsed, and refilled the washbasin two-thirds full of warm water and ensured the water temperature was suitable.	_____	_____	_____
46. Provided the patient a clean, soapy washcloth to clean the genital area or performed perineal care.	_____	_____	_____
47. Assisted with dressing.	_____	_____	_____
48. Ensured the bed wheels were locked and bed was in low position before repositioning the patient.	_____	_____	_____
49. Raised or lowered bed side rails according to plan of care.	_____	_____	_____
50. Removed, cleaned, and stored equipment properly.	_____	_____	_____
51. Removed soiled linens and discarded disposable equipment.	_____	_____	_____

Date of Completion: _____   Instructor's Initials:_____

Follow-Up	**S**	**U**	**Comments**
52. Removed and discarded your gloves.	_____	_____	_____
53. Practiced hand hygiene.	_____	_____	_____
54. Ensured patient comfort and placed the call light and personal items within reach.	_____	_____	_____
55. Conducted a safety check before leaving the room.	_____	_____	_____
56. Practiced hand hygiene.	_____	_____	_____
Reporting and Documentation			
57. Communicated any concerns to the licensed nursing staff.	_____	_____	_____
58. Documented care provided in the chart or EMR.	_____	_____	_____

Date of Completion: _____   Instructor's Initials:_____

Name: _____ Date: _____

Procedure: Providing Assistance with Hair Care

Preparation

		S	U	Comments

Preparation

1. Consulted the licensed nursing staff or plan of care for special instructions and precautions.
2. Practiced hand hygiene.
3. Knocked before entering the room.
4. Introduced yourself using your name and title. Explained that you worked with the licensed nursing staff and would be providing care.
5. Greeted the patient and confirmed the patient's identification.
6. Addressed the patient as Mr., Mrs., or Ms. and the last name.
7. Explained the procedure in simple terms and asked permission to perform the procedure.
8. Assembled the necessary equipment.

The Procedure

9. Provided privacy to the patient.
10. Raised the bed to hip height and locked the wheels.
11. Raised and secured side rails on the opposite side of the bed from where you would be working.
12. Practiced hand hygiene and put on disposable gloves.
13. Combed, brushed, or used your fingers to gently remove tangles from the patient's hair.
14. Covered the ear canals with a cotton ball or gauze bandage.
15. Loosened the patient's gown at the neck, helped into a supine position, and lowered the head of the bed.
16. Covered the patient with a bath blanket and fanfolded the top linens to the foot of the bed without exposing the patient.
17. Removed the pillow from under the patient's head and placed the head on the bed.
18. Placed a disposable protective pad or plastic trash bag and then a towel on the bed beneath the patient's head and upper body.
19. Placed the pillow with a waterproof cover under the shoulders and a bath towel around the head and shoulders.
20. Slid the shampoo tray or basin under the patient's head and ensured the basin tubing was connected to the catch basin.
21. Placed a protective pad on the floor near the head of the bed and set the catch basin atop it.
22. Placed a washcloth over the patient's eyes.
23. Ensured the water was a suitable temperature, used a pitcher to pour enough water to wet the hair, and refilled the pitcher as needed.
24. Formed a lather with your hands and massaged shampoo into the patient's scalp, working outward and from front to back.
25. Rinsed the hair thoroughly from the hairline and down the strands using warm water from the pitcher.
26. Applied and rinsed conditioner, if appropriate.
27. Removed, discarded, and replaced your gloves.
28. Dried the patient's forehead, ears, and neck with a clean towel and removed cotton or gauze from both ear canals.

Date of Completion: _____ Instructor's Initials: _____

	S	U	Comments
29. Removed the shampoo basin, ensured there was a dry towel under the patient's head, and raised the head of the bed.	_____	_____	_____
30. Dried the patient's hair by blotting, not rubbing.	_____	_____	_____
31. Parted the hair into sections and combed each using downward motions from underneath, if the hair was wet.	_____	_____	_____
32. Brushed the hair slowly and gently if dry and not tangled.	_____	_____	_____
33. Styled the patient's hair and used a hair dryer, if permitted.	_____	_____	_____
34. Removed all equipment and used towels.	_____	_____	_____
35. Assisted with changing the patient's gown if it got wet.	_____	_____	_____
36. Removed the bath blanket and replaced the linens.	_____	_____	_____
37. Removed the waterproof cover, put on a clean pillowcase, and put the pillow under the patient's head.	_____	_____	_____
38. Ensured the bed wheels were locked and bed was in low position before repositioning the patient.	_____	_____	_____
39. Raised or lowered bed side rails according to plan of care.	_____	_____	_____
40. Removed, cleaned, and stored equipment properly.	_____	_____	_____
41. Cleaned the brush and comb appropriately and let them air-dry before storing them.	_____	_____	_____
42. Removed soiled linens and discarded disposable equipment.	_____	_____	_____

Follow-Up

	S	U	Comments
43. Removed and discarded your gloves.	_____	_____	_____
44. Practiced hand hygiene.	_____	_____	_____
45. Ensured patient comfort and placed the call light and personal items within reach.	_____	_____	_____
46. Conducted a safety check before leaving the room.	_____	_____	_____
47. Practiced hand hygiene.	_____	_____	_____

Reporting and Documentation

	S	U	Comments
48. Communicated any concerns to the licensed nursing staff.	_____	_____	_____
49. Documented care provided in the chart or EMR.	_____	_____	_____

Date of Completion: _____   Instructor's Initials:_____

Name: _____ Date: _____

	S	U	Comments

Preparation

1. Consulted the licensed nursing staff or plan of care for special instructions and precautions.

2. Practiced hand hygiene.

3. Knocked before entering the room.

4. Introduced yourself using your name and title. Explained that you worked with the licensed nursing staff and would be providing care.

5. Greeted the patient and confirmed the patient's identification.

6. Addressed the patient as Mr., Mrs., or Ms. and the last name.

7. Explained the procedure in simple terms and asked permission to perform the procedure.

8. Assembled the necessary equipment.

The Procedure

9. Provided privacy to the patient.

10. Assisted the patient to a chair and positioned the overbed table comfortably with the necessary equipment and linens so the patient could brush the teeth.

11. Raised the bed to hip height and locked the wheels, if the patient would remain in bed during the procedure.

12. Raised and secured side rails on the opposite side of the bed from where you would be working.

13. Raised the head of the bed and ensured sufficient lighting.

14. Practiced hand hygiene and put on disposable gloves.

15. Protected the patient's clothing and linens by spreading a towel across the chest.

16. Mixed water and mouthwash in a disposable cup using a spoon or tongue blade, had the patient swish a mouthful of the mixture, held the emesis basin under the patient's chin for spitting the mixture, and wiped the mouth and chin dry.

17. Wet the toothbrush in a disposable cup half-filled with water and put toothpaste on the wet toothbrush.

18. Allowed the patient to brush the teeth, if able.

19. Brushed teeth from the back of the mouth forward using gentle, circular motions; cleaned the inside surfaces of the front teeth holding the brush vertically and using up-and-down strokes; and brushed the tongue.

20. Had the patient spit toothpaste and excess saliva into the emesis basin during brushing.

21. Helped the patient rinse the mouth using the mouthwash solution or fresh water and wiped the mouth after.

22. Allowed the patient to floss, if able.

23. Put on a mask, cut an 18-inch long piece of floss, wrapped the ends around your middle fingers and stretched tight, inserted the floss between each pair of teeth, and slid the floss across both sides of each tooth.

24. Discarded the floss and offered the patient the mouthwash solution or fresh water to rinse the mouth.

Date of Completion: _____ Instructor's Initials: _____

	S	U	Comments

25. Ensured the bed wheels were locked and bed was in low position before repositioning the patient.

26. Raised or lowered bed side rails according to plan of care. _____ _____ _____

27. Removed, cleaned, and stored equipment properly. _____ _____ _____

28. Removed soiled linens and discarded disposable equipment. _____ _____ _____

Follow-Up

29. Removed and discarded your gloves. _____ _____ _____

30. Practiced hand hygiene. _____ _____ _____

31. Ensured patient comfort and placed the call light and personal items within reach. _____ _____ _____

32. Conducted a safety check before leaving the room. _____ _____ _____

33. Practiced hand hygiene. _____ _____ _____

Reporting and Documentation

34. Communicated any concerns to the licensed nursing staff. _____ _____ _____

35. Documented care provided in the chart or EMR. _____ _____ _____

Date of Completion: _____ Instructor's Initials:_____

Name: _____   Date: _____

	S	U	Comments

Preparation

1. Consulted the licensed nursing staff or plan of care for special instructions and precautions.
2. Practiced hand hygiene.
3. Knocked before entering the room.
4. Introduced yourself using your name and title. Explained that you worked with the licensed nursing staff and would be providing care.
5. Greeted the patient and confirmed the patient's identification.
6. Addressed the patient as Mr., Mrs., or Ms. and the last name.
7. Explained the procedure in simple terms and asked permission to perform the procedure.
8. Assembled the necessary equipment.

The Procedure

9. Provided privacy to the patient.
10. Assisted the patient to a chair and positioned the overbed table with the necessary equipment and linens atop it so the patient may clean the dentures.
11. Raised the bed to hip height and locked the wheels, if the patient would remain in bed during the procedure.
12. Raised and secured side rails on the opposite side of the bed from where you would be working.
13. Raised the head of the bed.
14. Practiced hand hygiene and put on disposable gloves.
15. Protected the patient's clothing and linens by spreading a towel across the chest.
16. Placed a washcloth in the bottom of the emesis basin.
17. Asked the patient to remove dentures and place them in the emesis basin.
18. If removing dentures, grasped each denture with gauze, eased the upper denture downward and forward and the lower denture upward and forward, and removed each from the mouth.
19. Placed the dentures in the emesis basin atop the washcloth and took the basin and necessary equipment to the sink.
20. Cleaned the patient's oral cavity with oral swabs and half-strength mouthwash for full dentures.
21. Placed a washcloth in the bottom of the clean sink; did not put the dentures in the sink.
22. Took a denture out of the basin, applied toothpaste or denture cleaner, wet the toothbrush in running water, held the denture in your palm low in the sink, brushed all surfaces until clean, and rinsed thoroughly.
23. Repeated the procedure for the other denture.
24. Placed the dentures in the labeled denture cup with cool water, mouthwash, or denture solution and left the covered cup on the bedside table and within reach.
25. Ensured dentures were moist, if reinserting, and either instructed the patient to reinsert the dentures or assisted with reinsertion.
26. Removed and discarded your gloves.

Date of Completion: _____   Instructor's Initials: _____

	S	U	Comments

27. Practiced hand hygiene and put on a new pair of gloves.

28. Ensured the bed wheels were locked and bed was in low position before repositioning the patient.

29. Raised or lowered bed side rails according to plan of care.

30. Removed, cleaned, and stored equipment properly.

31. Disinfected the emesis basin.

32. Removed soiled linens and discarded disposable equipment.

Follow-Up

33. Removed and discarded your gloves.

34. Practiced hand hygiene.

35. Ensured patient comfort and placed the call light and personal items within reach.

36. Conducted a safety check before leaving the room.

37. Practiced hand hygiene.

Reporting and Documentation

38. Communicated any concerns to the licensed nursing staff.

39. Documented care provided in the chart or EMR.

Date of Completion: _____ Instructor's Initials: _____

Name: _____ Date: _____

Procedure: Providing Fingernail Care

	S	U	Comments
Preparation			
1. Consulted the licensed nursing staff or plan of care for special instructions and precautions.	____	____	_____
2. Practiced hand hygiene.	____	____	_____
3. Knocked before entering the room.	____	____	_____
4. Introduced yourself using your name and title. Explained that you worked with the licensed nursing staff and would be providing care.	____	____	_____
5. Greeted the patient and confirmed the patient's identification.	____	____	_____
6. Addressed the patient as Mr., Mrs., or Ms. and the last name.	____	____	_____
7. Explained the procedure in simple terms and asked permission to perform the procedure.	____	____	_____
8. Assembled the necessary equipment.	____	____	_____
The Procedure			
9. Provided privacy to the patient.	____	____	_____
10. Assisted the patient to a chair and positioned the overbed table with the necessary equipment and linens atop it so the patient may care for the fingernails.			
A. Assisted the patient as needed.	____	____	_____
B. Offered the patient a finger and hand massage afterward.	____	____	_____
11. Raised the bed to hip height and locked the wheels, if the patient would remain in bed during the procedure.	____	____	_____
12. Raised and secured side rails on the opposite side of the bed from where you would be working.	____	____	_____
13. Raised the head of the bed.	____	____	_____
14. Practiced hand hygiene and put on disposable gloves.	____	____	_____
15. Placed a washbasin of warm water on the overbed table in front of the patient, ensured the water was a suitable temperature, and added a small amount of soap.	____	____	_____
16. Helped the patient position the fingers in the washbasin, covered the basin and the patient's hands with a dry hand towel, and supported the wrists with a rolled-up towel.	____	____	_____
17. Soaked the patient's fingernails for 5–10 minutes, adding more warm water if needed.	____	____	_____
18. Washed the patient's hands and fingernails, pushed the cuticles back, and cleaned under each nail with an orangewood stick, wiping the stick clean after each nail.	____	____	_____
19. Removed the washbasin and dried the patient's hands.	____	____	_____
20. Cut each fingernail straight across with a nail clipper.	____	____	_____
21. Shaped and smoothed the fingernails with an emery board.	____	____	_____
22. Applied lotion, gently massaged the fingers and hands, and removed excess lotion with a towel.	____	____	_____
23. Ensured the bed wheels were locked and bed was in low position before repositioning the patient.	____	____	_____
24. Raised or lowered bed side rails according to plan of care.	____	____	_____
25. Removed, cleaned, and stored equipment properly.	____	____	_____
26. Disinfected the nail clippers.	____	____	_____
27. Removed soiled linens and discarded disposable equipment.	____	____	_____

Date of Completion: _____ Instructor's Initials: _____

Follow-Up   S   U   **Comments**

28. Removed and discarded your gloves.

29. Practiced hand hygiene.   _____ _____ _____

30. Ensured patient comfort and placed the call light and personal   _____ _____ _____
    items within reach.

31. Conducted a safety check before leaving the room.   _____ _____ _____

32. Practiced hand hygiene.   _____ _____ _____

Reporting and Documentation   _____ _____ _____

33. Communicated any concerns to the licensed nursing staff.

34. Documented care provided in the chart or EMR.   _____ _____ _____

                                                                    _____ _____ _____

Date of Completion: _____   Instructor's Initials:_____

Procedure: Providing Foot Care ▶ Video

	S	U	Comments
Preparation			
1. Consulted the licensed nursing staff or plan of care for special instructions and precautions.	_____	_____	_____
2. Practiced hand hygiene.	_____	_____	_____
3. Knocked before entering the room.	_____	_____	_____
4. Introduced yourself using your name and title. Explained that you worked with the licensed nursing staff and would be providing care.	_____	_____	_____
5. Greeted the patient and confirmed the patient's identification.	_____	_____	_____
6. Addressed the patient as Mr., Mrs., or Ms. and the last name.	_____	_____	_____
7. Explained the procedure in simple terms and asked permission to perform the procedure.	_____	_____	_____
8. Assembled the necessary equipment.	_____	_____	_____
The Procedure			
9. Provided privacy to the patient.	_____	_____	_____
10. Assisted the patient to a chair and positioned a disposable protective pad in front of the chair.	_____	_____	_____
11. Raised the bed to hip height and locked the wheels, if the patient would remain in bed during the procedure.	_____	_____	_____
12. Raised and secured side rails on the opposite side of the bed from where you would be working.	_____	_____	_____
13. Raised the head of the bed.	_____	_____	_____
14. Practiced hand hygiene and put on disposable gloves.	_____	_____	_____
15. Placed a washbasin or foot bath of warm water on top of the protective pad, ensured the water was a suitable temperature, and added a small amount of soap.	_____	_____	_____
16. Helped the patient position feet in the washbasin or foot bath; soaked one foot at a time for the patient in bed or both feet together for the patient in a chair.	_____	_____	_____
17. Ensured the feet were completely covered with water and covered the feet and washbasin with a dry hand towel.	_____	_____	_____
18. Soaked the feet for 10–15 minutes.	_____	_____	_____
19. Lifted, washed, and rinsed one foot at a time, paying attention to the area between the toes and under the fingernails.	_____	_____	_____
20. Pushed the cuticles back gently.	_____	_____	_____
21. Removed the washbasin or foot bath and dried the feet, especially between the toes.	_____	_____	_____
22. Cut the toenails with a nail clipper.	_____	_____	_____
23. Shaped and smoothed any rough toenail edges with an emery board.	_____	_____	_____
24. Applied and massaged lotion on the tops and soles of the feet, avoided the area between the toes, and removed any excess lotion with a towel.	_____	_____	_____
25. Removed and discarded your gloves, practiced hand hygiene, and put on a new pair of gloves.	_____	_____	_____
26. Ensured the bed wheels were locked and bed was in low position before repositioning the patient.	_____	_____	_____

Date of Completion: _____ Instructor's Initials:_____

	S	U	Comments
27. Raised or lowered bed side rails according to plan of care.			
28. Removed, cleaned, and stored equipment properly.	___	___	_____
29. Disinfected the nail clippers.	___	___	_____
30. Removed soiled linens and discarded disposable equipment.	___	___	_____

Follow-Up

31. Removed and discarded your gloves.	___	___	_____
32. Practiced hand hygiene.	___	___	_____
33. Ensured patient comfort and placed the call light and personal items within reach.	___	___	_____
34. Conducted a safety check before leaving the room.	___	___	_____
35. Practiced hand hygiene.	___	___	_____

Reporting and Documentation

36. Communicated any concerns to the licensed nursing staff.	___	___	_____
37. Documented care provided in the chart or EMR.	___	___	_____

Date of Completion: _____   Instructor's Initials:_____

Procedure: Providing Female Perineal Care ▶ Video

Preparation	S	U	Comments
1. Consulted the licensed nursing staff or plan of care for special instructions and precautions.	____	____	_____
2. Practiced hand hygiene.	____	____	_____
3. Knocked before entering the room.	____	____	_____
4. Introduced yourself using your name and title. Explained that you worked with the licensed nursing staff and would be providing care.	____	____	_____
5. Greeted the patient and confirmed the patient's identification.	____	____	_____
6. Addressed the patient as Mr., Mrs., or Ms. and the last name.	____	____	_____
7. Explained the procedure in simple terms and asked permission to perform the procedure.	____	____	_____
8. Assembled the necessary equipment.	____	____	_____

The Procedure

	S	U	Comments
9. Provided privacy to the patient.	____	____	_____
10. Raised the bed to hip height and locked the wheels.	____	____	_____
11. Raised and secured side rails on the opposite side of the bed from where you would be working.	____	____	_____
12. Practiced hand hygiene and put on disposable gloves.	____	____	_____
13. Positioned the patient on her back and placed a disposable protective pad under her buttocks.	____	____	_____
14. Covered the patient with a bath blanket and asked her to hold it in place while you fanfolded the bed linens at the foot of the bed.	____	____	_____
15. Offered the patient a bedpan, emptied the contents, and washed the bedpan after use.	____	____	_____
16. Removed and discarded your gloves.	____	____	_____
17. Practiced hand hygiene and put on a new pair of gloves.	____	____	_____
18. Filled a washbasin with warm water and ensured the water was a suitable temperature.	____	____	_____
19. Asked the patient to bend her knees and separate her legs.	____	____	_____
20. Moved the linens down to the foot of the bed, exposing only the perineal area and keeping the legs covered.	____	____	_____
21. Wet a washcloth in the washbasin and applied a small amount of soap.	____	____	_____
22. Separated the labia and washed the inner and outer folds using single, downward strokes from top to bottom or front to back.	____	____	_____
23. Turned the washcloth to a clean side or replaced it with each downward stroke and avoided placing fingers on an area after washing it.	____	____	_____
24. Used a new washcloth with a small amount of soap to clean down the center from the clitoris to the anus.	____	____	_____
25. Replaced the water in the washbasin and changed your gloves, if needed.	____	____	_____
26. Rinsed the area using fresh water and a clean washcloth and patted the area dry with a towel.	____	____	_____
27. Turned the patient onto her side away from you.	____	____	_____
28. Lifted the upper buttock; washed the anal area using a wet, soapy washcloth and gentle front-to-back strokes from vagina to anus; rinsed; and patted the area dry.	____	____	_____

Date of Completion: _____ Instructor's Initials: _____

	S	U	Comments
29. Repositioned the patient on her back.			
30. Removed and disposed of the protective pad and your gloves.	_____	_____	_____
31. Practiced hand hygiene and put on a new pair of gloves.	_____	_____	_____
32. Replaced the top covers and removed the bath blanket.	_____	_____	_____
33. Ensured the bed wheels were locked and bed was in low position before repositioning the patient.	_____	_____	_____
34. Raised or lowered bed side rails according to plan of care.	_____	_____	_____
35. Removed, cleaned, and stored equipment properly.	_____	_____	_____
36. Removed soiled linens and discarded disposable equipment.	_____	_____	_____

Follow-Up

	S	U	Comments
37. Removed and discarded your gloves.	_____	_____	_____
38. Practiced hand hygiene.	_____	_____	_____
39. Ensured patient comfort and placed the call light and personal items within reach.	_____	_____	_____
40. Conducted a safety check before leaving the room.	_____	_____	_____
41. Practiced hand hygiene.	_____	_____	_____

Reporting and Documentation

	S	U	Comments
42. Communicated any concerns to the licensed nursing staff.	_____	_____	_____
43. Documented care provided in the chart or EMR.	_____	_____	_____

Date of Completion: _____ Instructor's Initials:_____

Procedure: Providing Male Perineal Care ▶ Video

Preparation

	S	U	Comments

1. Consulted the licensed nursing staff or plan of care for special instructions and precautions.

2. Practiced hand hygiene.

3. Knocked before entering the room.

4. Introduced yourself using your name and title. Explained that you worked with the licensed nursing staff and would be providing care.

5. Greeted the patient and confirmed the patient's identification.

6. Addressed the patient as Mr., Mrs., or Ms. and the last name.

7. Explained the procedure in simple terms and asked permission to perform the procedure.

8. Assembled the necessary equipment.

The Procedure

9. Provided privacy to the patient.

10. Raised the bed to hip height and locked the wheels.

11. Raised and secured side rails on the opposite side of the bed from where you would be working.

12. Practiced hand hygiene and put on disposable gloves.

13. Positioned the patient on his back and placed a disposable protective pad under his buttocks.

14. Covered the patient with a bath blanket and asked him to hold it in place while you fanfolded the bed linens at the foot of the bed.

15. Offered the patient a bedpan or urinal, emptied the contents, and washed the bedpan or urinal after use.

16. Removed and discarded your gloves.

17. Practiced hand hygiene and put on a new pair of gloves.

18. Filled a washbasin with warm water and ensured the water was a suitable temperature.

19. Asked the patient to bend his knees and separate his legs.

20. Moved the linens down to the foot of the bed, exposing only the perineal area and keeping the legs covered.

21. Wet a washcloth in the washbasin and applied a small amount of soap.

22. Washed each side of the penis in a circular motion from tip to base.

23. Pulled back the foreskin while washing, rinsing, and drying; reported if the foreskin would not retract.

24. Washed the scrotum and inner thighs.

25. Replaced the water in the washbasin and changed your gloves, if needed.

26. Rinsed the area using fresh water and a clean washcloth and patted the area dry with a towel.

27. Turned the patient onto his side away from you.

28. Lifted the upper buttock; washed the anal area using a wet, soapy washcloth and gentle front-to-back strokes; rinsed; and patted the area dry.

29. Repositioned the patient on his back.

Date of Completion: _____   Instructor's Initials: _____

	S	U	Comments
30. Removed and disposed of the protective pad and your gloves.	___	___	_____
31. Practiced hand hygiene and put on a new pair of gloves.	___	___	_____
32. Replaced the top covers and removed the bath blanket.	___	___	_____
33. Ensured the bed wheels were locked and bed was in low position before repositioning the patient.	___	___	_____
34. Raised or lowered bed side rails according to plan of care.	___	___	_____
35. Removed, cleaned, and stored equipment properly.	___	___	_____
36. Removed soiled linens and discarded disposable equipment.	___	___	_____

Follow-Up

37. Removed and discarded your gloves.	___	___	_____
38. Practiced hand hygiene.	___	___	_____
39. Ensured patient comfort and placed the call light and personal items within reach.	___	___	_____
40. Conducted a safety check before leaving the room.	___	___	_____
41. Practiced hand hygiene.	___	___	_____

Reporting and Documentation

42. Communicated any concerns to the licensed nursing staff.	___	___	_____
43. Documented care provided in the chart or EMR.	___	___	_____

Date of Completion: _____ Instructor's Initials: _____

Procedure: Dressing and Undressing ▶️ Video

	S	U	Comments
Preparation			
1. Consulted the licensed nursing staff or plan of care for special instructions and precautions.	___	___	_____
2. Practiced hand hygiene.	___	___	_____
3. Knocked before entering the room.	___	___	_____
4. Introduced yourself using your name and title. Explained that you worked with the licensed nursing staff and would be providing care.	___	___	_____
5. Greeted the patient and confirmed the patient's identification.	___	___	_____
6. Addressed the patient as Mr., Mrs., or Ms. and the last name.	___	___	_____
7. Explained the procedure in simple terms and asked permission to perform the procedure.	___	___	_____
8. Assembled the necessary equipment.	___	___	_____
9. Provided privacy to the patient.	___	___	_____
10. Raised the bed to hip height and locked the wheels, if the patient would remain in bed during the procedure.	___	___	_____
11. Raised and secured side rails on the opposite side of the bed from where you would be working.	___	___	_____
12. Assisted the patient into a Fowler's position, a chair, or a sitting position at the edge of the bed.	___	___	_____
13. Raised the head of the bed to a comfortable height.	___	___	_____
14. Covered the patient with a bath blanket and fanfolded the top linens to the foot of the bed without exposing the patient.	___	___	_____
The Procedure: Dressing			
15. Asked the patient to put arms through the bra straps, place breasts in the breast cups, and lean forward while you secured her bra in the back.	___	___	_____
16. If the upper garment opened in the back, you:			
A. slipped the clothing over the arm of the patient's weak side first	___	___	_____
B. positioned it on the shoulders	___	___	_____
C. closed the garment and any fasteners	___	___	_____
17. If the upper garment opened in the front, you:			
A. slid the clothing over the arm and shoulder of the patient's weak side first	___	___	_____
B. brought the garment around the back	___	___	_____
C. asked the patient to lower the head to easily slide the stronger arm through the garment	___	___	_____
D. closed the garment and any fasteners	___	___	_____
18. If the upper garment slipped over the head, you:			
A. put the neck of the garment over the patient's head	___	___	_____
B. slid the weaker arm and shoulder into the garment	___	___	_____
C. raised the patient's head and shoulders and pulled the garment toward the waist	___	___	_____
D. slid the arm and shoulder of the stronger arm through the garment	___	___	_____
E. closed any fasteners	___	___	_____

Date of Completion: _____   Instructor's Initials:_____

	S	U	Comments

19. To put on the patient's lower garments, you:

    A. started with the weaker side first

    B. slid the patient's underwear and then pants over the feet and up the legs

    C. asked the patient to bend at the knees and lift the buttocks off the bed

    D. grasped the top of the garment with both hands and slid the garment up toward the waist

    E. closed any fasteners

20. Pulled the patient's socks or stockings over each foot and adjusted the length until smooth.

21. Put on the patient's footwear, if leaving bed.

22. Replaced top bed linens and discarded the bath blanket, if the patient was staying in bed.

23. Ensured the bed wheels were locked and bed was in low position before repositioning the patient.

24. Raised or lowered bed side rails according to plan of care.

The Procedure: Undressing

25. Raised the patient's head and shoulders or turned the patient slightly to the side away from you and undid any fasteners.

26. Removed the clothing from the patient's arms and pulled upper garments that opened in the back or front to the patient's sides.

27. If the upper garment slipped over the head, brought the clothing up to the neck and removed over the head.

28. Removed the patient's socks, stockings, and footwear.

29. Removed the patient's belt, undid any fasteners, and asked the patient to lift the buttocks.

30. Grasped the top of the lower garment, slid the pants down the legs, and removed the pants from the stronger leg first, asking the patient to roll from side to side.

31. Replaced top bed linens and discarded the bath blanket.

32. Ensured the bed wheels were locked and bed was in low position before repositioning the patient.

33. Raised or lowered bed side rails according to plan of care.

Follow-Up

34. Practiced hand hygiene.

35. Ensured patient comfort and placed the call light and personal items within reach.

36. Conducted a safety check before leaving the room.

37. Practiced hand hygiene.

Reporting and Documentation

38. Communicated any concerns to the licensed nursing staff.

39. Documented care provided in the chart or EMR.

Date of Completion: _____ Instructor's Initials: _____

Name: _____ Date: _____

	S	U	Comments

Procedure: Changing a Hospital Gown with an IV Catheter

Preparation

1. Consulted the licensed nursing staff or plan of care for special instructions and precautions. _____ _____ _____

2. Practiced hand hygiene. _____ _____ _____

3. Knocked before entering the room. _____ _____ _____

4. Introduced yourself using your name and title. Explained that you worked with the licensed nursing staff and would be providing care. _____ _____ _____

5. Greeted the patient and confirmed the patient's identification. _____ _____ _____

6. Addressed the patient as Mr., Mrs., or Ms. and the last name. _____ _____ _____

7. Explained the procedure in simple terms and asked permission to perform the procedure. _____ _____ _____

8. Assembled the necessary equipment. _____ _____ _____

The Procedure

9. Provided privacy to the patient. _____ _____ _____

10. Raised the bed to hip height and locked the wheels. _____ _____ _____

11. Raised and secured side rails on the opposite side of the bed from where you would be working. _____ _____ _____

12. Practiced hand hygiene and put on disposable gloves. _____ _____ _____

13. Assisted the patient into Fowler's position and raised the head of the bed based on patient comfort. _____ _____ _____

14. Covered the patient with a bath blanket and fanfolded the top linens to the foot of the bed. _____ _____ _____

15. Undid the gown fasteners or ties, freed the gown from underneath the body, and slipped the gown down the patient's arms while the bath blanket stayed in place. _____ _____ _____

16. Removed the gown from the arm without the IV catheter and tubing first, moved the gown across the chest, and laid it next to the other arm. _____ _____ _____

17. Gathered the sleeve, slid the gown over the IV site and tubing, and carefully removed the patient's arm and hand from the sleeve. _____ _____ _____

18. Kept the sleeve gathered and slid your hand along the tubing to the IV bag, removed the IV bag from the IV pole, and did not disconnect the IV tubing. _____ _____ _____

19. Slid the IV bag and tubing through the sleeve and hung the IV bag back on the pole. _____ _____ _____

20. Gathered the sleeve of a clean gown, removed the IV bag from the pole, slipped the gathered sleeve over the IV bag and tubing, and slid the gown up the arm and onto the shoulder. _____ _____ _____

21. Put the patient's opposite arm through the other sleeve and fastened the gown. _____ _____ _____

22. Replaced top bed linens and discarded the bath blanket. _____ _____ _____

23. Ensured the bed wheels were locked and bed was in low position before repositioning the patient. _____ _____ _____

24. Raised or lowered bed side rails according to plan of care. _____ _____ _____

25. Removed, cleaned, and stored equipment properly. _____ _____ _____

26. Removed soiled linens and discarded disposable equipment. _____ _____ _____

Date of Completion: _____ Instructor's Initials: _____

Follow-Up

                                                 S   **U**   **Comments**

27. Removed and discarded your gloves.

28. Practiced hand hygiene.

29. Ensured patient comfort and placed the call light and personal items within reach.

30. Conducted a safety check before leaving the room.

31. Practiced hand hygiene.

Reporting and Documentation

32. Communicated any concerns to the licensed nursing staff.

33. Documented care provided in the chart or EMR.

Date of Completion: _____ Instructor's Initials: _____

Name: _____ Date: _____

Procedure: Using Warm, Moist Compresses

	S	U	Comments

Preparation

1. Consulted the licensed nursing staff or plan of care for special instructions and precautions. _____ _____ _____

2. Practiced hand hygiene. _____ _____ _____

3. Knocked before entering the room. _____ _____ _____

4. Introduced yourself using your name and title. Explained that you worked with the licensed nursing staff and would be providing care. _____ _____ _____

5. Greeted the patient and confirmed the patient's identification. _____ _____ _____

6. Addressed the patient as Mr., Mrs., or Ms. and the last name. _____ _____ _____

7. Explained the procedure in simple terms and asked permission to perform the procedure. _____ _____ _____

8. Assembled the necessary equipment. _____ _____ _____

The Procedure

9. Provided privacy to the patient. _____ _____ _____

10. Raised the bed to hip height and locked the wheels. _____ _____ _____

11. Raised and secured side rails on the opposite side of the bed from where you would be working. _____ _____ _____

12. Positioned the patient properly, placed a disposable protective pad under the body part, and covered the patient with the bath blanket. _____ _____ _____

13. Filled a washbasin with warm water and ensured the water was a suitable temperature. _____ _____ _____

14. Practiced hand hygiene and put on disposable gloves. _____ _____ _____

15. Used a washcloth or gauze pad as a compress, placed it in the warm water, and squeezed out any excess moisture. _____ _____ _____

16. Observed the application site for inflammation and redness, alerted the licensed nursing staff of any concerns, and proceeded only by direction. _____ _____ _____

17. Noted the time you applied the compress; covered it with plastic wrap and a bath towel; and secured the towel with ties, tape, or rolled gauze. _____ _____ _____

18. Placed the call light, personal items, and a glass of fresh water within reach. _____ _____ _____

19. Ensured the bed wheels were locked and bed was in low position before repositioning the patient. _____ _____ _____

20. Raised or lowered bed side rails according to plan of care and unscreened the patient or opened the door to the room. _____ _____ _____

21. Removed and discarded your gloves. _____ _____ _____

22. Practiced hand hygiene. _____ _____ _____

23. Checked on the patient every five minutes and ended the treatment after 20 minutes unless otherwise ordered. _____ _____ _____

24. Raised the bed to hip height and locked the wheels when the compress was to be removed. _____ _____ _____

25. Raised and secured side rails on the opposite side of the bed from where you would be working. _____ _____ _____

26. Practiced hand hygiene and put on disposable gloves. _____ _____ _____

27. Noted the time while carefully removing the compress and observed the patient's response. _____ _____ _____

Date of Completion: _____ Instructor's Initials: _____

	S	U	Comments
28. Appropriately discarded the compress, removed the protective pad, and changed any wet linens.			
29. Assisted with any further treatment as instructed.	____	____	_____
30. Ensured the bed wheels were locked and bed was in low position before repositioning the patient.	____	____	_____
31. Raised or lowered bed side rails according to plan of care.	____	____	_____
32. Removed, cleaned, and stored equipment properly.	____	____	_____
33. Removed soiled linens and discarded disposable equipment.	____	____	_____

Follow-Up

	S	U	Comments
34. Removed and discarded your gloves.	____	____	_____
35. Practiced hand hygiene.	____	____	_____
36. Ensured patient comfort and placed the call light and personal items within reach.	____	____	_____
37. Conducted a safety check before leaving the room.	____	____	_____
38. Practiced hand hygiene.	____	____	_____

Reporting and Documentation

	S	U	Comments
39. Communicated any concerns to the licensed nursing staff.	____	____	_____
40. Documented care provided in the chart or EMR.	____	____	_____

Date of Completion: _____ Instructor's Initials:_____

Name: _____ Date: _____

Procedure: Using Warm Soaks

	S	U	Comments

Preparation

1. Consulted the licensed nursing staff or plan of care for special instructions and precautions. _____ _____ _____
2. Practiced hand hygiene. _____ _____ _____
3. Knocked before entering the room. _____ _____ _____
4. Introduced yourself using your name and title. Explained that you worked with the licensed nursing staff and would be providing care. _____ _____ _____
5. Greeted the patient and confirmed the patient's identification. _____ _____ _____
6. Addressed the patient as Mr., Mrs., or Ms. and the last name. _____ _____ _____
7. Explained the procedure in simple terms and asked permission to perform the procedure. _____ _____ _____
8. Assembled the necessary equipment. _____ _____ _____

The Procedure

9. Provided privacy to the patient. _____ _____ _____
10. Raised the bed to hip height and locked the wheels. _____ _____ _____
11. Raised and secured side rails on the opposite side of the bed from where you would be working. _____ _____ _____
12. Practiced hand hygiene and put on disposable gloves. _____ _____ _____
13. Positioned the patient and body part for the procedure. _____ _____ _____
14. Covered the patient with a bath blanket. _____ _____ _____
15. Filled a washbasin with warm water and ensured the water was a suitable temperature. _____ _____ _____
16. Put a disposable protective pad under the washbasin. _____ _____ _____
17. Noted the time while placing the affected body part in the warm water and padded the edge of the washbasin with a towel. _____ _____ _____
18. Placed the call light, personal items, and a glass of fresh water within reach. _____ _____ _____
19. Ensured the bed wheels were locked and bed was in low position. _____ _____ _____
20. Raised or lowered bed side rails according to plan of care and unscreened the patient or opened the door to the room. _____ _____ _____
21. Ensured all safety precautions were in place if the patient was sitting in a chair or at the edge of the bed. _____ _____ _____
22. Removed and discarded your gloves. _____ _____ _____
23. Practiced hand hygiene. _____ _____ _____
24. Checked on the patient every five minutes, ended the treatment after 15–20 minutes unless otherwise ordered, and refreshed the water to maintain warmth. _____ _____ _____
25. Raised the bed to hip height and locked the wheels when the soak was complete. _____ _____ _____
26. Raised and secured side rails on the opposite side of the bed from where you would be working. _____ _____ _____
27. Practiced hand hygiene and put on disposable gloves. _____ _____ _____
28. Noted the time while removing the body part from the water and patted it dry with a towel. _____ _____ _____
29. Assisted with any further treatment as instructed. _____ _____ _____

Date of Completion: _____ Instructor's Initials: _____

	S	U	Comments
30. Discarded the water and protective pad and changed any wet linens.			
31. Ensured the bed wheels were locked and bed was in low position before repositioning the patient.	___	___	_____
32. Raised or lowered bed side rails according to plan of care.	___	___	_____
33. Removed, cleaned, and stored equipment properly.	___	___	_____
34. Removed soiled linens and discarded disposable equipment.	___	___	_____

Follow-Up

	S	U	Comments
35. Removed and discarded your gloves.			
36. Practiced hand hygiene.	___	___	_____
37. Ensured patient comfort and placed the call light and personal items within reach.	___	___	_____
38. Conducted a safety check before leaving the room.	___	___	_____
39. Practiced hand hygiene.	___	___	_____

Reporting and Documentation

	S	U	Comments
40. Communicated any concerns to the licensed nursing staff.	___	___	_____
41. Documented care provided in the chart or EMR.	___	___	_____

Date of Completion: _____   Instructor's Initials: _____

Name: _____ Date: _____

Procedure: Using Cold, Moist Compresses

	S	U	Comments
Preparation			
1. Consulted the licensed nursing staff or plan of care for special instructions and precautions.	_____	_____	_____
2. Practiced hand hygiene.	_____	_____	_____
3. Knocked before entering the room.	_____	_____	_____
4. Introduced yourself using your name and title. Explained that you worked with the licensed nursing staff and would be providing care.	_____	_____	_____
5. Greeted the patient and confirmed the patient's identification.	_____	_____	_____
6. Addressed the patient as Mr., Mrs., or Ms. and the last name.	_____	_____	_____
7. Explained the procedure in simple terms and asked permission to perform the procedure.	_____	_____	_____
8. Assembled the necessary equipment.	_____	_____	_____
The Procedure			
9. Provided privacy to the patient.	_____	_____	_____
10. Raised the bed to hip height and locked the wheels.	_____	_____	_____
11. Raised and secured side rails on the opposite side of the bed from where you would be working.	_____	_____	_____
12. Positioned the patient and body part for the procedure.	_____	_____	_____
13. Placed a disposable protective pad under the body part and covered the patient with a bath blanket.	_____	_____	_____
14. Poured cold water from a small basin into a large basin with ice.	_____	_____	_____
15. Used a washcloth or gauze pad as a compress, placed it in the cold water, and squeezed out any excess moisture.	_____	_____	_____
16. Noted the time while applying the compress and wrapped it with a towel, working as quickly as possible.	_____	_____	_____
17. Changed the compress frequently and continued treatment for the ordered amount of time.	_____	_____	_____
18. Appropriately discarded each compress, removed the protective pad, and changed any wet linens.	_____	_____	_____
19. Assisted with any further treatment as instructed.	_____	_____	_____
20. Ensured the bed wheels were locked and bed was in low position before repositioning the patient.	_____	_____	_____
21. Raised or lowered bed side rails according to plan of care.	_____	_____	_____
22. Removed, cleaned, and stored equipment properly.	_____	_____	_____
23. Removed soiled linens and discarded disposable equipment.	_____	_____	_____
Follow-Up			
24. Practiced hand hygiene.	_____	_____	_____
25. Ensured patient comfort and placed the call light and personal items within reach.	_____	_____	_____
26. Conducted a safety check before leaving the room.	_____	_____	_____
27. Practiced hand hygiene.	_____	_____	_____
Reporting and Documentation			
28. Communicated any concerns to the licensed nursing staff.	_____	_____	_____
29. Documented care provided in the chart or EMR.	_____	_____	_____

Date of Completion: _____ Instructor's Initials: _____

Name: _____ Date: _____

Procedure: Using Ice Packs

Preparation

	S	U	Comments
1. Consulted the licensed nursing staff or plan of care for special instructions and precautions.			
2. Practiced hand hygiene.	___	___	_____
3. Knocked before entering the room.	___	___	_____
4. Introduced yourself using your name and title. Explained that you worked with the licensed nursing staff and would be providing care.	___	___	_____
5. Greeted the patient and confirmed the patient's identification.	___	___	_____
6. Addressed the patient as Mr., Mrs., or Ms. and the last name.	___	___	_____
7. Explained the procedure in simple terms and asked permission to perform the procedure.	___	___	_____
8. Assembled the necessary equipment.	___	___	_____

The Procedure

	S	U	Comments
9. Provided privacy to the patient.	___	___	_____
10. Raised the bed to hip height and locked the wheels.	___	___	_____
11. Raised and secured side rails on the opposite side of the bed from where you would be working.	___	___	_____
12. Positioned the patient and body part for the procedure.	___	___	_____
13. Placed a disposable protective pad under the body part and covered the patient with a bath blanket.	___	___	_____
14. If you not using a disposable cold pack, you:			
A. filled an ice pack halfway with ice using a spoon, cup, or ice scooper	___	___	_____
B. squeezed the pack to remove excess air	___	___	_____
C. placed a cap or stopper on the pack tightly	___	___	_____
D. dried the ice pack with a towel	___	___	_____
E. placed it in its cover	___	___	_____
15. Noted the time while applying the pack and secured it with ties, tape, or rolled gauze.	___	___	_____
16. Ensured the bed wheels were locked and bed was in low position.	___	___	_____
17. Raised or lowered bed side rails according to plan of care and unscreened the patient or opened the door to the room.	___	___	_____
18. Ensured all safety precautions were in place if the patient was sitting in a chair or at the edge of the bed.	___	___	_____
19. Checked on the patient every five minutes, ended the treatment after 20 minutes unless otherwise ordered, and changed the pack if the ice started melting.	___	___	_____
20. Raised the bed to hip height and locked the wheels when the application was to be removed.	___	___	_____
21. Raised and secured side rails on the opposite side of the bed from where you would be working.	___	___	_____
22. Noted the time while removing the ice pack and patted the body part dry with a towel.	___	___	_____
23. Assisted with any further treatment as instructed.	___	___	_____
24. Discarded the water and protective pad and changed any wet linens.	___	___	_____

Date of Completion: _____ Instructor's Initials: _____

Name: _____   Date: _____

	S	U	Comments

25. Ensured the bed wheels were locked and bed was in low position before repositioning the patient. _____ _____ _____

26. Raised or lowered bed side rails according to plan of care. _____ _____ _____

27. Removed, cleaned, and stored equipment properly. _____ _____ _____

28. Removed soiled linens and discarded disposable equipment. _____ _____ _____

Follow-Up

29. Practiced hand hygiene. _____ _____ _____

30. Ensured patient comfort and placed the call light and personal items within reach. _____ _____ _____

31. Conducted a safety check before leaving the room. _____ _____ _____

32. Practiced hand hygiene. _____ _____ _____

Reporting and Documentation

33. Communicated any concerns to the licensed nursing staff. _____ _____ _____

34. Documented care provided in the chart or EMR. _____ _____ _____

Date of Completion: _____   Instructor's Initials:_____

Name: _____ Date: _____

Procedure: Assisting with Meals in the Room ▶ Video

Preparation

	S	U	Comments
1. Consulted the licensed nursing staff or plan of care for special instructions and precautions.			
2. Practiced hand hygiene.			
3. Knocked before entering the room.			
4. Introduced yourself using your name and title. Explained that you worked with the licensed nursing staff and would be providing care.			
5. Greeted the patient and confirmed the patient's identification.			
6. Addressed the patient as Mr., Mrs., or Ms. and the last name.			
7. Explained the procedure in simple terms and asked permission to perform the procedure.			
8. Assembled the necessary equipment.			

The Procedure

	S	U	Comments
9. Provided privacy to the patient.			
10. Raised the bed to hip height and locked the wheels.			
11. Raised and secured side rails on the opposite side of the bed from where you would be working.			
12. Positioned the patient lying in bed, sitting at the edge of the bed, or sitting in a chair.			
13. Assisted with dressing and provided before-meal hygiene.			
14. Cleared the overbed table, checked the name on the tray, and ensured all appropriate foods were there and represented the correct diet.			
15. Covered the patient's chest with a cloth or paper clothing protector.			
16. Sat at eye level next to the patient, prepared the meal tray, and helped as needed.			
17. Arranged finger foods within the patient's reach, described foods to patients with poor eyesight, helped the patient locate food by describing in terms of a clock face, and named each mouthful of food as you offered it.			
18. Fed a weak patient or patient with paralysis on the strong side.			
19. Alternated between solid foods and liquids, offered liquids frequently between bites, did not rush feeding, and served food in order of patient preference.			
20. Allowed the patient enough time for chewing and swallowing, encouraged the patient to swallow twice between each bite, and checked that the mouth was empty before offering more food or fluids.			
21. Provided a straw for each liquid.			
22. Encouraged the patient to eat as much as possible with verbal cues, demonstrations, hand-over-hand guidance, or praise.			
23. Wiped the patient's hands, face, and mouth during and after the meal and discarded the napkin when done.			
24. Removed the meal tray and observed intake, asking the patient for explanation.			
25. Provided privacy and post-meal hygiene.			

Date of Completion: _____ Instructor's Initials:_____

	S	U	Comments
26. Recorded the amount of food eaten according to facility policy and notified the licensed nursing staff if less than two-thirds of the meal was eaten.	_____	_____	_____
27. Ensured the bed wheels were locked and bed was in low position before repositioning the patient.	_____	_____	_____
28. Raised or lowered bed side rails according to plan of care.	_____	_____	_____
29. Took the used meal tray to the meal cart.	_____	_____	_____
30. Removed, cleaned, and stored equipment properly.	_____	_____	_____
31. Removed soiled linens and discarded disposable equipment.	_____	_____	_____

Follow-Up

	S	U	Comments
32. Practiced hand hygiene.	_____	_____	_____
33. Ensured patient comfort and placed the call light and personal items within reach.	_____	_____	_____
34. Conducted a safety check before leaving the room.	_____	_____	_____
35. Practiced hand hygiene.	_____	_____	_____

Reporting and Documentation

	S	U	Comments
36. Communicated any concerns to the licensed nursing staff.	_____	_____	_____
37. Documented care provided in the chart or EMR.	_____	_____	_____

Date of Completion: _____   Instructor's Initials: _____

Name: _____ Date: _____

	S	U	Comments
Preparation			
1. Consulted the licensed nursing staff or plan of care for special instructions and precautions.			
2. Practiced hand hygiene.			
3. Knocked before entering the room.			
4. Introduced yourself using your name and title. Explained that you worked with the licensed nursing staff and would be providing care.			
5. Greeted the patient and confirmed the patient's identification.			
6. Addressed the patient as Mr., Mrs., or Ms. and the last name.			
7. Explained the procedure in simple terms and asked permission to perform the procedure.			
8. Assembled the necessary equipment.			
The Procedure: Measuring Oral Fluid Intake			
9. Provided privacy to the patient.			
10. Practiced hand hygiene.			
11. Noted the amount of liquid the patient was served, poured remaining liquid into a measuring cup or graduate, and measured the amount left in each leveled container.			
12. Subtracted each amount measured from the full amount the patient was served, noted the amount the patient actually drank, added all amounts to get total intake, and recorded this total on the I&O form.			
13. Asked the licensed nursing staff who was responsible for measuring intake from IV fluids or tubes.			
The Procedure: Measuring Urinary Output			
14. Provided privacy to the patient.			
15. Practiced hand hygiene and put on disposable gloves.			
16. If the patient was ambulatory, you:			
A. placed a urinary hat in the commode or toilet and instructed the patient to urinate into it			
B. asked the patient not to put toilet paper into the commode or toilet			
C. provided a bag or waste container for toilet paper			
D. asked the patient not to remove the urinary hat			
E. instructed the patient to use the call light when the urinary hat was ready to be emptied			
17. Used a urinal, bedpan, or urinary catheter with a drainage bag to collect fluids from a patient in bed.			
18. If using a urinary drainage bag, you:			
A. placed a protective pad with a graduate atop it on the floor beneath the drainage bag			
B. cleaned the tubing with an antiseptic wipe			
C. opened the drain at the bottom of the bag to empty urine into the graduate			
D. ensured the urine did not splash and the drainage tube did not touch the sides of the graduate			
E. closed the drain and cleaned it according to facility policy			
F. replaced the drain in the holder on the drainage bag			

Date of Completion: _____ Instructor's Initials: _____

Procedural

	S	U	Comments

19. If using a bedpan or urinal, you:
    A. placed a paper towel on a level surface and set a graduate on top _____ _____ _____
    B. poured the urine into the graduate carefully _____ _____ _____
    C. measured the amount at eye level _____ _____ _____
    D. made note of the amount in the graduate _____ _____ _____
20. Noted the color, odor, clarity, or presence of any particles in the urine. _____ _____ _____
21. Disposed of urine in the toilet, avoiding splashes. _____ _____ _____
22. Rinsed the graduate and poured the rinse water into the toilet. _____ _____ _____
23. Asked the licensed nursing staff who was responsible for measuring all other output. _____ _____ _____
24. Removed, cleaned, and stored equipment properly. _____ _____ _____
25. Removed soiled linens and discarded disposable equipment. _____ _____ _____
26. Removed and discarded your gloves. _____ _____ _____
27. Practiced hand hygiene. _____ _____ _____
28. Recorded the output amount on the I&O form and the total output amount at the end of your shift or as ordered. _____ _____ _____
29. Ensured the bed wheels were locked and bed was in low position before repositioning the patient. _____ _____ _____
30. Raised or lowered bed side rails according to plan of care. _____ _____ _____

Follow-Up

31. Ensured patient comfort and placed the call light and personal items within reach. _____ _____ _____
32. Conducted a safety check before leaving the room. _____ _____ _____
33. Practiced hand hygiene. _____ _____ _____

Reporting and Documentation

34. Communicated any concerns to the licensed nursing staff. _____ _____ _____
35. Documented care provided in the chart or EMR. _____ _____ _____

tion: _____ Instructor's Initials:_____

g Assistant

Name: _____ Date: _____

Procedure: Assisting to a Toilet

	S	U	Comments

Preparation

1. Consulted the licensed nursing staff or plan of care for special instructions and precautions. _____ _____ _____

2. Practiced hand hygiene. _____ _____ _____

3. Knocked before entering the room. _____ _____ _____

4. Introduced yourself using your name and title. Explained that you worked with the licensed nursing staff and would be providing care. _____ _____ _____

5. Greeted the patient and confirmed the patient's identification. _____ _____ _____

6. Addressed the patient as Mr., Mrs., or Ms. and the last name. _____ _____ _____

7. Explained the procedure in simple terms and asked permission to perform the procedure. _____ _____ _____

8. Assembled the necessary equipment. _____ _____ _____

The Procedure

9. Provided privacy to the patient. _____ _____ _____

10. Raised the bed to hip height and locked the wheels. _____ _____ _____

11. Raised and secured side rails on the opposite side of the bed from where you would be working. _____ _____ _____

12. Practiced hand hygiene and put on disposable gloves. _____ _____ _____

13. Helped the patient dangle at the edge of the bed and put on robe and slippers. _____ _____ _____

14. Helped the patient to the bathroom, using a gait belt if necessary. _____ _____ _____

15. Removed and adjusted the patient's clothing so the patient could sit comfortably on the toilet, using a seat extension if needed. _____ _____ _____

16. If the patient was on I&O, you:

    A. placed a urinary hat in the toilet _____ _____ _____

    B. instructed the patient to discard any toilet paper in the provided bag or waste container _____ _____ _____

    C. asked the patient not to flush the toilet _____ _____ _____

17. Stayed with the patient if needed. _____ _____ _____

18. If the patient could be left alone, you:

    A. placed the toilet paper and call light within reach _____ _____ _____

    B. instructed the patient to use the call light once finished _____ _____ _____

    C. removed and discarded your gloves and practiced hand hygiene before leaving the patient _____ _____ _____

    D. returned to the room upon signal or within five minutes _____ _____ _____

    E. practiced hand hygiene and put on disposable gloves _____ _____ _____

19. Assisted with wiping and perineal care, as needed. _____ _____ _____

20. Removed and discarded your gloves. _____ _____ _____

21. Practiced hand hygiene and put on a new pair of gloves. _____ _____ _____

22. Helped the patient put on a new gown and undergarments. _____ _____ _____

23. Assisted the patient with hand hygiene. _____ _____ _____

24. Helped the patient back to bed and removed robe and slippers. _____ _____ _____

25. Ensured the bed wheels were locked and bed was in low position before repositioning the patient. _____ _____ _____

Date of Completion: _____ Instructor's Initials:_____

Procedu

	S	U	Comments

26. Raised or lowered bed side rails according to plan of care. _____ _____ _____

27. Returned to the bathroom; observed the urine for color, odor, and clarity; and checked stool for unusual appearance or odor. _____ _____ _____

28. Measured urinary output or any liquid stool and recorded it properly, if the patient was on I&O. _____ _____ _____

29. Recorded any bowel movements appropriately. _____ _____ _____

30. Emptied the urinary hat into the toilet, rinsed it, poured the rinse water into the toilet, and flushed. _____ _____ _____

31. Cleaned, dried, and stored the urinary hat properly. _____ _____ _____

Follow-Up

32. Removed and discarded your gloves. _____ _____ _____

33. Practiced hand hygiene. _____ _____ _____

34. Ensured patient comfort and placed the call light and personal items within reach. _____ _____ _____

35. Conducted a safety check before leaving the room. _____ _____ _____

36. Practiced hand hygiene. _____ _____ _____

Reporting and Documentation

37. Communicated any concerns to the licensed nursing staff. _____ _____ _____

38. Documented care provided in the chart or EMR. _____ _____ _____

Instructor's Initials:_____

ssistant

Name: _____ Date: _____

Procedure: Assisting to a Bedside Commode

Preparation

	S	U	Comments
1. Consulted the licensed nursing staff or plan of care for special instructions and precautions.			
2. Practiced hand hygiene.			
3. Knocked before entering the room.			
4. Introduced yourself using your name and title. Explained that you worked with the licensed nursing staff and would be providing care.			
5. Greeted the patient and confirmed the patient's identification.			
6. Addressed the patient as Mr., Mrs., or Ms. and the last name.			
7. Explained the procedure in simple terms and asked permission to perform the procedure.			
8. Assembled the necessary equipment.			

The Procedure

	S	U	Comments
9. Provided privacy to the patient.			
10. Raised the bed to hip height and locked the wheels.			
11. Raised and secured side rails on the opposite side of the bed from where you would be working.			
12. Practiced hand hygiene and put on disposable gloves.			
13. Helped the patient dangle at the edge of the bed, removed the patient's undergarments, and put on robe and slippers.			
14. Helped the patient to the commode using a gait belt if needed and ensured any clothing was out of the way.			
15. Asked the patient to discard toilet paper in the provided bag or waste container if the patient was on I&O.			
16. Stayed with the patient if needed.			
17. If the patient could be left alone, you:			
A. placed the toilet paper and call light within reach			
B. instructed the patient to use the call light once finished			
C. removed and discarded your gloves and practiced hand hygiene before leaving the patient			
D. returned to the room upon signal or within five minutes			
E. practiced hand hygiene and put on disposable gloves			
18. Assisted with wiping and perineal care and covered the commode.			
19. Removed and discarded your gloves.			
20. Practiced hand hygiene and put on a new pair of gloves.			
21. Helped the patient back to bed, removed robe and slippers, and changed the patient's gown and undergarments.			
22. Filled a washbasin with warm water and ensured the water was a suitable temperature.			
23. Placed the washbasin and some towels on the bedside stand and assisted the patient with hand hygiene.			
24. Removed the washbasin and used towels and straightened or changed bed linens.			
25. Ensured the bed wheels were locked and bed was in low position before repositioning the patient.			

Date of Completion: _____ Instructor's Initials:_____

Procedu

Name: _____   Date: _____

	S	U	Comments

26. Raised or lowered bed side rails according to plan of care.

27. Took the container from the commode into the bathroom; observed the urine for color, odor, and clarity; and checked stool for unusual appearance or odor.

28. Measured urinary output or any liquid stool and recorded it properly, if the patient was on I&O.

29. Recorded any bowel movements appropriately.

30. Emptied the container's contents into the toilet, rinsed it, poured the rinse water into the toilet, and flushed.

31. Cleaned, dried, and stored the commode properly.

Follow-Up

32. Removed and discarded your gloves.

33. Practiced hand hygiene.

34. Ensured patient comfort and placed the call light and personal items within reach.

35. Conducted a safety check before leaving the room.

36. Practiced hand hygiene.

Reporting and Documentation

37. Communicated any concerns to the licensed nursing staff.

38. Documented care provided in the chart or EMR.

Instructor's Initials: _____

ssistant

Name: _____ Date: _____

Procedure: Assisting with a Standard or Fracture Bedpan ▶ Video

Preparation	S	U	Comments
1. Consulted the licensed nursing staff or plan of care for special instructions and precautions.	_____	_____	_____
2. Practiced hand hygiene.	_____	_____	_____
3. Knocked before entering the room.	_____	_____	_____
4. Introduced yourself using your name and title. Explained that you worked with the licensed nursing staff and would be providing care.	_____	_____	_____
5. Greeted the patient and confirmed the patient's identification.	_____	_____	_____
6. Addressed the patient as Mr., Mrs., or Ms. and the last name.	_____	_____	_____
7. Explained the procedure in simple terms and asked permission to perform the procedure.	_____	_____	_____
8. Assembled the necessary equipment.	_____	_____	_____

The Procedure

	S	U	Comments
9. Provided privacy to the patient.	_____	_____	_____
10. Raised the bed to hip height and locked the wheels.	_____	_____	_____
11. Raised and secured side rails on the opposite side of the bed from where you would be working.	_____	_____	_____
12. Practiced hand hygiene and put on disposable gloves.	_____	_____	_____
13. Folded the top linens back and raised the patient's gown, keeping it out of the way of the bedpan.	_____	_____	_____
14. Asked the patient to bend the knees with both feet flat on the mattress and raise the hips.	_____	_____	_____
15. Put a protective pad on the bed under the hips and positioned the bedpan under the buttocks.	_____	_____	_____
16. If using a standard bedpan, you:			
A. positioned it like a regular toilet seat	_____	_____	_____
B. placed the buttocks on the wide, rounded shelf	_____	_____	_____
C. ensured the open end pointed toward the foot of the bed	_____	_____	_____
17. If using a fracture bedpan, you:			
A. had the patient lift the hips	_____	_____	_____
B. faced the thin edge of the bedpan toward the head of the bed	_____	_____	_____
C. placed the bedpan under the patient's buttocks	_____	_____	_____
18. If the patient was unable to lift the hips, rolled the patient onto the side facing away from you, placed the bedpan against the buttocks, and had the patient roll back with the bedpan beneath.	_____	_____	_____
19. Covered the patient with a bath blanket, raised the head of the bed, and propped pillows behind the patient's back for comfort.	_____	_____	_____
20. Instructed the patient to discard any toilet paper in the provided bag or waste container, if on I&O.	_____	_____	_____
21. Stayed with the patient if needed.			
22. If the patient could be left alone, you:			
A. placed the toilet paper and call light within reach	_____	_____	_____
B. instructed the patient to use the call light once finished	_____	_____	_____
C. removed and discarded your gloves and practiced hand hygiene before leaving the patient	_____	_____	_____
D. returned to the room upon signal or within five minutes	_____	_____	_____
E. practiced hand hygiene and put on disposable gloves	_____	_____	_____

Date of Completion: _____ Instructor's Initials: _____

Proce

	S	U	Comments
23. Assisted with wiping and perineal care and covered the bedpan.	_____	_____	_____
24. Removed and discarded your gloves.	_____	_____	_____
25. Practiced hand hygiene and put on a new pair of gloves.	_____	_____	_____
26. Helped the patient raise the hips or roll to the side, removed the bedpan, and removed and discarded the protective pad.	_____	_____	_____
27. Covered the bedpan immediately and placed it on top of a paper towel in a secure place.	_____	_____	_____
28. Removed and discarded your gloves.	_____	_____	_____
29. Practiced hand hygiene and put on a new pair of gloves.	_____	_____	_____
30. Filled a washbasin with warm water and ensured the water was a suitable temperature.	_____	_____	_____
31. Placed the washbasin and some towels on the bedside stand and assisted the patient with hand hygiene.	_____	_____	_____
32. Removed the washbasin and used towels and discarded the towels in the laundry hamper.	_____	_____	_____
33. Changed the patient's gown and undergarments.	_____	_____	_____
34. Covered the patient with the top linens, removed the bath blanket and discarded it in the hamper, and straightened or changed the bed linens.	_____	_____	_____
35. Ensured the bed wheels were locked and bed was in low position before repositioning the patient.	_____	_____	_____
36. Raised or lowered bed side rails according to plan of care.	_____	_____	_____
37. Took the bedpan into the bathroom; observed the urine for color, odor, and clarity; and checked stool for unusual appearance or odor.	_____	_____	_____
38. Emptied the bedpan into the toilet, rinsed it, poured the rinse water into the toilet, and flushed.	_____	_____	_____
39. Cleaned, dried, and stored the bedpan properly.	_____	_____	_____
40. Removed and discarded your gloves.	_____	_____	_____
41. Practiced hand hygiene and put on a new pair of gloves.	_____	_____	_____
42. Measured urinary output or any liquid stool and recorded it properly, if the patient was on I&O.	_____	_____	_____
43. Recorded any bowel movements appropriately.	_____	_____	_____

Follow-Up

44. Ensured patient comfort and placed the call light and personal items within reach.	_____	_____	_____
45. Conducted a safety check before leaving the room.	_____	_____	_____
46. Practiced hand hygiene.	_____	_____	_____

Reporting and Documentation

47. Communicated any concerns to the licensed nursing staff.	_____	_____	_____
48. Documented care provided in the chart or EMR.	_____	_____	_____

_____   Instructor's Initials:_____

...sistant

Name: _____ Date: _____

Procedure: Assisting with a Urinal

Preparation

                                                                   S   U   Comments

1. Consulted the licensed nursing staff or plan of care for special instructions and precautions.

2. Practiced hand hygiene.

3. Knocked before entering the room.

4. Introduced yourself using your name and title. Explained that you worked with the licensed nursing staff and would be providing care.

5. Greeted the patient and confirmed the patient's identification.

6. Addressed the patient as Mr., Mrs., or Ms. and the last name.

7. Explained the procedure in simple terms and asked permission to perform the procedure.

8. Assembled the necessary equipment.

The Procedure

9. Provided privacy to the patient.

10. Raised the bed to hip height and locked the wheels.

11. Raised and secured side rails on the opposite side of the bed from where you would be working.

12. Practiced hand hygiene and put on disposable gloves.

13. Gave the patient the urinal, positioned the urinal so the penis was well inside the opening, ensured the urinal did not spill, and placed a disposable protective pad under the patient.

14. Stayed with the patient if needed.

15. If the patient could be left alone, you:

    A. placed the call light within reach

    B. instructed the patient to use the call light once finished

    C. asked the patient not to place the urinal on the overbed table or bedside stand

    D. raised or lowered side rails according to plan of care

    E. removed and discarded your gloves and practiced hand hygiene before leaving the patient

    F. returned to the room upon signal or within five minutes

    G. practiced hand hygiene and put on disposable gloves

16. Assisted with any cleansing and perineal care.

17. Removed, covered, and placed the urinal on top of a paper towel in a secure location.

18. Removed and discarded your gloves.

19. Practiced hand hygiene and put on a new pair of gloves.

20. Filled a washbasin with warm water and ensured the water was a suitable temperature.

21. Assisted the patient with hand hygiene.

22. Removed the washbasin and used towels and straightened or changed the bed linens.

23. Changed the patient's gown and undergarments.

24. Ensured the bed wheels were locked and bed was in low position before repositioning the patient.

Date of Completion: _____ Instructor's Initials: _____

Proc

Name: _____   Date: _____

	S	U	Comments

25. Raised or lowered bed side rails according to plan of care.

26. Took the urinal into the bathroom and observed the urine for color, odor, and clarity.

27. Measured urinary output or any liquid stool and recorded it properly, if the patient was on I&O.

28. Emptied the urinal's contents into the toilet, rinsed it, poured the rinse water into the toilet, and flushed.

29. Cleaned, dried, and stored the commode properly.

Follow-Up

30. Removed and discarded your gloves.

31. Practiced hand hygiene.

32. Ensured patient comfort and placed the call light and personal items within reach.

33. Conducted a safety check before leaving the room.

34. Practiced hand hygiene.

Reporting and Documentation

35. Communicated any concerns to the licensed nursing staff.

36. Documented care provided in the chart or EMR.

Instructor's Initials:_____

stant

Name: _____ Date: _____

Procedure: Providing Male Catheter Care

	S	U	Comments

Preparation

1. Consulted the licensed nursing staff or plan of care for special instructions and precautions.

2. Practiced hand hygiene.

3. Knocked before entering the room.

4. Introduced yourself using your name and title. Explained that you worked with the licensed nursing staff and would be providing care.

5. Greeted the patient and confirmed the patient's identification.

6. Addressed the patient as Mr., Mrs., or Ms. and the last name.

7. Explained the procedure in simple terms and asked permission to perform the procedure.

8. Assembled the necessary equipment.

The Procedure

9. Provided privacy to the patient.

10. Raised the bed to hip height and locked the wheels.

11. Raised and secured side rails on the opposite side of the bed from where you would be working.

12. Practiced hand hygiene and put on disposable gloves.

13. Positioned the patient on his back.

14. Covered the patient with a bath blanket and fanfolded the top linens to the foot of the bed.

15. Checked the catheter insertion area for crusting, lesions, discharge, or abnormalities and notified the licensed nursing staff if needed.

16. Placed a protective pad under the patient's buttocks.

17. Removed the applicators from the kit or prepared a washcloth and soap in a washbasin filled with warm water.

18. Applied the antiseptic solution to the entire insertion area in circular motions using the applicators or cleansed the area using a clean part of a washcloth for each stroke.

19. Pulled the foreskin back and applied antiseptic solution to the insertion site or cleaned it with a washcloth and soap.

20. Held the catheter tubing near the opening of the penis.

21. Cleaned the catheter using circular motions, started near the penis and moved down the catheter 4 inches, and used a clean part of the washcloth.

22. Patted the perineal area dry, moving from front to back.

23. Secured the catheter tubing to the upper thigh, left slack in the catheter tubing, coiled the remaining tubing, and ensured it was not bent or twisted.

24. Secured the bag to an immovable part of the bedframe away from the wheels and below the patient.

25. Discarded the disposable protective pad, covered the patient with the top linens, and removed the bath blanket.

26. Changed the patient's gown or clothing.

27. Raised or lowered bed side rails according to plan of care.

28. Removed, cleaned, and stored equipment properly.

29. Removed soiled linens and discarded disposable equipment.

Date of Completion: _____ Instructor's Initials:_____

	S	U	Comments
Follow-Up			
30. Removed and discarded your gloves.	_____	_____	_____
31. Practiced hand hygiene.	_____	_____	_____
32. Ensured patient comfort and placed the call light and personal items within reach.	_____	_____	_____
33. Conducted a safety check before leaving the room.	_____	_____	_____
34. Practiced hand hygiene.	_____	_____	_____
Reporting and Documentation			
35. Communicated any concerns to the licensed nursing staff.	_____	_____	_____
36. Documented care provided in the chart or EMR.	_____	_____	_____

Date of Completion: _____ Instructor's Initials: _____

Name: _____ Date: _____

Preparation

	S	U	Comments
1. Consulted the licensed nursing staff or plan of care for special instructions and precautions.			
2. Practiced hand hygiene.			
3. Knocked before entering the room.			
4. Introduced yourself using your name and title. Explained that you worked with the licensed nursing staff and would be providing care.			
5. Greeted the patient and confirmed the patient's identification.			
6. Addressed the patient as Mr., Mrs., or Ms. and the last name.			
7. Explained the procedure in simple terms and asked permission to perform the procedure.			
8. Assembled the necessary equipment.			

The Procedure

	S	U	Comments
9. Provided privacy to the patient.			
10. Raised the bed to hip height and locked the wheels.			
11. Raised and secured side rails on the opposite side of the bed from where you would be working.			
12. Practiced hand hygiene and put on disposable gloves.			
13. Positioned the patient on her back.			
14. Covered the patient with a bath blanket and fanfolded the top linens to the foot of the bed.			
15. Checked the catheter insertion area for crusting, lesions, discharge, or abnormalities and notified the licensed nursing staff if needed.			
16. Placed a protective pad under the patient's buttocks.			
17. Removed the applicators from the kit or prepared a washcloth and soap in a washbasin filled with warm water.			
18. Separated the labia with one gloved hand and cleansed the perineal area from front to back using a new applicator or a clean part of the washcloth for each stroke.			
19. Began at the center of the perineal area, cleansed each side, and discarded the used applicator in a plastic bag or used a clean part of the washcloth for each stroke.			
20. Held the catheter tubing near the opening of the urethra.			
21. Cleaned the catheter two to three times in a circular motion from the meatus down the catheter about 4 inches.			
22. Patted the perineal area dry, moving from front to back.			
23. Secured the catheter tubing to the upper thigh, left slack in the catheter tubing, coiled the remaining tubing, and ensured it was not bent or twisted.			
24. Secured the bag to an immovable part of the bedframe away from the wheels and below the patient.			
25. Discarded the disposable protective pad, covered the patient with the top linens, and removed the bath blanket.			
26. Changed the patient's gown or clothing.			
27. Ensured the bed wheels were locked and bed was in low position before repositioning the patient.			

Date of Completion: _____ Instructor's Initials:_____

	S	U	Comments
28. Raised or lowered bed side rails according to plan of care.	_____	_____	_____
29. Removed, cleaned, and stored equipment properly.	_____	_____	_____
30. Removed soiled linens and discarded disposable equipment.	_____	_____	_____

Follow-Up

31. Removed and discarded your gloves.	_____	_____	_____
32. Practiced hand hygiene.	_____	_____	_____
33. Ensured patient comfort and placed the call light and personal items within reach.	_____	_____	_____
34. Conducted a safety check before leaving the room.	_____	_____	_____
35. Practiced hand hygiene.	_____	_____	_____

Reporting and Documentation

36. Communicated any concerns to the licensed nursing staff.	_____	_____	_____
37. Documented care provided in the chart or EMR.	_____	_____	_____

Date of Completion: _____   Instructor's Initials: _____

Name: _____ Date: _____

Procedure: Changing a Urinary Drainage Bag

	S	U	Comments

Preparation

1. Consulted the licensed nursing staff or plan of care for special instructions and precautions.
2. Practiced hand hygiene.
3. Knocked before entering the room.
4. Introduced yourself using your name and title. Explained that you worked with the licensed nursing staff and would be providing care.
5. Greeted the patient and confirmed the patient's identification.
6. Addressed the patient as Mr., Mrs., or Ms. and the last name.
7. Explained the procedure in simple terms and asked permission to perform the procedure.
8. Assembled the necessary equipment.

The Procedure

9. Provided privacy to the patient.
10. Raised the bed to hip height and locked the wheels.
11. Raised and secured side rails on the opposite side of the bed from where you would be working.
12. Practiced hand hygiene and put on disposable gloves.
13. Positioned the patient on the back, covered the patient with a bath blanket, and fanfolded the top linens to the foot of the bed.
14. Folded the blanket to form a triangle on the side of the drainage bag and turned the triangle over to expose the catheter and drainage bag tubing.
15. Clamped the catheter to prevent urine drainage and allowed the urine below the clamp to drain into the bag.
16. Placed a protective pad under the patient's leg where the catheter and tubing connect.
17. Opened the antiseptic wipes and the package with the sterile cap and catheter plug and placed them atop paper towels on the overbed table.
18. Attached the new drainage bag to the bedframe with the tubing end on top of the protective pad.
19. Disconnected the catheter from the old drainage bag tubing without allowing anything to touch the end of the catheter and wiped the area with an antiseptic wipe if there was contact.
20. Inserted the sterile catheter plug into the end of the catheter without touching the end of the plug.
21. Placed the sterile cap on the end of the old drainage bag tubing without touching the end of the tubing.
22. Removed the cap from the end of the new drainage bag tubing and the sterile plug from the catheter.
23. Inserted the end of the new drainage bag tubing into the catheter and removed the clamp.
24. Coiled and secured the remaining tubing without twisting or bending it.
25. Removed the old drainage bag and placed it in the bedpan.
26. Discarded the disposable protective pad, covered the patient with the top linens, and removed the bath blanket.

Date of Completion: _____ Instructor's Initials:_____

	S	U	Comments
27. Ensured the bed wheels were locked and bed was in low position before repositioning the patient.	_____	_____	_____
28. Raised or lowered bed side rails according to plan of care.	_____	_____	_____
29. Took the old drainage bag and tubing into the bathroom, opened the clamp at the bottom of the bag, drained the urine into a graduate, and closed the clamp.	_____	_____	_____
30. Measured the amount of urine in the graduate and recorded it properly on the I&O form.	_____	_____	_____
31. Discarded the old drainage bag and tubing according to facility policy.	_____	_____	_____
32. Removed, cleaned, and stored equipment properly.	_____	_____	_____
33. Removed soiled linens and discarded disposable equipment.	_____	_____	_____

Follow-Up

	S	U	Comments
34. Removed and discarded your gloves.	_____	_____	_____
35. Practiced hand hygiene.	_____	_____	_____
36. Ensured patient comfort and placed the call light and personal items within reach.	_____	_____	_____
37. Conducted a safety check before leaving the room.	_____	_____	_____
38. Practiced hand hygiene.	_____	_____	_____

Reporting and Documentation

	S	U	Comments
39. Communicated any concerns to the licensed nursing staff.	_____	_____	_____
40. Documented care provided in the chart or EMR.	_____	_____	_____

Date of Completion: _____   Instructor's Initials: _____

Name: _____ Date: _____

Procedure: Inserting a Rectal Tube

	S	U	Comments

Preparation

1. Consulted the licensed nursing staff or plan of care for special instructions and precautions.

2. Practiced hand hygiene.

3. Knocked before entering the room.

4. Introduced yourself using your name and title. Explained that you worked with the licensed nursing staff and would be providing care.

5. Greeted the patient and confirmed the patient's identification.

6. Addressed the patient as Mr., Mrs., or Ms. and the last name.

7. Explained the procedure in simple terms and asked permission to perform the procedure.

8. Assembled the necessary equipment.

The Procedure

9. Provided privacy to the patient.

10. Raised the bed to hip height and locked the wheels.

11. Raised and secured side rails on the opposite side of the bed from where you would be working.

12. Practiced hand hygiene and put on disposable gloves.

13. Covered the patient with a bath blanket and fanfolded the top linens to the foot of the bed.

14. Helped the patient onto the left side and bent the right knee toward the chest in Sims' position.

15. Raised the lower corner of the blanket to expose the patient's buttocks.

16. Squeezed lubricant onto a tissue or toilet paper and rubbed the gel on the tip of the rectal tube.

17. Lifted the upper buttock to expose the anus and inserted the rectal tube 2–4 inches into the rectum.

18. Attached the tube to the buttocks according to facility policy or plan of care, reminding the patient to lie still.

19. Stayed with the patient if needed.

20. If the patient could be left alone, you:

　　A. placed the call light in reach and instructed the patient how to use it

　　B. raised or lowered side rails according to plan of care

　　C. removed and discarded your gloves and practiced hand hygiene before leaving the patient

　　D. returned to the room upon signal or after 20 minutes

　　E. practiced hand hygiene and put on disposable gloves

21. Asked if the patient was able to pass flatus and was feeling relieved and checked for drainage.

22. Removed the rectal tube slowly; cleansed the anal area from front to back using a warm, wet washcloth or cleansing wipe; and assisted with any additional hygiene.

23. Ensured the bed wheels were locked and bed was in low position before repositioning the patient.

Date of Completion: _____ Instructor's Initials:_____

	S	U	Comments
24. Raised or lowered bed side rails according to plan of care.	_____	_____	_____
25. Removed, cleaned, and stored equipment properly.	_____	_____	_____
26. Removed soiled linens and discarded disposable equipment.	_____	_____	_____

Follow-Up

27. Removed and discarded your gloves.	_____	_____	_____
28. Practiced hand hygiene.	_____	_____	_____
29. Ensured patient comfort and placed the call light and personal items within reach.	_____	_____	_____
30. Conducted a safety check before leaving the room.	_____	_____	_____
31. Practiced hand hygiene.	_____	_____	_____

Reporting and Documentation

32. Communicated any concerns to the licensed nursing staff.	_____	_____	_____
33. Documented care provided in the chart or EMR.	_____	_____	_____

Date of Completion: _____ Instructor's Initials:_____

Name: _____   Date: _____

Procedure: Inserting a Rectal Suppository

Preparation	S	U	Comments
1. Consulted the licensed nursing staff or plan of care for special instructions and precautions.			
2. Practiced hand hygiene.	___	___	_____
3. Knocked before entering the room.	___	___	_____
4. Introduced yourself using your name and title. Explained that you worked with the licensed nursing staff and would be providing care.	___	___	_____
5. Greeted the patient and confirmed the patient's identification.	___	___	_____
6. Addressed the patient as Mr., Mrs., or Ms. and the last name.	___	___	_____
7. Explained the procedure in simple terms and asked permission to perform the procedure.	___	___	_____
8. Assembled the necessary equipment.	___	___	_____

The Procedure

	S	U	Comments
9. Provided privacy to the patient.	___	___	_____
10. Raised the bed to hip height and locked the wheels.	___	___	_____
11. Raised and secured side rails on the opposite side of the bed from where you would be working.	___	___	_____
12. Practiced hand hygiene and put on disposable gloves.	___	___	_____
13. Covered the patient with a bath blanket and fanfolded the top linens to the foot of the bed.	___	___	_____
14. Helped the patient onto the left side and bent the right knee toward the chest in Sims' position.	___	___	_____
15. Unwrapped the suppository.	___	___	_____
16. Raised the lower corner of the blanket to expose the patient's buttocks and lifted the upper buttock to expose the anus.	___	___	_____
17. Applied a lubricating gel to the anus and suppository before inserting the suppository into the rectum 2 inches beyond the sphincter and wiped off any excess lubricant.	___	___	_____
18. Encouraged the patient to breathe deeply and relax until the need to have a bowel movement.	___	___	_____
19. Stayed with the patient if needed.	___	___	_____
20. If the patient could be left alone, you:			
A. placed the call light in reach and instructed the patient to use it when the need to have a bowel movement is felt	___	___	_____
B. raised or lowered the side rails according to plan of care	___	___	_____
C. removed and discarded your gloves and practiced hand hygiene before leaving the patient	___	___	_____
D. returned to the room upon signal or every five minutes	___	___	_____
E. practiced hand hygiene and put on disposable gloves	___	___	_____
21. Assisted the patient to the bathroom or commode or positioned the patient on a bedpan.	___	___	_____
22. Provided privacy, assisted back to bed, and helped with hygiene as needed.	___	___	_____
23. Ensured the bed wheels were locked and bed was in low position before repositioning the patient.	___	___	_____
24. Raised or lowered bed side rails according to plan of care.	___	___	_____

Date of Completion: _____   Instructor's Initials: _____

	S	U	Comments

25. Checked stool for unusual appearance and alerted the licensed nursing staff of any abnormalities. _____ _____ _____

26. Discarded the stool in the toilet or followed special instructions. _____ _____ _____

27. Removed, cleaned, and stored equipment properly. _____ _____ _____

28. Removed soiled linens and discarded disposable equipment. _____ _____ _____

Follow-Up

29. Removed and discarded your gloves. _____ _____ _____

30. Practiced hand hygiene. _____ _____ _____

31. Ensured patient comfort and placed the call light and personal items within reach. _____ _____ _____

32. Conducted a safety check before leaving the room. _____ _____ _____

33. Practiced hand hygiene. _____ _____ _____

Reporting and Documentation

34. Communicated any concerns to the licensed nursing staff. _____ _____ _____

35. Documented care provided in the chart or EMR. _____ _____ _____

Date of Completion: _____ Instructor's Initials: _____

Name: _____ Date: _____

Procedure: Administering a Cleansing Enema

Preparation

	S	U	Comments

1. Consulted the licensed nursing staff or plan of care for special instructions and precautions.

2. Practiced hand hygiene.

3. Knocked before entering the room.

4. Introduced yourself using your name and title. Explained that you worked with the licensed nursing staff and would be providing care.

5. Greeted the patient and confirmed the patient's identification.

6. Addressed the patient as Mr., Mrs., or Ms. and the last name.

7. Explained the procedure in simple terms and asked permission to perform the procedure.

8. Assembled the necessary equipment.

The Procedure

9. Prepared the enema solution in the bathroom or utility room.

10. Clamped the enema bag tubing, filled the bag with the ordered amount of solution, and sealed the bag.

11. Unclamped the tubing, ran a small amount of solution through the tubing, checked the temperature of the solution, clamped the tubing, and brought the bag into the room.

12. Hung the enema bag on the IV pole about 18 inches above the mattress.

13. Provided privacy to the patient.

14. Raised the bed to hip height and locked the wheels.

15. Raised and secured side rails on the opposite side of the bed from where you would be working.

16. Practiced hand hygiene and put on disposable gloves.

17. Covered the patient with a bath blanket, fanfolded the top linens to the foot of the bed, and placed a protective pad under the patient's buttocks.

18. Helped the patient onto the left side and bent the right knee toward the chest in Sims' position.

19. Raised the lower corner of the blanket to expose the patient's buttocks.

20. Lubricated the enema tubing 2–4 inches from the tip.

21. Lifted the upper buttock to expose the anus and inserted the tubing 2–4 inches into the rectum, immediately stopping and reporting if pain, resistance, or bleeding occurred.

22. Unclamped the tubing, allowed the solution to flow slowly, and instructed the patient to breathe deeply.

23. Closed the clamp before the bag was empty and when most of the solution had flowed into the rectum.

24. Held paper towel around the tubing and against the anus, withdrew the tubing slowly and wrapped the tubing in paper towels before placing it in the empty kit container.

25. Asked the patient to squeeze the buttocks to hold the solution in.

26. Assisted the patient to the bathroom, commode, or bedpan, asked the patient not to flush, stayed nearby, and ensured the call light was within reach.

Date of Completion: _____ Instructor's Initials: _____

	S	U	Comments
27. Removed and discarded your gloves.	_____	_____	_____
28. Practiced hand hygiene.	_____	_____	_____
29. Checked on the patient every few minutes.	_____	_____	_____
30. Disposed of the enema equipment according to facility policy.	_____	_____	_____
31. Practiced hand hygiene and put on a new pair of gloves.	_____	_____	_____
32. Assisted the patient back to bed and with hygiene care.	_____	_____	_____
33. Removed the protective pad and bath blanket, changed any soiled linens, and covered the patient with the top linens.	_____	_____	_____
34. Ensured the bed wheels were locked and bed was in low position before repositioning the patient.	_____	_____	_____
35. Raised or lowered bed side rails according to plan of care.	_____	_____	_____
36. Removed and discarded your gloves.	_____	_____	_____
37. Practiced hand hygiene and put on a new pair of gloves.	_____	_____	_____
38. Removed, cleaned, and stored equipment properly.	_____	_____	_____
39. Removed soiled linens and discarded disposable equipment.	_____	_____	_____

Follow-Up

40. Removed and discarded your gloves.	_____	_____	_____
41. Practiced hand hygiene.	_____	_____	_____
42. Ensured patient comfort and placed the call light and personal items within reach.	_____	_____	_____
43. Conducted a safety check before leaving the room.	_____	_____	_____
44. Practiced hand hygiene.	_____	_____	_____

Reporting and Documentation

45. Communicated any concerns to the licensed nursing staff.	_____	_____	_____
46. Documented care provided in the chart or EMR.	_____	_____	_____

Date of Completion: _____   Instructor's Initials:_____

Name: _____ Date: _____

Preparation	S	U	Comments
1. Consulted the licensed nursing staff or plan of care for special instructions and precautions.			
2. Practiced hand hygiene.			
3. Knocked before entering the room.			
4. Introduced yourself using your name and title. Explained that you worked with the licensed nursing staff and would be providing care.			
5. Greeted the patient and confirmed the patient's identification.			
6. Addressed the patient as Mr., Mrs., or Ms. and the last name.			
7. Explained the procedure in simple terms and asked permission to perform the procedure.			
8. Assembled the necessary equipment.			

The Procedure

	S	U	Comments
9. Provided privacy to the patient.			
10. Raised the bed to hip height and locked the wheels.			
11. Raised and secured side rails on the opposite side of the bed from where you would be working.			
12. Practiced hand hygiene and put on disposable gloves.			
13. Covered the patient with a bath blanket, fanfolded the top linens to the foot of the bed, and placed a protective pad under the patient's buttocks.			
14. Helped the patient onto the left side and bent the right knee toward the chest in Sims' position.			
15. Opened the box, removed the enema, and placed the solution container in warm water.			
16. Moved the linens to expose the patient's buttocks.			
17. Removed the cover from the prelubricated enema tip and gently squeezed the container to ensure the tip was open.			
18. Raised the upper buttock to expose the anus.			
19. Asked the patient to breathe deeply and inserted the enema tip 2 inches into the rectum upon exhalation.			
20. Squeezed from the bottom and rolled the container until only a small amount remained in the container.			
21. Removed the enema tip from the anus and placed the container in the box.			
22. Asked the patient to hold the solution in the rectum for 20 minutes and to alert you when the insistent urge to defecate was felt.			
23. Stayed with the patient if needed.			
24. Positioned the patient safely with the call light within reach if left alone.			
25. Discarded the enema container, removed your gloves, and practiced hand hygiene.			
26. Assisted the patient to the bathroom, commode, or bedpan, asked the patient not to flush, stayed nearby, ensured the call light was within reach, and returned when signaled.			
27. Checked on the patient every few minutes.			
28. Practiced hand hygiene and put on a new pair of gloves.			

Date of Completion: _____ Instructor's Initials: _____

	S	U	Comments
29. Assisted the patient back to bed and with hygiene care.	_____	_____	_____
30. Removed the protective pad and bath blanket, changed any soiled linens, and covered the patient with the top linens.	_____	_____	_____
31. Ensured the bed wheels were locked and bed was in low position before repositioning the patient.	_____	_____	_____
32. Raised or lowered bed side rails according to plan of care.	_____	_____	_____
33. Removed, cleaned, and stored equipment properly.	_____	_____	_____
34. Removed soiled linens and discarded disposable equipment.	_____	_____	_____

Follow-Up

35. Removed and discarded your gloves.	_____	_____	_____
36. Practiced hand hygiene.	_____	_____	_____
37. Ensured patient comfort and placed the call light and personal items within reach.	_____	_____	_____
38. Conducted a safety check before leaving the room.	_____	_____	_____
39. Practiced hand hygiene.	_____	_____	_____

Reporting and Documentation

40. Communicated any concerns to the licensed nursing staff.	_____	_____	_____
41. Documented care provided in the chart or EMR.	_____	_____	_____

Date of Completion: _____   Instructor's Initials:_____

Name: _____ Date: _____

Procedure: Providing Ostomy Care

Preparation

                                                                    S   U   Comments

1. Consulted the licensed nursing staff or plan of care for special instructions and precautions.

2. Practiced hand hygiene.   _____ _____ _____

3. Knocked before entering the room.   _____ _____ _____

4. Introduced yourself using your name and title. Explained that you worked with the licensed nursing staff and would be providing care.   _____ _____ _____

5. Greeted the patient and confirmed the patient's identification.   _____ _____ _____

6. Addressed the patient as Mr., Mrs., or Ms. and the last name.   _____ _____ _____

7. Explained the procedure in simple terms and asked permission to perform the procedure.   _____ _____ _____

8. Assembled the necessary equipment.   _____ _____ _____

The Procedure

9. Provided privacy to the patient.   _____ _____ _____

10. Raised the bed to hip height and locked the wheels.   _____ _____ _____

11. Raised and secured side rails on the opposite side of the bed from where you would be working.   _____ _____ _____

12. Practiced hand hygiene and put on disposable gloves.   _____ _____ _____

13. Positioned the patient on the back with a protective pad under the buttocks.   _____ _____ _____

14. Covered the patient with a bath blanket, fanfolded the top linens to the foot of the bed, and moved clothing to expose the stoma.   _____ _____ _____

15. Placed another protective pad alongside the patient's body and covered the patient with a bath blanket from the waist down.   _____ _____ _____

16. Removed the clamp at the bottom of the ostomy bag, let the stool drain into a graduate, ensured the drain and bag end did not touch the graduate, and avoided any splashing.   _____ _____ _____

17. Wiped the open end of the ostomy bag with an antiseptic wipe, folded the end of the bag, and clamped it shut.   _____ _____ _____

18. Noted the color, amount, consistency, and odor of the stool and measured stool and drainage appropriately if recording I&O.   _____ _____ _____

19. Emptied the stool and drainage into the toilet or bedpan.   _____ _____ _____

20. Removed and discarded your gloves.   _____ _____ _____

21. Practiced hand hygiene and put on a new pair of gloves.   _____ _____ _____

22. Disconnected the bag from the ostomy belt before removing and inspecting the belt and disposed of the belt appropriately if soiled.   _____ _____ _____

23. Removed the bag and skin barrier by gently stretching the skin and pulling the bag away, using warm water or adhesive remover if necessary.   _____ _____ _____

24. Placed the ostomy bag in a bedpan, covered it, and neutralized any odor.   _____ _____ _____

25. Wiped the stoma with a gauze pad or toilet paper to remove any stool or drainage and discarded the gauze and your gloves afterward.   _____ _____ _____

26. Practiced hand hygiene and put on a new pair of gloves.   _____ _____ _____

27. Washed the stoma and surrounding skin with a gauze pad or washcloth mitt, soap, and water or a cleansing agent.   _____ _____ _____

Date of Completion: _____ Instructor's Initials: _____

	S	U	Comments

28. Rinsed and dried the skin around the stoma. _____ _____ _____

29. Observed the stoma and surrounding skin and reported any skin irritation, breakdown, or bleeding immediately. _____ _____ _____

30. Applied the correctly sized skin barrier. _____ _____ _____

31. Positioned the clean ostomy belt, removed the adhesive backing from the ostomy bag, ensured the drain or end was pointing downward, and centered the bag over the stoma. _____ _____ _____

32. Sealed the bag to the skin by gently pressing around the edges, added deodorant, and closed the bag at the bottom using either clips or the clamp. _____ _____ _____

33. Attached the ostomy belt and ensured it was not too tight. _____ _____ _____

34. Removed the protective pads and bath blanket, changed any soiled linens, and replaced the top linens. _____ _____ _____

35. Ensured the bed wheels were locked and bed was in low position before repositioning the patient. _____ _____ _____

36. Raised or lowered bed side rails according to plan of care. _____ _____ _____

37. Removed, cleaned, and stored equipment properly. _____ _____ _____

38. Removed soiled linens and discarded disposable equipment. _____ _____ _____

Follow-Up

39. Removed and discarded your gloves. _____ _____ _____

40. Practiced hand hygiene. _____ _____ _____

41. Ensured patient comfort and placed the call light and personal items within reach. _____ _____ _____

42. Conducted a safety check before leaving the room. _____ _____ _____

43. Practiced hand hygiene. _____ _____ _____

Reporting and Documentation

44. Communicated any concerns to the licensed nursing staff. _____ _____ _____

45. Documented care provided in the chart or EMR. _____ _____ _____

Date of Completion: _____   Instructor's Initials:_____

Procedure: Bathing Infants

Preparation

	S	U	Comments
1. Consulted the licensed nursing staff or the mother for special instructions and precautions.			
2. Practiced hand hygiene.			
3. Knocked before entering the room.			
4. Introduced yourself using your name and title. Explained that you worked with the licensed nursing staff and would be providing care.			
5. Greeted the mother and confirmed the infant's identification.			
6. Explained the procedure in simple terms and asked permission to perform the procedure.			
7. Assembled the necessary equipment.			

The Procedure

	S	U	Comments
8. Provided privacy to the patient.			
9. Practiced hand hygiene.			
10. Filled the bathtub with 1–2 inches of warm water and ensured the water was a suitable temperature.			
11. Placed a towel or paper towel on a safe, flat surface; placed the bathtub atop it; and lined the bottom of the tub with a foam liner or towel.			
12. Laid a bath towel on the counter next to the tub, kept one hand on the infant at all times, undressed the infant, and laid the infant on the bath towel.			
13. Moistened a cotton ball with warm water, squeezed out the excess water, and wiped the infant's eyes and eyelids outward from nose to ears using a clean cotton ball for each eye.			
14. Lowered the infant feet first into the tub.			
15. Held the infant in an upright position with the head and chest out of the water and supported the head at all times.			
16. Wet a washcloth, put a small amount of baby shampoo on the infant's head, washed the infant's hair and scalp in a circular motion, rinsed by squeezing water from the washcloth, and ensured suds did not get into the eyes.			
17. Washed the neck and behind the ears with soap and a washcloth and rinsed.			
18. Cleaned the gums and tongue with a clean washcloth.			
19. Washed the chest, arms, hands, legs, folds, creases, and between the fingers and toes thoroughly and rinsed the washcloth and infant.			
20. Cleaned the umbilical cord with a disposable wipe or cotton ball and ensured it was dry afterward.			
21. If the infant was female, you:			
A. gently spread the labia			
B. washed from front to back			
C. used warm water and no soap			
22. If the infant was male, you:			
A. gently washed from the urethra to the scrotum with warm water			
B. avoided pulling back the foreskin if the infant was uncircumcised			
C. gently cleaned the penis with a disposable wipe or cotton ball wet with warm water and applied any ordered dressings if the infant was circumcised			

Date of Completion: _____ Instructor's Initials: _____

	S	U	Comments
23. Cleaned the anal area with soap and water and washed the back and buttocks with a clean washcloth.	_____	_____	_____
24. Lifted the infant out of the tub, wrapped in a towel, patted the infant dry, ensured that all folds and creases were dry, and kept the infant covered and warm.	_____	_____	_____
25. Trimmed the infant's nails with baby scissors or clippers right after the bath, following the natural shape for the fingernails and trimming straight across for the toenails.	_____	_____	_____
26. Applied lotion or cream to the skin.	_____	_____	_____
27. Diapered and dressed the infant and ensured safety and comfort.	_____	_____	_____
28. Removed, cleaned, and stored equipment properly.	_____	_____	_____
29. Removed soiled linens and discarded disposable equipment.	_____	_____	_____

Follow-Up

30. Practiced hand hygiene.	_____	_____	_____
31. Conducted a safety check before leaving the room.	_____	_____	_____
32. Practiced hand hygiene.	_____	_____	_____

Reporting and Documentation

33. Communicated any concerns to the licensed nursing staff.	_____	_____	_____
34. Documented care provided in the chart or EMR.	_____	_____	_____

Date of Completion: _____   Instructor's Initials:_____

Name: _____ Date: _____

Procedure: Diapering

Preparation

	S	U	Comments
1. Consulted the licensed nursing staff or the mother for special instructions and precautions.			
2. Practiced hand hygiene.	____	____	_____
3. Knocked before entering the room.	____	____	_____
4. Introduced yourself using your name and title. Explained that you worked with the licensed nursing staff and would be providing care.	____	____	_____
5. Greeted the mother and confirmed the infant's identification.	____	____	_____
6. Explained the procedure in simple terms and asked permission to perform the procedure.	____	____	_____
7. Assembled the necessary equipment.	____	____	_____

The Procedure

	S	U	Comments
8. Provided privacy to the patient.	____	____	_____
9. Practiced hand hygiene and put on disposable gloves.	____	____	_____
10. Placed a disposable protective pad under the infant and unfastened the tabs or pins of the dirty diaper.	____	____	_____
11. Wiped the perineal area from front to back with the front of the diaper, removing as much stool as possible.	____	____	_____
12. Rolled the soiled diaper so urine and stool were inside and set the diaper aside.	____	____	_____
13. Cleaned the infant with disposable wipes, cotton balls wet with soap and water, or a washcloth and checked for skin irritation, rashes, or lesions.			
14. Rinsed thoroughly and patted dry.	____	____	_____
15. Removed, discarded, and replaced your gloves.	____	____	_____
16. Cleaned the umbilical cord and the circumcision with a disposable wipe or a cotton ball wet with soap and water.	____	____	_____
17. Applied cream or lotion to the perineal area and buttocks.	____	____	_____
18. Raised the infant's legs, slid a diaper under the buttocks, and folded a cloth diaper appropriately.	____	____	_____
19. Brought the diaper up between the legs to cover the lower abdomen, ensured the diaper was snug at the hips and abdomen, and ensured the diaper was below the umbilicus if the cord stump was not yet healed.			
20. Secured the diaper with tape strips or pins and inserted pins sideways with points away from the abdomen.	____	____	_____
21. Covered a cloth diaper with a diaper cover.	____	____	_____
22. Ensured the infant was safe and comfortable.	____	____	_____
23. Rinsed stool from a cloth diaper into the toilet and stored the used diaper in a covered pail or wet bag.	____	____	_____
24. Disposed of a disposable diaper in a covered waste container.	____	____	_____
25. Removed and discarded your gloves.	____	____	_____
26. Practiced hand hygiene and put on a new pair of gloves.	____	____	_____
27. Removed, cleaned, and stored equipment properly.	____	____	_____
28. Removed soiled linens and discarded disposable equipment.	____	____	_____

Date of Completion: _____ Instructor's Initials: _____

Follow-Up   S   U   **Comments**

29. Removed and discarded your gloves.   _____   _____   _____

30. Practiced hand hygiene.   _____   _____   _____

31. Conducted a safety check before leaving the room.   _____   _____   _____

32. Practiced hand hygiene.   _____   _____   _____

Reporting and Documentation

33. Communicated any concerns to the licensed nursing staff.   _____   _____   _____

34. Documented care provided in the chart or EMR.   _____   _____   _____

Date of Completion: _____   Instructor's Initials:_____

Procedure: Clearing an Infant's Obstructed Airway

Preparation

                                                                      S   U   **Comments**

1. Practiced hand hygiene, if time permitted.

The Procedure: Infant Is Conscious

2. Observed the infant for difficulty breathing, a weak or absent cry, choking, wheezing, and inability to cough.

3. Called for help or activated the emergency system.

4. Exposed the infant's upper body, positioned the infant over your forearm facedown with the head lower than the trunk, supported the head and neck with one hand with your forearm resting on your thigh, and delivered five back blows between the infant's shoulder blades.

5. Checked for an object obstructing the airway and stopped if it was dislodged.

6. Supported the infant on your arm, turned the infant faceup with the head lower than the trunk, and used your index and middle finger to perform five chest thrusts in the midsternal region at a rate of one thrust per second.

7. Checked for an object obstructing the airway and stopped if it was dislodged.

8. Repeated steps 4 through 7 until item was dislodged or infant became unconscious.

The Procedure: Infant Is Unconscious

9. Observed the infant for difficulty breathing and called for help or activated the emergency system.

10. Placed the infant on the back and opened the airway by tilting the head and lifting the chin without hyperextending the neck.

11. Breathed in and placed your mouth over the infant's mouth and nose, forming an airtight seal; blew one small puff of air into the infant's mouth and nose; observed if the chest rose; and removed your mouth to hear or feel an exhaled breath.

12. Replaced your mouth over the infant's mouth and nose and repositioned the infant with head tilted back and chin lifted if the chest did not rise with each breath.

13. Observed for breathing, coughing, or movement in response to rescue breaths and checked the brachial pulse.

14. Performed CPR if pulse was absent:

    A. placed two fingers on the sternum just below an imaginary line between the two nipples

    B. gave 30 chest compressions to one-third the depth of the chest

    C. opened the airway by tilting the infant's head and lifting the chin without hyperextending the neck

    D. gave two breaths so the chest rose

    E. continued the cycle of 30 compressions and two breaths

    F. removed the foreign object from the infant's mouth

    G. continued CPR until the object was expelled or until medical professionals arrived

Follow-Up

15. Practiced hand hygiene.

16. Ensured the infant was safe and comfortable.

Reporting and Documentation

17. Communicated any concerns to the licensed nursing staff.

18. Documented care provided in the chart or EMR.

Date of Completion: _____ Instructor's Initials: _____

Name: _____   Date: _____

Procedure: Applying Antiembolism Stockings ▶ Video

	S	U	Comments

Preparation

1. Consulted the licensed nursing staff or plan of care for special instructions and precautions. _____ _____ _____

2. Practiced hand hygiene. _____ _____ _____

3. Knocked before entering the room. _____ _____ _____

4. Introduced yourself using your name and title. Explained that you worked with the licensed nursing staff and would be providing care. _____ _____ _____

5. Greeted the patient and confirmed the patient's identification. _____ _____ _____

6. Addressed the patient as Mr., Mrs., or Ms. and the last name. _____ _____ _____

7. Explained the procedure in simple terms and asked permission to perform the procedure. _____ _____ _____

8. Assembled the necessary equipment. _____ _____ _____

The Procedure

9. Provided privacy to the patient. _____ _____ _____

10. Raised the bed to hip height and locked the wheels. _____ _____ _____

11. Raised and secured side rails on the opposite side of the bed from where you would be working. _____ _____ _____

12. Practiced hand hygiene and put on disposable gloves. _____ _____ _____

13. Assisted the patient into a supine position, exposed one leg by fanfolding the linens toward the opposite leg, and ensured the exposed leg was dry and free from lotions, ointments, or oils. _____ _____ _____

14. Gathered or turned one stocking inside out to the heel and slipped the foot of the stocking over the patient's toes, foot, and heel. _____ _____ _____

15. Rolled the stocking up the leg to the knee or thigh and ensured proper placement. _____ _____ _____

16. Repeated steps 13–15 on the other leg. _____ _____ _____

17. Ensured the bed wheels were locked and bed was in low position before repositioning the patient. _____ _____ _____

18. Raised or lowered bed side rails according to plan of care. _____ _____ _____

Follow-Up

19. Practiced hand hygiene. _____ _____ _____

20. Ensured patient comfort and placed the call light and personal items within reach. _____ _____ _____

21. Conducted a safety check before leaving the room. _____ _____ _____

22. Practiced hand hygiene. _____ _____ _____

Reporting and Documentation

23. Communicated any concerns to the licensed nursing staff. _____ _____ _____

24. Documented care provided in the chart or EMR. _____ _____ _____

Date of Completion: _____   Instructor's Initials: _____

Name: _____ Date: _____

Procedure: Responding to Choking Using the Heimlich Maneuver

Preparation   S   U   **Comments**

1. Followed first aid guidelines and remained calm.   _____   _____   _____

2. Called or had someone else call for help.   _____   _____   _____

The Procedure: Choking—Conscious Adult or Child
(Over One Year of Age)

3. Reassured the choking person you were there to help, checked
   ability to breathe, and waited to see if coughing dislodged the object.   _____   _____   _____

4. Stood or knelt behind the choking person and wrapped your arms
   around the waist, if coughing did not dislodge the object.   _____   _____   _____

5. Made a fist with one hand, placed the thumb side against the
   abdomen slightly above the navel and well below the sternum,
   grasped your fist with your other hand, did not tuck your thumb
   inside your fist, and avoided pressing on the person's ribs with
   your forearms.   _____   _____   _____

6. Pressed forcefully into the abdomen with the thumb side of your
   fist, performed five quick inward and upward abdominal thrusts,
   and checked to see if the item was visible or expelled.   _____   _____   _____

7. Titled the person's head back and lifted the chin to open the airway,
   looked into the mouth, and grasped and removed the object if it
   was visible and reachable.   _____   _____   _____

8. Kept performing abdominal thrusts until the object could be
   removed or until the person became unconscious.   _____   _____   _____

The Procedure: Choking—Unconscious Adult or Child
(Over One Year of Age)

9. Put on disposable gloves, if available.   _____   _____   _____

10. Laid the person in a supine position, checked for a pulse, opened
    the airway by tilting the head and lifting the chin, delivered one
    breath, watched to see if chest rose, and delivered one more breath
    if the chest did not rise.   _____   _____   _____

11. Began conventional or Hands-Only™ CPR according to your level
    of training if the rescue breaths did not cause the chest to rise.   _____   _____   _____

12. Opened the airway and checked for the object after every
    30 compressions.   _____   _____   _____

13. Removed the foreign object without pushing it farther down the
    throat or continued performing CPR and checking the airway until
    the object was expelled or trained healthcare professionals arrived.   _____   _____   _____

Follow-Up

14. Reported observations and actions to the trained healthcare
    providers when they arrived, if not in a healthcare facility.   _____   _____   _____

15. Recorded the person's vital signs once the object was expelled
    and alerted the licensed nursing staff, if in a healthcare facility.   _____   _____   _____

16. Removed and discarded your gloves, if used.   _____   _____   _____

17. Practiced hand hygiene.   _____   _____   _____

18. Ensured the patient's comfort and placed the call light
    and personal items within reach.   _____   _____   _____

19. Removed, cleaned, and stored equipment properly.   _____   _____   _____

20. Removed soiled linens and discarded disposable equipment.   _____   _____   _____

21. Conducted a safety check before leaving the room.   _____   _____   _____

22. Practiced hand hygiene.   _____   _____   _____

Date of Completion: _____ Instructor's Initials: _____

Name: _____ Date: _____

Reporting and Documentation

	S	U	Comments
23. Updated a licensed nursing staff member with the person's vital signs.	_____	_____	_____
24. Communicated any concerns to the licensed nursing staff.	_____	_____	_____
25. Documented care provided in the chart or EMR.	_____	_____	_____

Date of Completion: _____ Instructor's Initials:_____

Name: _____ Date: _____

Procedure: Responding to Fainting

	S	U	Comments
Preparation			
1. Followed first aid guidelines and remained calm.	_____	_____	_____
2. Called or had someone else call for help.	_____	_____	_____
The Procedure			
3. Reassured the person that you were there to help, assisted to a safe position, helped the person sit or lie down, and did not leave the person unattended.	_____	_____	_____
4. Had the person bend forward and place the head between both knees for at least five minutes, if sitting.	_____	_____	_____
5. Placed the person on the back and raised or elevated both legs approximately 12 inches so they were above the heart, if lying down.	_____	_____	_____
6. Ensured the clothing around the person's neck, chest, and abdomen was not too tight and loosened any restrictive clothing.	_____	_____	_____
7. Lowered the person to the floor using your body as an incline if the person fainted while not lying down.	_____	_____	_____
8. Turned the person's head to the side, checked breathing and pulse, called for help, and stayed with the person.	_____	_____	_____
9. Did not let the person get up for at least five minutes after fainting and did not give the person anything to eat or drink unless directed.	_____	_____	_____
10. Did not leave the person alone as you waited for trained healthcare providers to arrive.	_____	_____	_____
Follow-Up			
11. Reported observations and actions to the trained healthcare providers when they arrived, if not in a healthcare facility.	_____	_____	_____
12. Practiced hand hygiene.	_____	_____	_____
13. Alerted the licensed nursing staff, if in a healthcare facility.	_____	_____	_____
14. Ensured the patient's comfort and placed the call light and personal items within reach.	_____	_____	_____
15. Removed, cleaned, and stored equipment properly.	_____	_____	_____
16. Removed soiled linens and discarded disposable equipment.	_____	_____	_____
17. Conducted a safety check before leaving the room.	_____	_____	_____
18. Practiced hand hygiene.	_____	_____	_____
Reporting and Documentation			
19. Communicated any concerns to the licensed nursing staff.	_____	_____	_____
20. Documented care provided in the chart or EMR.	_____	_____	_____

Date of Completion: _____   Instructor's Initials: _____

Name: _____ Date: _____

	S	U	Comments

Preparation

1. Followed first aid guidelines and remained calm.

2. Called or had someone else call for help.

The Procedure

3. Reassured the person you were there to help.

4. Did not attempt to stop the seizure and noted the time the seizure started.

5. Lowered the person to the floor using your body as an incline, if the person was not already lying down.

6. Maintained an open airway, turned the person on the side, and ensured the person's head was turned to promote drainage of any saliva or vomit.

7. Protected the head by placing something soft between it and the floor or by cradling it in your lap.

8. Loosened any tight clothing or jewelry around the neck and cleared the area of equipment or sharp objects.

9. Did not force the mouth open, put any objects or your fingers between the teeth, or attempt to restrain or control movements.

10. Noted the time the seizure ended and placed the person in a recovery position.

Follow-Up

11. Reported observations and actions to the trained healthcare providers when they arrived, if not in a healthcare facility.

12. Practiced hand hygiene.

13. Alerted the licensed nursing staff, if in a healthcare facility.

14. Ensured the patient's comfort and placed the call light and personal items within reach.

15. Removed, cleaned, and stored equipment properly.

16. Removed soiled linens and discarded disposable equipment.

17. Conducted a safety check before leaving the room.

18. Practiced hand hygiene.

Reporting and Documentation

19. Communicated any concerns to the licensed nursing staff.

20. Documented care provided in the chart or EMR.

Date of Completion: _____ Instructor's Initials:_____

Name: _____ Date: _____

Procedure: Responding to and Controlling Bleeding

	S	U	Comments

Preparation

1. Followed first aid guidelines and remained calm. _____ _____ _____

2. Called or had someone else call for help. _____ _____ _____

The Procedure: Internal Hemorrhage

3. Reassured the person you were there to help. _____ _____ _____

4. Kept the person flat, warm, and quiet. _____ _____ _____

5. Did not give the person any fluids or remove any objects that may have caused the hemorrhage. _____ _____ _____

6. Waited with the person for trained healthcare professionals to arrive. _____ _____ _____

The Procedure: External Hemorrhage

7. Reassured the person you were there to help. _____ _____ _____

8. Did not remove any objects that may have caused the hemorrhage. _____ _____ _____

9. Put on disposable gloves, if available. _____ _____ _____

10. Applied firm, steady, direct pressure to the bleeding site until the bleeding stopped. _____ _____ _____

11. Used a sterile dressing or a clean material and secured it with a bandage or tape. _____ _____ _____

12. Elevated the affected area and bound the wound when the bleeding stopped. _____ _____ _____

13. Watched for bleeding through the bandage and applied indirect pressure on a pressure point. _____ _____ _____

14. Covered the person with a blanket and did not provide anything to eat or drink. _____ _____ _____

15. Did not leave the person alone as you waited for trained healthcare providers to arrive. _____ _____ _____

Follow-Up

16. Reported observations and actions to the trained healthcare providers when they arrived, if not in a healthcare facility. _____ _____ _____

17. Practiced hand hygiene. _____ _____ _____

18. Alerted the licensed nursing staff, if in a healthcare facility. _____ _____ _____

19. Ensured the patient's comfort and placed the call light and personal items within reach. _____ _____ _____

20. Removed, cleaned, and stored equipment properly. _____ _____ _____

21. Removed soiled linens and discarded disposable equipment. _____ _____ _____

22. Conducted a safety check before leaving the room. _____ _____ _____

23. Practiced hand hygiene. _____ _____ _____

Reporting and Documentation

24. Communicated any concerns to the licensed nursing staff. _____ _____ _____

25. Documented care provided in the chart or EMR. _____ _____ _____

Date of Completion: _____ Instructor's Initials: _____

Name: _____ Date: _____

Procedure: Providing Postmortem Care

Preparation	S	U	Comments
1. Consulted the licensed nursing staff or plan of care for special instructions and precautions.	___	___	_____
2. Practiced hand hygiene.	___	___	_____
3. Knocked before entering the room.	___	___	_____
4. Introduced yourself to the deceased patient's family using your name and title. Explained that you worked with the licensed nursing staff and would be providing care.	___	___	_____
5. Confirmed the deceased patient's identification.	___	___	_____
6. Addressed the family members as Mr., Mrs., or Ms. and the last name.	___	___	_____
7. Determined if the family would stay in the room for the procedure and explained the procedure in simple terms.	___	___	_____
8. Assembled the necessary equipment.	___	___	_____

The Procedure

	S	U	Comments
9. Provided privacy to the patient.	___	___	_____
10. Raised the bed to hip height and locked the wheels.	___	___	_____
11. Raised and secured side rails on the opposite side of the bed from where you would be working.	___	___	_____
12. Practiced hand hygiene and put on disposable gloves.	___	___	_____
13. Flattened the bed, placed a pillow under the patient's head and shoulders for body alignment, and fanfolded the linens to the foot of the bed.	___	___	_____
14. Straightened the arms and legs and placed both arms at the sides.	___	___	_____
15. Undressed the patient and covered with a bath blanket.	___	___	_____
16. Grasped the eyelashes, pulled the lids down, held the eyes shut for a few seconds, and placed moistened cotton balls over the eyes if they wouldn't stay shut.	___	___	_____
17. Cleaned and inserted the patient's dentures or placed them in a labeled denture cup.	___	___	_____
18. Closed the patient's mouth, requesting instructions from the licensed nursing staff if it would not stay shut.	___	___	_____
19. Removed all jewelry except the wedding ring unless instructed otherwise and placed a cotton ball and tape over any rings left in place.	___	___	_____
20. Placed all jewelry and personal belongings into an envelope or bag and attached an identification tag.	___	___	_____
21. Emptied and replaced any drainage bags, removed tubing and appliances, and asked for guidance if the patient was wearing a prosthetic.	___	___	_____
22. Removed and discarded your gloves.	___	___	_____
23. Practiced hand hygiene and put on a new pair of gloves.	___	___	_____
24. Filled a washbasin with warm water, placed it on the overbed table, washed the patient's body, dried it thoroughly, and placed and taped gauze in any areas that needed drainage absorbed.	___	___	_____
25. Changed any wet or soiled linens and placed a disposable protective pad under the patient's buttocks.	___	___	_____
26. Put a clean gown on the patient and fixed hair if the family requested to view the patient.	___	___	_____

Date of Completion: _____ Instructor's Initials: _____

	S	U	Comments

27. Placed a pillow behind the patient's head, raised the bed to supine or Fowler's position, covered the patient's body up to the shoulders with a sheet, and did not cover the face.   _____ _____ _____

28. Disposed of any soiled linens, dressings, and tubing and prepared the room for the family's arrival.   _____ _____ _____

29. Removed and discarded your gloves.   _____ _____ _____

30. Practiced hand hygiene and put on a new pair of gloves.   _____ _____ _____

31. Closed the door and removed the sheet covering the body after the family left.   _____ _____ _____

32. Filled out identification tags and tied one to the ankle or right big toe.   _____ _____ _____

33. Positioned the shroud or body bag under the patient's body.   _____ _____ _____

34. If using a shroud, you:

    A. brought the top of the shroud over the patient's head   _____ _____ _____

    B. folded the bottom of the shroud up over the feet   _____ _____ _____

    C. folded the sides of the shroud over the body   _____ _____ _____

    D. pinned or taped the shroud in place   _____ _____ _____

    E. attached one identification tag to the shroud   _____ _____ _____

35. Gathered all personal belongings and the denture cup and listed and labeled these items.   _____ _____ _____

36. Inquired whether the body should stay in the room or be moved to the morgue and checked facility transport policy.   _____ _____ _____

37. Removed, cleaned, and stored equipment properly.   _____ _____ _____

38. Removed soiled linens and discarded disposable equipment.   _____ _____ _____

39. Closed the door to the room or pulled the privacy curtain around the bed if the patient was to remain in the room.   _____ _____ _____

Follow-Up

40. Removed and discarded your gloves.   _____ _____ _____

41. Practiced hand hygiene.   _____ _____ _____

42. Followed the steps for cleaning a room after discharge after the body was removed.   _____ _____ _____

Reporting and Documentation

43. Communicated the date and time that the body was transported.   _____ _____ _____

44. Reported how the patient's belongings were handled and secured and if dentures or any other artificial body parts accompanied the patient.   _____ _____ _____

45. Documented care provided in the chart or EMR.   _____ _____ _____

Date of Completion: _____   Instructor's Initials: _____

Practice Examinations

Name: _____ Date: _____

On completion of a nursing assistant education and training program, prospective nursing assistants take the certification competency examination to become certified as nursing assistants. The certification competency exam tests an individual's *knowledge* (in a written or oral exam) and *skills* (as part of a hands-on demonstration). The written exam usually consists of 50 or more multiple-choice questions. The skills demonstration requires prospective nursing assistants to show how well they can perform procedures. To become certified, one must pass both parts of the exam with a state-determined score.

Knowing what to expect is an important part of taking the certification competency exam. Reviewing the certification competency exam handbook will provide information about how to apply for the exam, what to prepare for and bring, and what topics to study.

Learning how to study and prepare for the exam can make a difference in the outcome. Building excellent study habits and skills is essential. Some techniques to help you study include

- knowing your learning style (visual, auditory, or kinesthetic);
- designating a study space in which you can concentrate;
- scheduling study times, frequent breaks, and rewards for studying;
- taking good notes;
- using acronyms, pictures, smells, and flash cards to improve memory; and
- forming a study group.

The night before the exam, quickly review the material, make a checklist of items to bring, and go to bed early. On the day of the exam, eat a healthy breakfast, dress neatly, and bring needed supplies. Get to the exam site early and go to the bathroom before entering the exam room.

It is normal to feel nervous about taking the certification competency exam, but using good test-taking strategies can help reduce anxiety and support your success:

- Listen closely to directions and read instructions slowly and carefully. Ask for explanations if you do not understand.
- Take a few slow, deep breaths to relax yourself and visualize yourself being successful.
- Before answering questions on the written exam, scan the exam so you can budget your time.
- Answer questions you are sure about first. Come back to more challenging questions later.
- Think of the answer to a question before looking at the options. Then, choose the option that most closely matches your answer.
- If you are unsure of the answer, eliminate any answer options that appear totally wrong. If you must guess, choose the longest, most detailed answer.
- Don't keep changing your answer. Your first choice is usually the correct answer. If you finish with time left, review your answers.

Practice Certification Competency Examination 1

Select the *best* answer.

_____ 1. Which of the following is an example of violating a professional boundary?
   A. graciously refusing a gift from a family member of a resident
   B. admiring pictures a resident shares of his or her children
   C. bringing a resident a milkshake on a day off work
   D. advocating for a resident's bathing preference

_____ 2. What must a nursing assistant do to be placed on a state's nursing assistant registry?
   A. complete a state-approved education and training program and pass the certification competency exam
   B. work in a long-term care facility
   C. be in good standing on the state's board of medical ethics
   D. pay a fine and submit an application to the state's training program

_____ 3. Nursing assistants work under the supervision of a
   A. medical doctor
   B. licensed nursing staff member
   C. lead nursing assistant
   D. social worker

_____ 4. Which of the following is useful in the prevention of epidemics?
   A. injected antibodies
   B. alternative herbals
   C. vaccines
   D. pasteurization of serum

_____ 5. What is a skilled nursing facility?
   A. a facility that provides 24-hour, supervised care
   B. a building in which people who have had a stroke regain all function
   C. an acute care setting for people who have suffered a traumatic brain injury
   D. a college in which nursing students learn their skills

_____ 6. A resident who retired from teaching at age 65 will receive what type of public insurance?
   A. Medicaid
   B. Affordable Care
   C. Retirecare
   D. Medicare

_____ 7. A nursing assistant unintentionally failed to lock the wheels of a resident's bed, and when the resident tried to sit down, the bed rolled away. The resident suffered a fractured hip. This is an example of
   A. negligence
   B. abuse
   C. malpractice
   D. ethics

_____ 8. A nursing assistant inserted a urinary catheter after watching a licensed nursing staff member perform the procedure multiple times. He did not have the training or education to perform the procedure and was violating
   A. scope of practice
   B. accreditation
   C. assault
   D. liability

_____ 9. A nursing assistant gives a back rub to a resident and notes three large contusions. The resident states, "My son hit me with a broom." The nursing assistant should immediately report to the licensed nursing staff with the suspicion of
   A. malpractice
   B. libel
   C. slander
   D. abuse

_____ 10. To which person in the chain of command should the nursing assistant report concerns first?
   A. the charge nurse
   B. the doctor
   C. the director of nursing
   D. the nurse manager

_____ 11. Which of the following promotes an effective healthcare team?
   A. spending time together at social functions
   B. making decisions collaboratively
   C. spending work time talking about things in common
   D. working for a long time in healthcare

_____ 12. Nursing assistants provide objective information during which step of the nursing process?
   A. medical diagnosis
   B. evaluating
   C. planning
   D. diagnosing

_____ 13. Why are facility procedures important for nursing assistants?
   A. Procedures provide nonessential information.
   B. Procedures prevent questions.
   C. Nursing assistants need a complex guide.
   D. Procedures ensure that all healthcare providers give consistent care.

_____ 14. Which of the following is one of the five rights of delegation?
A. right away
B. right person
C. right equipment
D. right order

_____ 15. A resident refuses to go to a polka band social activity and says, "Nobody wants me around." What need is the resident expressing?
A. love and belonging
B. self-esteem
C. self-actualization
D. basic and physiological

_____ 16. When a nursing assistant enters a resident's room to give morning care, the resident hysterically shouts at her roommate, "Get out, get out, get out!" How should the nursing assistant respond?
A. by telling the roommate to get out of the room
B. by performing morning care as if nothing happened
C. by introducing himself or herself, drawing the privacy curtain, sitting down at eye level, and listening
D. by entering the room smiling and telling the resident to calm down

_____ 17. An example of health promotion is
A. paying attention to stressors and finding appropriate ways to manage them
B. asking a doctor for a prescription to manage anxiety
C. setting a weekly goal to lose 10 pounds, quit smoking, and run 6 miles daily
D. discouraging vaccination because of the risks

_____ 18. What are illness and wellness?
A. Illness and wellness cannot be described.
B. Illness and wellness are two unattainable goals.
C. Illness and wellness are represented by a line separating the ventral and anterior body.
D. Illness and wellness are represented by a line with illness on one end and wellness on the other.

_____ 19. What is the smallest structural and functional unit of the human body?
A. prion
B. cell
C. dendrite
D. axon

_____ 20. What happens to skin during the aging process?
A. Skin becomes less sensitive to pain.
B. Skin becomes supple and elastic.
C. Skin becomes resistant to injury.
D. Skin becomes a decubitus ulcer.

_____ 21. A nursing assistant asks for help to logroll a resident who is obese. The nursing assistant uses her strong leg and hip muscles to successfully care for the resident. What type of muscle is involved in this process?
A. synovial muscle
B. involuntary muscle
C. skeletal muscle
D. smooth muscle

_____ 22. A resident twisted his ankle playing golf, but when a nursing assistant applied cool compresses, the pain went away quickly. What type of pain did the resident have?
A. chronic
B. throbbing
C. radiating
D. acute

_____ 23. A nursing assistant knows that urinary catheters provide a portal of entry for pathogens. What can a nursing assistant do to prevent a urinary tract infection?
A. remember to wipe from the dirtiest area to the cleanest area
B. force oral fluids to wash natural flora from the bladder
C. provide excellent catheter and perineal care
D. dress a resident in an incontinence brief, even if the resident refuses

_____ 24. About 90 percent of communication is
A. nonverbal
B. verbal
C. jargon
D. slang

_____ 25. A nursing assistant is explaining an enema procedure to a resident. What should the nursing assistant do to be sure the resident understands?
A. have the resident repeat back what was heard
B. have the resident tell his or her family
C. have the resident send an e-mail
D. have the resident ask questions

_____ 26. A nursing assistant can show active listening by
A. interrupting to get other work done
B. using good eye contact and responding appropriately
C. using active body movements
D. cupping the ear to indicate the message was not heard

_____ 27. When a nursing assistant is prejudiced,
A. he or she is impatient with another person
B. an opinion is formed before getting the facts
C. special attention is given to another person
D. rumors are spread about another person

_____ 28. A nursing assistant is caring for a resident who has unfamiliar worship practices. What should the nursing assistant know about cultural humility?
A. Food has no significance in worship practices.
B. Cultural humility focuses on the facility's customs.
C. Each resident should be treated as an individual.
D. Residents should respect others by keeping their practices private.

_____ 29. The purpose of a plan of care is to provide
A. necessary directions for delivering individualized, holistic care
B. the family with a plan of action for the resident
C. the doctor with a plan for ordering care
D. the resident with instructions for discharge

_____ 30. What is the purpose of a change-of-shift report?
  A. to let staff talk with each other about staffing issues and problems
  B. to meet and connect with staff from other shifts
  C. to talk with a resident's doctor about important issues
  D. to transfer essential resident information from one shift to the next

_____ 31. When documenting critical observations, a nursing assistant should include
  A. logical and factual opinions
  B. objective observations and the resident's subjective comments
  C. subjective observations and care other staff members have performed
  D. observations from the doctor and director of nursing

_____ 32. How should a nursing assistant answer the telephone in a long-term care facility?
  A. by identifying the work area and first name and asking, "How can I help you?"
  B. by identifying his or her full name and title
  C. by pleasantly saying hello; identifying work area, name, and title; and asking, "How can I help you?"
  D. by asking, "How can I help you?"

_____ 33. After a resident falls and sustains a serious head injury, the charge nurse is occupied with calling the doctor and delegates documentation of the unseen events to a nursing assistant. What should the nursing assistant tell the charge nurse?
  A. "I will do that after I talk to the director of nursing."
  B. "I will include that in my progress notes."
  C. "I will check facility policy to see if I can document things I didn't do."
  D. "I understand you are busy, but I can only document what I have seen or done."

_____ 34. During a telephone call, a nursing assistant should
  A. take notes after the doctor gives an order
  B. take notes during the call and confirm accuracy with the caller
  C. put the caller on hold and find the director of nursing
  D. take notes after the phone call to avoid interrupting the caller

_____ 35. What microorganisms cause infection?
  A. natural flora
  B. fomites
  C. pathogens
  D. nuclei

_____ 36. How is pneumonia transmitted?
  A. through red blood cells
  B. through feces
  C. through the oral-fecal route
  D. through droplets

_____ 37. The microorganism that causes hepatitis is
  A. spread through sneezing
  B. a parasite
  C. spread through the soil
  D. a bloodborne pathogen

_____ 38. Which of the following standard precautions does a nursing assistant use most frequently?
  A. proper hand washing
  B. isolation gowns
  C. sterile dressings
  D. care of draining wounds

_____ 39. What is the first thing a nursing assistant should do if exposed to a resident's blood?
  A. call the director of nursing
  B. alert the resident's family
  C. follow the healthcare facility's exposure control plan
  D. go to the nearest emergency room

_____ 40. A nursing assistant is helping an RN with a sterile dressing change. The nursing assistant should
  A. only use sterile items in the sterile field
  B. keep all nonsterile items 1 inch inside the sterile field
  C. wear clean, disposable gloves
  D. carefully reach over the sterile field

_____ 41. How can a nursing assistant prevent falls?
  A. by restraining a resident to prevent a fall
  B. by putting a fall risk sign outside the door according to facility policy
  C. by telling a resident not to get out of bed
  D. by advising the family that a resident is a fall risk

_____ 42. What should a nursing assistant do to ensure a resident is receiving oxygen as ordered?
  A. check the oxygen tubing for kinks
  B. increase the oxygen flow rate and observe the resident's reaction
  C. turn off the oxygen and observe the resident's response
  D. remove the oxygen cannula and encourage coughing and deep breathing

_____ 43. A nursing assistant ensures safety by
  A. turning off oxygen before shaving a resident with a safety razor
  B. keeping doors fully open during procedures
  C. placing the call light on the bedside stand
  D. making sure the call light is accessible to the resident

_____ 44. How should a nursing assistant help a resident with active ROM exercises?
  A. by secretly watching the resident perform the exercises
  B. by performing the exercises on both sides of the body
  C. by telling the resident to exercise independently in bed at night
  D. by giving instructions and observing while the resident performs the exercises

_____ 45. During the transfer process, a nursing assistant can include a resident by asking the resident to
  A. move on the count of five
  B. move on the count of three
  C. move on the count of two
  D. move on the count of four

_____ 46. A nursing assistant can help a mobile resident reposition in bed by
  A. lifting the resident up under the arms
  B. using a gait or transfer belt to pull the resident toward the head of the bed
  C. asking the resident to bend the knees and push up with the feet
  D. having the resident use a draw sheet to slide up in bed

_____ 47. Which of the following pulse rates should be reported to the licensed nursing staff?
  A. 85 bpm
  B. 65 bpm
  C. 82 bpm
  D. 54 bpm

_____ 48. What is the first thing a nursing assistant should do prior to obtaining a resident's weight?
  A. fully dress the resident for warmth
  B. move the lower and upper weights until the balance pointer is balanced
  C. move the weights on the balance scale bar to zero
  D. add the amounts shown on the two bars to determine weight

_____ 49. What does an oral temperature of 102.6°F indicate?
  A. hyperthermia and possible infection
  B. hypothermia
  C. body temperature in the normal range
  D. body temperature that is high, but not concerning

_____ 50. An anxious resident is having stitches removed from the abdomen. How can a holistic nursing assistant comfort the resident?
  A. by encouraging the resident to be independent during the procedure
  B. by draping the resident properly for privacy and warmth
  C. by keeping the resident from touching the area
  D. by repeating all instructions given to the resident

_____ 51. What position is typical for a well-woman exam?
  A. lithotomy position
  B. Fowler's position
  C. prone position
  D. knee-chest position

_____ 52. For an enema, a nursing assistant should position a resident in
  A. prone position
  B. supine position
  C. Fowler's position
  D. Sims' position

_____ 53. What test is used to detect blood in the stool?
  A. sputum specimen
  B. fecal occult blood test
  C. 24-hour collection
  D. complete blood count (CBC)

_____ 54. A nursing assistant prepares a resident's bed at 2200. What kind of bed will await the resident when he or she returns from walking?
  A. surgical bed
  B. occupied bed
  C. closed, occupied bed
  D. open, unoccupied bed

_____ 55. In a facility's call light system, white indicates a resident room, and red indicates a resident bathroom. Two red call lights are illuminated, and other staff members are involved with a change-of-shift report. What should the nursing assistant do?
  A. go to the closest resident and rush him or her along
  B. immediately check both bathrooms for safety
  C. turn off both call lights to stop the noise and seek another staff member
  D. check both residents' EMRs to determine which resident is more likely to get up without help

_____ 56. When a new resident is admitted to a long-term care facility, a nursing assistant should safeguard the resident's personal items by
  A. waiting for the social worker to complete the labeling process
  B. documenting the items according to facility policy and labeling as necessary
  C. unpacking the resident's belongings and putting them in logical places
  D. asking the resident's husband to complete the facility checklist

_____ 57. A resident with a tremor related to Parkinson's disease requests assistance with oral care. To what angle should the head of his bed be raised?
  A. at least 120°
  B. at least 60°
  C. at least 40°
  D. at least 20°

_____ 58. A resident has recovered from a stroke and has a weak right side. A nursing assistant should remove the resident's blouse from which side last?
  A. left arm
  B. stronger arm
  C. weaker right arm
  D. unaffected arm

_____ 59. When helping residents with some or all ADLs, holistic nursing assistants should
  A. encourage resident independence to promote self-esteem
  B. do everything for a resident to save the resident's energy
  C. ask the family for help bonding with a resident
  D. have a resident help with activities that cause pain

_____ 60. The body builds tissue using
  A. healthy fats consumed
  B. calories
  C. energy
  D. protein

_____ 61. When caring for a resident receiving enteral feeding, a nursing assistant should
A. provide frequent oral and nasal care
B. logroll the resident to change his or her brief within 30 minutes of the feeding
C. keep the bed supine
D. perform ROM exercises during the feeding to make good use of time

_____ 62. A resident has dysphagia, and the doctor has ordered that all liquids should be extremely thick. What consistency should a nursing assistant expect to see?
A. nectar
B. honey
C. pudding
D. thin

_____ 63. A nursing assistant reports that a resident has a dry mouth and complains of thirst. What condition is suspected?
A. hypoglycemia
B. hypertension
C. dehydration
D. arthritis

_____ 64. A resident has an indwelling urinary catheter. A nursing assistant should carefully measure intake and output (I&O) amounts in
A. milliliters
B. ounces
C. centimeters
D. milligrams

_____ 65. A resident is instructing a nursing assistant to search for his lost hearing aid battery. What can the nursing assistant do while communicating with the resident?
A. tell the resident to ask the staff to replace batteries in the future
B. face the resident when talking to him
C. talk loudly while searching under the bed
D. leave the resident and immediately inform the charge nurse

_____ 66. A resident has recovered from a stroke in the brain's left hemisphere. A nursing assistant notes that the resident understands words, but cannot form them. What type of aphasia does the resident have?
A. receptive
B. expressive
C. depressive
D. progressive

_____ 67. A nursing assistant receives a change-of-shift report noting that a resident shows cognitive changes related to dementia. What is an example of a cognitive change?
A. fecal incontinence
B. memory loss and confusion
C. a motor change
D. a brief improvement with ambulation

_____ 68. What is the most common mental health condition?
A. schizophrenia among older adults
B. agoraphobia
C. suicide
D. depression

_____ 69. A resident has recovered from a left total knee surgery. What can a nursing assistant do to prevent postoperative infection?
A. encourage the family to wait a few weeks before visiting
B. keep the head of the bed elevated 30°
C. maintain excellent hand hygiene
D. discourage ambulation until the site heals

_____ 70. A nursing assistant notes a change in a resident's wound dressing. What change should be reported immediately to the licensed nursing staff?
A. increased amount of purulent drainage and blood
B. decreased amount of clear, yellow fluid
C. small amount of dry tissue
D. small amount of clear, pink fluid

_____ 71. A resident is spending a lot of time in bed recovering from the flu. What should a nursing assistant do to prevent complications due to immobility?
A. perform passive ROM exercises every 30 minutes
B. increase the flow rate of the resident's oxygen
C. encourage the resident to regularly cough and breathe deeply
D. encourage the resident to stay in bed

_____ 72. Cardiopulmonary resuscitation (CPR) is a lifesaving procedure, and odds of survival are increased further by the use of a(n)
A. pulse oximeter
B. sphygmomanometer
C. thermometer
D. automated external defibrillator (AED)

_____ 73. An ambulatory resident is choking on a grape. What should a nursing assistant immediately do?
A. perform cardiopulmonary resuscitation (CPR)
B. give 20 back blows with an open palm
C. give abdominal thrusts, known as the *Heimlich maneuver*
D. lower the resident to the floor

_____ 74. Which of the following is an example of an advance directive?
A. living will
B. funeral arrangements
C. Health Insurance Portability and Accountability Act (HIPAA)
D. Resident Bill of Rights

_____ 75. A nursing assistant is helping the charge nurse give palliative care to a resident who is dying. What kind of care is provided?
A. holistic medicines to cure the disease
B. the relief of uncomfortable symptoms
C. perioperative care
D. the cessation of personal care to give the resident peace

Practice Certification Competency Examination 2

Select the *best* answer.

_____ 1. A nursing assistant is caring for a group of residents. Where is the nursing assistant working?
   A. in a long-term care facility
   B. in hospice
   C. in a subacute care center
   D. in a person's home

_____ 2. A nursing assistant practices holistic care. This means his or her care addresses
   A. the resident's most important physiological needs above all
   B. body, nurse, and doctor
   C. body, mind, and spirit
   D. ethics, morals, and law

_____ 3. What is the Omnibus Budget Reconciliation Act (OBRA)?
   A. a COBRA insurance benefit
   B. an OSHA law that protects workers from unsafe conditions
   C. a policy that varies from facility to facility
   D. a law that standardizes nursing assistant training and education requirements

_____ 4. A resident in a long-term care facility falls and is transferred via ambulance to the emergency room. What type of care transition has occurred?
   A. chronic care to subacute care
   B. subacute care to chronic care
   C. hospice care to trauma care
   D. chronic care to acute care

_____ 5. A person living at home has been diagnosed with a terminal illness. From what type of care would the person benefit?
   A. rehabilitation to regain function and abilities
   B. hospice to receive care and comfort
   C. subacute care to recuperate from the illness
   D. inpatient mental health care to cope with the diagnosis

_____ 6. A resident with moderate dementia cannot live alone, and the family is seeking direct services for long-term chronic care. What type of facility would provide this care?
   A. nursing home
   B. rehabilitation facility
   C. hospital
   D. asylum

_____ 7. A resident is expecting a visit from a friend and is afraid to miss his visitor, so he refuses his scheduled shower. The nursing assistant wants the resident to look his best and gently forces him to undress for the shower. Which resident right is being violated?
   A. freedom from neglect
   B. freedom from physical abuse
   C. freedom from psychological abuse
   D. freedom from verbal abuse

_____ 8. A busy nurse delegates the removal of an IV to an experienced nursing assistant. What should the nursing assistant do to make sure this task is within the scope of practice?
   A. ask the resident for permission
   B. ask the lead nursing assistant to watch
   C. consult the healthcare facility's procedure manual
   D. consult the resident's plan of care

_____ 9. What is the Health Insurance Portability and Accountability Act (HIPAA)?
   A. a law that protects the privacy of healthcare information
   B. a law that protects healthcare staff from injury
   C. a law that protects the rights of family members to access a resident's information
   D. a law that protects the privacy of the healthcare team

_____ 10. How can a nursing assistant demonstrate critical thinking?
   A. by being on time for the work shift
   B. by stopping and thinking carefully about a situation before acting
   C. by reacting anxiously during critical moments
   D. by completing one task at a time and not integrating tasks

_____ 11. What can a new nursing assistant do to be an effective member of the healthcare team?
   A. explain what it means to be an effective member of the team
   B. demonstrate dependability, be respectful, and be present
   C. smile and get work done
   D. plan on socializing with the team every weekend

_____ 12. A doctor has written orders for a patient's discharge and transfer to a facility for cardiac rehabilitation. What must be obtained before the transfer?
   A. an ambulance
   B. a wheelchair
   C. the patient's valuables
   D. the patient's permission

_____ 13. A charge nurse has delegated a new nursing assistant the task of changing a clean dressing for a resident. The nursing assistant cannot remember how to do the procedure. What should the nursing assistant do?
   A. express willingness, but request supervision and training
   B. delegate the task to an experienced nursing assistant
   C. ask another nurse to assist so the charge nurse doesn't know and look up the procedure
   D. tell the charge nurse that the task is outside scope of practice

_____ 14. A resident is alone and is crying in her room. What should the nursing assistant do?
   A. knock, go in, gently take the resident's hand, and ask why she is crying
   B. do not go in the room and give the resident privacy
   C. go in the room, sit on the bed, and sing the resident a song
   D. go in the room and encourage the resident to come out and play cards

_____ 15. Which of the following is true about stress?
   A. Residents react to stress in ways that are different from family members.
   B. Stress management is easy for healthcare staff.
   C. Stress and stress management are different for everyone.
   D. Stress is beneficial and promotes change if it manages the person.

_____ 16. A nursing assistant should report symptoms of resident stress to the licensed nursing staff because
   A. reporting is important, but not necessary with good documentation
   B. reporting is important; mandatory; and essential for providing safe, quality care
   C. reporting helps the nurse talk to the family of the resident
   D. reporting is important for teaching nursing assistants in staff meetings

_____ 17. The cell's activities are directed by
   A. cytoplasm
   B. the cell membrane
   C. organelles
   D. the nucleus

_____ 18. A resident has not had a bowel movement in four days. Which part of the gastrointestinal tract is likely affected?
   A. pancreas
   B. jejunum
   C. small intestine
   D. large intestine

_____ 19. A nursing assistant receives a shift report about a resident with a condition affecting the front cavity of the body. Which cavity is affected?
   A. dorsal cavity
   B. spinal cavity
   C. ventral cavity
   D. cranial cavity

_____ 20. A resident has rheumatoid arthritis, which is a(n)
   A. endocrine disease
   B. degenerative disease
   C. infectious disease
   D. chronic obstructive pulmonary disease

_____ 21. A resident has difficulty speaking after a cerebrovascular accident. What is this symptom called?
   A. dysplasia
   B aphasia
   C. hemiplegia
   D. malaysia

_____ 22. A resident's coccyx has one small blister filled with fluid, and the surrounding area is irritated and red. What stage of decubitus ulcer does the resident have?
   A. stage 1
   B. stage 2
   C. stage 3
   D. stage 4

_____ 23. How should a nursing assistant communicate with an older resident who has a hearing impairment?
   A. use short sentences and simple words
   B. shout louder than the television volume
   C. stand far from the person while talking
   D. talk fast and with a high tone

_____ 24. What four components are needed to communicate a message?
   A. listener, receiver, communicator, and observer
   B. observer, mode of communication, receiver, and participant
   C. sender, observer, strategy, and feedback
   D. sender, mode of communication, recipient, and feedback

_____ 25. A resident has terminal acquired immunodeficiency syndrome (AIDS) and is in his final days. He states, "I can't believe I'm here. I have to get back to my lake house. The fishing is great this time of year." What stage of grief is the resident experiencing?
   A. pain and guilt
   B. anger and bargaining
   C. depression
   D. shock and denial

_____ 26. What is ethnicity?
   A. racist roots, customs, and rituals as a group
   B. a group's identification with common social, cultural, and traditional practices
   C. a group's decision about practicing rituals
   D. a group's religious ideas

_____ 27. Which of the following demonstrates cross-cultural communication skills?
   A. providing clean linens during morning care
   B. providing comfortable chairs
   C. being present and using active listening skills
   D. keeping the curtains closed during a procedure

_____ 28. A nursing assistant reviews a resident's new plan of care. The plan of care is based on identification of the resident's health problems, called the
A. nursing goal
B. nursing intervention
C. nursing evaluation
D. nursing diagnosis

_____ 29. A nursing assistant uses objective and subjective observations to document a resident's care. Which of the following is an objective observation?
A. The resident says, "My urine is dark and cloudy."
B. The resident states, "I have a fever and chills."
C. Urine is dark yellow, foul smelling, cloudy, 350 mL.
D. The resident has given up ambulating with a sore back.

_____ 30. What does the healthcare team use to ensure continuity of care?
A. assignment sheet
B. plan of care
C. doctor's orders
D. subjective documentation

_____ 31. A nursing assistant documents in an electronic medical record (EMR). What does an EMR contain?
A. information about a specific patient's single stay
B. information for the family to review at the bedside
C. health information from multiple doctors for nursing assistant followup
D. medical records since the birth of the resident

_____ 32. An important responsibility of a nursing assistant is maintaining confidentiality. What is an example of confidentiality?
A. keeping a resident's name and birth date from a healthcare provider
B. sharing a resident's personal information with the family
C. making resident information available to neighbors
D. keeping a resident's personal information private

_____ 33. A nursing assistant changes a resident's position 15 minutes after midnight. What time is this on the 24-hour clock?
A. 0115
B. 1215
C. 2315
D. 0015

_____ 34. A nursing assistant gives quality care to break the chain of infection. The chain of infection includes a(n)
A. resistant host and mode of transmission
B. portal of entry and portal of exit
C. reservoir and infectious chain
D. mode of entry and bacteria

_____ 35. While he lived at home, a resident spilled a boiling pot of soup and burned 18 percent of his body. The nursing assistant is concerned because the first line of defense against infection is
A. intact skin
B. low temperature
C. adequate hydration
D. good nutrition

_____ 36. A resident has a urinary tract infection (UTI) caused by the most common microorganism. Which microorganism most commonly causes infection?
A. fungus
B. natural flora
C. bacterium
D. virus

_____ 37. A nursing assistant caring for a resident in isolation should
A. touch the resident with sterile gloves
B. wear proper PPE when caring for the resident
C. dispose of PPE after leaving the resident's room
D. transport the resident without a mask to prevent embarrassment

_____ 38. A resident is battling cancer and taking chemotherapy medication. Because the resident's resistance to microorganisms is low, the resident should be in
A. protective isolation
B. contact isolation
C. airborne isolation
D. droplet isolation

_____ 39. When removing personal protective equipment (PPE), a nursing assistant is careful to
A. remove protective eyewear first
B. remove the gown first
C. remove the mask first
D. remove gloves first

_____ 40. A resident is secretively smoking a cigarette in her bathroom, and a paper towel ignites. The resident pulls the bathroom call light cord. What should a nursing assistant do first?
A. safely remove the resident from the room
B. extinguish the fire
C. run down the hall and pull the fire alarm
D. inform the charge nurse

_____ 41. What can a nursing assistant do to prevent back strains?
A. wear expensive shoes for good support
B. ask other, stronger nursing assistants to do the heavy lifting
C. avoid frequent bed changes
D. always ask for help when transferring heavy residents

_____ 42. A busy nursing assistant forgets that a resident's status is nothing by mouth (NPO), and a procedure had to be canceled. The surgeon is angry. The nursing assistant works in a facility with a culture of safety. What is the focus in this facility?
   A. punishing whoever made the error
   B. how many times the error was made
   C. what happened and how to prevent it, not who did it
   D. the person who supervises the nursing assistant

_____ 43. Proper body mechanics include
   A. keeping the resident's weight close to the nursing assistant's center of gravity
   B. bending over to lift a resident
   C. pulling and not pushing a resident
   D. ordering a mechanical lift for a tired resident

_____ 44. A nursing assistant consistently uses a gait or transfer belt. What is the primary purpose of a gait belt?
   A. to reduce the nursing assistant's liability in a court of law
   B. to be used as a safety hold and prevent falls
   C. to be worn in the dining room in case of a fall
   D. to logroll a resident

_____ 45. A resident recovering from pneumonia sleeps most of the day. How often should the resident be repositioned?
   A. every shift
   B. every 30 minutes
   C. every hour
   D. every two hours

_____ 46. A nursing assistant is obtaining vital signs (VS) for an entire wing in a long-term care facility. When are respirations best measured in the process?
   A. right after measuring pulse when the resident is unaware
   B. right before measuring temperature
   C. right after measuring blood pressure
   D. right before measuring pulse

_____ 47. A nursing assistant reviews a resident's plan of care and notes that the doctor has ordered weekly weight measurements. How should the nursing assistant position the ambulatory resident on a stand-up scale?
   A. facing sideways on the platform
   B. on the center of the scale with the arm resting on the nursing assistant's shoulder for safety
   C. safely on the center of the scale with the arms down
   D. fully dressed with 1-inch heels placed on the edge of the scale platform for stability

_____ 48. A nursing assistant is caring for an infant with an infection of unknown cause. How should the nursing assistant measure the infant's rectal temperature?
   A. insert the thermometer 4 inches into the anus and hold in place for five minutes
   B. insert the thermometer 3 inches into the anus and hold in place for one to three minutes
   C. insert the thermometer 2 inches into the anus and hold in place for two to four minutes
   D. insert the thermometer 1 inch or less into the anus and hold in place for three to five minutes

_____ 49. A licensed nurse delegates the procedure of obtaining a resident's sputum specimen to a nursing assistant. How should the sputum be collected from the resident?
   A. deep coughing
   B. bowel movement
   C. blood specimen
   D. tissue biopsy

_____ 50. A resident has burning, painful urination. The doctor orders a midstream urine specimen for urinalysis and culture. How should the nursing assistant prepare and collect the specimen?
   A. The nursing assistant will select a container, but it does not need to be sterile.
   B. The resident's perineal area will not need to be cleansed.
   C. The resident will start to urinate, and only the last part of the stream will be collected.
   D. The sample will be collected at bedtime.

_____ 51. A resident's soiled linens can spread pathogens. As a result, a nursing assistant should
   A. keep soiled linens close to the body during transport
   B. push a dirty linen cart into a resident's room to receive soiled bed linens
   C. avoid shaking linens and roll the dirty side in when removing from the bed
   D. replace full dirty linen bags every other day to avoid touching them

_____ 52. A nursing assistant is concerned that a resident with a vision impairment will stumble and fall in his cluttered room. How should the nursing assistant communicate this concern?
   A. ask the family to take the items before an accident happens
   B. ask to help the resident organize his belongings
   C. put risky items away while the resident sleeps
   D. talk to the charge nurse because this is beyond the nursing assistant's scope of practice

_____ 53. What is the most important consideration when working with beds?
   A. bed placement
   B. bed firmness
   C. bed position
   D. bed safety, including locking wheels

_____ 54. A nursing assistant checks the plan of care for instructions about a resident's warm, moist compress. The doctor has not specified a length of time. How long should the compress be applied?
   A. 5 minutes
   B. 10 minutes
   C. 20 minutes
   D. 30 minutes

_____ 55. A resident's feet need foot care. What should a nursing assistant do?
   A. wash the feet, rinse them well, let them air-dry, and avoid lotion
   B. wash, rinse, and dry the feet and apply lotion between the toes
   C. use water to rinse the feet, avoid soap, and apply lotion, but not between the toes
   D. wash, rinse, and dry the feet and apply lotion, but not between the toes

_____ 56. An incontinent resident requires perineal care four times daily. A nursing assistant helps her stay clean and dry. How should the nursing assistant perform female perineal care?
   A. wash, rinse, and dry the perineal area using front-to-back strokes with a clean area of cloth
   B. wash, rinse, and dry the buttocks first and then clean the vulva
   C. wash, rinse, and dry the thighs and then perform perineal care with the same water
   D. wash, rinse, and dry the perineal area using back-to-front strokes with a clean area of cloth

_____ 57. Which of the following are metric units of measurement?
   A. inch, millimeter, and liter
   B. ounce, centimeter, and gram
   C. centimeter, kilogram, and milliliter
   D. milliliter, ounce, and meter

_____ 58. A nursing assistant notices that an independent resident is having difficulty eating vegetable soup. The resident pushes the soup away in frustration. What should the nursing assistant do?
   A. tell the kitchen to thicken the soup
   B. provide a spoon designed to maintain a resident's independence
   C. feed the resident the soup
   D. show the resident how to drink the soup from a cup

_____ 59. A resident is exhausted from a day out with family and requests a light dinner in bed. The nursing assistant delivers the meal and adjusts the bed to
   A. Fowler's position
   B. prone position
   C. Trendelenburg position
   D. Sims' position

_____ 60. A resident resting in bed has a Foley catheter. A nursing assistant checks the tubing for kinks and proper placement of the drainage bag. Where should the drainage bag be placed?
   A. on the bed
   B. out of sight of visitors
   C. hung on the bedframe
   D. hung on the bed side rail

_____ 61. A nursing assistant follows facility policy to provide catheter care. The nursing assistant should
   A. pull gently on the tubing to check proper placement
   B. keep the tubing unkinked
   C. flush the tubing with sterile water for blockages
   D. replace the drainage bag every six months

_____ 62. A resident's colostomy appliance is full and is pulling away from the skin. To provide colostomy care, a nursing assistant should
   A. wash, rinse, and dry the perineal area and apply barrier cream
   B. quickly tear off the remaining appliance to lessen discomfort
   C. gently wash, rinse, and dry the area around the stoma
   D. draw a line around the stoma to measure the size

_____ 63. A resident has a urinary tract infection (UTI) and sudden cognitive changes. What is this reversible cognitive disorder called?
   A. Lewy body dementia
   B. dementia
   C. Parkinson's disease
   D. delirium

_____ 64. A resident with Alzheimer's disease demonstrates a change in behavior when the sun goes down. What is most likely the cause of this change?
   A. The resident is bored and needs stimulating activity at the end of the day.
   B. The resident's medication is causing change at the end of the day.
   C. Due to sundowning, the resident becomes more confused at the end of the day.
   D. The resident needs to be left alone at the end of the day.

_____ 65. A holistic nursing assistant is helping an independent resident with a vision impairment. The nursing assistant should
   A. not tell the resident where obstacles are in the facility
   B. keep personal items in different places to stimulate the brain
   C. keep furniture in the center of the room and walls clear
   D. make sure there are no obstacles in the way to the bathroom

_____ 66. A resident has hip surgery and develops a blood clot in the right lower extremity due to immobility. What is another name for this condition?
A. pulmonary embolism (PE)
B. urinary tract infection (UTI)
C. deep vein thrombosis (DVT)
D. peripheral vascular disease (PVD)

_____ 67. A resident must understand, agree to, and sign a document prior to surgery. This document, which gives permission for a procedure, is called
A. informed consent
B. informed admission
C. informed insurance
D. informed proceed

_____ 68. A resident has a wound drain in her abdominal cavity. A nursing assistant is monitoring the site and should
A. keep the drain pinned to the resident's gown at all times
B. keep the drainage collection device below the incision site
C. keep a clean dressing over the site during visiting hours
D. rotate the drain site every two hours

_____ 69. A confused resident grasped a light bulb, causing a second-degree burn. What is a characteristic of this burn?
A. pink skin without pain
B. open, bleeding tissue
C. charred, black skin
D. blistering

_____ 70. A nursing assistant is helping residents in the dining room. A resident is clutching at his throat and cannot speak. The resident
A. has burned his mouth
B. is choking
C. is having a cerebrovascular accident
D. is having a myocardial infarction

_____ 71. A resident has slurred speech and left-side weakness. A nursing assistant immediately reports the change in condition to the charge nurse. The resident is most likely having
A. a myocardial infarction
B. a cerebrovascular accident
C. a seizure
D. deep vein thrombosis

_____ 72. A resident who is dying is receiving palliative care. Which of the following is common among residents who are dying?
A. increased ambulation and anxiety
B. increased fatigue and sleep
C. increased hunger and activity
D. increased pain and hunger

_____ 73. A resident's wife asks a nursing assistant to witness his do-not-resuscitate (DNR) order. How should the nursing assistant respond?
A. "This is not within my scope of practice. Let me get the charge nurse for you."
B. "Where do I sign?"
C. "I will check facility policy and sign it after lunch."
D. "Please make me a copy for my file."

_____ 74. A resident and her family feel well-informed and have requested hospice services. Why have they made this request?
A. The resident has limited finances.
B. The resident and her family want more information about curing the resident's disease.
C. The resident and her family understand the resident has a terminal illness and needs special care.
D. The resident and her family have given up all hope.

_____ 75. A nursing assistant feels emotional that a resident who has been in his care for three years is dying. What can the nursing assistant do for his emotional well-being?
A. take the resident out for one last meal together
B. talk with the charge nurse or another nurse in the facility
C. talk with the resident's family and friends
D. remain professional and deny feelings